Clinical and Neuropsychological Aspects of Closed Head Injury

Brain Damage, Behaviour and Cognition
Developments in Clinical Neuropsychology

Series editors: Chris Code, Scraptoft Campus, Leicester Polytechnic, and Dave Müller, Suffolk College of Higher and Further Education

Acquired Apraxia of Speech in Aphasic Adults
Edited by Paula Square-Storer

Neuropsychology and the Dementias
Siobhan Hart and James Semple

The Characteristics of Aphasia
Edited by Chris Code

Clinical and Neuropsychological Aspects of Closed Head Injury
John Richardson

Neuropsychology of Amnesic Syndromes
Alan Parkin and Nicholas Leng

Cognitive Rehabilitation using Microcomputers
Veronica Bradley

Cognitive Rehabilitation in Perspective
Edited by Roger Ll. Wood and Ian Fussey

Acquired Neurological Speech/Language Disorders in Childhood
Edited by Bruce Murdoch

Personality and Emotional Disturbance Following Brain Injury
Howard Jackson and Alan Hopewell

Introduction to Paediatric Neuropsychology
Peter Griffiths

Clinical and Neuropsychological Aspects of Closed Head Injury

John T. E. Richardson

Taylor & Francis

London · New York · Philadelphia

UK   Taylor & Francis Ltd. 4 John St., London WC1N 2ET

USA   Taylor & Francis Inc., 1900 Frost Road, Suite 101, Bristol, PA 19007

First published 1990

British Library Cataloguing in Publication Data
Richardson, John
    Clinical and neuropsychological aspects of closed head injury.
    1. Man. Brain. Brain damage. Neuropsychological aspects
    I. Title   II. Series
    616.84

    ISBN 0-85066-448-9
    ISBN 0-85066-468-7 pbk

Typeset in 11/13 Bembo
by Chapterhouse, The Cloisters, Formby

Printed in Great Britain by Burgess Science Press, Basingstoke on paper which has a specified pH value on final paper manufacture of not less than 7.5 and is therefore 'acid free'.

Contents

Series Preface

From being an area primarily on the periphery of mainstream behavioural and cognitive science, neuropsychology has developed in recent years into an area of central concern for a range of disciplines. We are witnessing not only a revolution in the way in which brain-behaviour-cognition relationships are viewed, but a widening of interest concerning developments in neuropsychology on the part of a range of workers in a variety of fields. Major advances in brain imaging techniques and the cognitive modelling of the impairments following brain damage promise a wider understanding of the nature of the representation of cognition and behaviour in the damaged and undamaged brain.

Neuropsychology is now centrally important for those working with brain damaged people, but the very rate of expansion in the area makes it difficult to keep up with findings from current research. The aim of the *Brain Damage, Behaviour and Cognition* series is to publish a wide range of books which present comprehensive and up-to-date overviews of current developments in specific areas of interest.

These books will be of particular interest to those working with the brain-damaged. It is the editors' intention that undergraduates, postgraduates, clinicians and researchers in psychology, speech pathology and medicine will find this series a useful source of information on important current developments. The authors and editors of the books in this series are experts in their respective fields working at the forefront of contemporary research. They have produced texts which are accessible and scholarly. We thank them for their contribution and their hard work in fulfilling the aims of the series.

Chris Code and Dave Müller
Leicester and Ipswich

Preface

My interest in the effects of closed head injury was initially stimulated more than 15 years ago while I was working with Dr Freda Newcombe in the Neuropsychology Unit of the Department of Clincial Neurology at the University of Oxford and attached to the Department of Neurological Surgery at the Radcliffe Infirmary. When I moved to Brunel University in 1975, I was fortunate to be able to develop my own research in this area, thanks to the encouragement of Mr J. T. Jackson and his fellow consultants at Hillingdon Hospital. That research was supported in part by the UK Medical Research Council, and was conducted with the assistance of my colleague Dr Chris Barry and my student Ms Wendy Snape.

This book began as a joint project with Dr Steven White, then of the Maudsley Hospital, London, and now of the Medical College of Virginia, Richmond. The broad structure of this book owes much to his understanding of the field, and I am very grateful to him for generously allowing me to make use of material which he had produced on the neuropathology of closed head injury. Subsequent contributions to the planning of this book were made by Dr Alan Sunderland of the Avon Stroke Unit at Frenchay Hospital, Bristol, and Dr Bill McKinlay of the Western General Hospital, Edinburgh, both of whom provided comments on early drafts of several chapters.

Much of the detailed preparation of this volume was carried out while I was a Visiting Scholar at St John's College, Oxford, during July and August 1986, and subsequently while I was on study leave from Brunel University as Honorary Senior Research Fellow at the Open University from January to September 1987. I am very grateful to all three institutions for their support. Acknowledgements are also due to the following individuals for their generous assistance: Dr Gerhard Baumann of Brunel University; Ms Ethel Black and Ms Linda Washington of the US National Center for Health Statistics; Mr Adrian Hobbs of the Transport and Road Research Laboratory, Crowthorne; Dr Narinder Kapur of the Wessex Neurological Centre, Southampton; Mrs G. Ladva of the Office of Population Censuses and Surveys, London; Professor Harvey Levin of the University of Texas Medical Branch at Galveston; Dr Martin Livingston of the University of Glasgow; Mr S. C. R. Maslen of the Statistics and Research Section of the Department of Health and Social Security,

London; and the librarians of Brunel University, the Cairns Library, Oxford, the Open University, the University of North Carolina at Greensboro, and the Reference Center of the US Embassy in London.

I am also grateful for the detailed comments, advice, and suggestions of the following colleagues who kindly devoted their own scarce time to reading the manuscript of this book in draft form: Dr Narinder Kapur of the Wessex Neurological Centre, Southampton; Professor Marc Marschark of the University of North Carolina at Greensboro; Mr Denis Salter of the Crichton Royal Hospital, Dumfries; and Dr Barbara Wilson of the University of Southampton. The comments of Professor Bryan Jennett of the University of Glasgow on an earlier version of Chapter 2 were also much appreciated. Obviously I am myself solely responsible for any inaccuracies or other infelicities that remain. Finally, I am grateful for the patience and encouragement shown over the last few years by the Series Editors, Dave Müller and Chris Code, and by my wife and daughter, Hilary and Katharine.

John T. E. Richardson

Abbreviations

BPRS	Brief Psychiatric Rating Scale
CT	Computerized tomography
GOAT	Galveston Orientation and Amnesia Test
ICD	*International Classification of Diseases*
ICD-8	ICD, Eighth Revision
ICD-9	ICD, Ninth Revision
ICD-9-CM	ICD-9, Clinical Modification
IQ	Intelligence Quotient
MAE	Multilingual Aphasia Examination
MQ	Memory Quotient
MRI	Magnetic resonance imaging
NCCEA	Neurosensory Center Comprehensive Examination for Aphasia
PASAT	Paced auditory serial addition task
PICA	Porch Index of Communicative Ability
PTA	Post-traumatic amnesia
RA	Retrograde amnesia
WAIS	Wechsler Adult Intelligence Scale
WAIS-R	Wechsler Adult Intelligence Scale — Revised
WISC	Wechsler Intelligence Scale for Children
WMS	Wechsler Memory Scale
WMS-R	Wechsler Memory Scale — Revised

Chapter 1

Definitions, Epidemiology and Causes

In all industrialized countries, closed head injuries are responsible for vast numbers of hospital admissions and days of work lost. For instance, about 150 000 patients are admitted to hospital in the United Kingdom each year with a diagnosis that reflects closed head injury. Such injuries are a major cause of deaths following accidents, especially those that involve children and young people, and they are also a major cause of handicap and morbidity among the survivors. The population of head-injured patients is a substantial one and one that is unlikely to decrease in the foreseeable future. A good deal of valuable research has been aimed at the prevention or reduction of brain damage following head injury, but this has tended to focus on problems to do with the design of vehicles and protective devices rather than on the control and management of human behaviour on the roads, at work and elsewhere. Moreover, the clinical problem of treating these vast numbers of patients is not going to be solved by any dramatic medical breakthrough. Rather, it must be tackled by seeking a better appreciation of the condition that these patients present.

This clinical condition is intrinsically a neurological one, but its proper evaluation demands an understanding of the associated psychology and psychopathology. At the same time, a major neurological condition with such a high level of incidence ought to be extremely informative about the functioning of the human brain, and hence provide a major focus for neuropsychological investigation. In this book I have tried to integrate these two different perspectives by reviewing the clinical and neuropsychological aspects of closed head injury in a manner that is equally intelligible to reasearchers who are interested in the effects of brain damage upon human behaviour and to practitioners who are responsible for the assessment, management and rehabilitation of head-injured patients.

Definitions

To begin with, it is important to be clear about what is to count as a closed head injury and the different ways of conceptualizing the severity of such an injury. Unfortunately, this is by no means a simple matter.

Closed and Open Head Injuries

Strictly speaking, a *closed head injury* is an injury to the head that does not expose the contents of the skull. Such an injury can be distinguished from an *open* head injury in which the dura mater (the membrane that lines the interior of the skull) is torn and consequently the contents of the skull are exposed. This distinction is obviously important with regard to questions of immediate management, but it is of limited value for present purposes because head injuries of both sorts can occur that are otherwise relatively similar both in terms of their biomechanics and in terms of their clinical and neuropsychological consequences. In particular, it is somewhat arbitrary from this point of view to differentiate between a head injury in which the skull is left intact, a head injury that gives rise to a depressed fracture of the vault of the skull in which fragments of bone penetrate the dura mater, and a head injury that gives rise to a depressed fracture of the base of the skull which is compound into the paranasal or middle-ear cavities (cf. Jennett and Teasdale, 1981, p. 13). It is more useful, if less precise, to use the term 'closed head injury' to denote an injury in which the primary mechanism of damage is one of *blunt* impact to the head (Levin *et al.*, 1976a). This usually arises either as the result of rapid *acceleration* of the head due to a physical blow from a relatively blunt object or as the result of rapid *deceleration* of the head due to contact with a blunt and relatively immovable object or surface, although compression injuries resulting from crushing of the head may occasionally be encountered.

In this sense, closed head injuries are conventionally distinguished from *penetrating* head injuries of the sort produced by sharp instruments, such as knives or umbrellas, or by explosively propelled missiles, such as bullets or fragments of shells. The latter account for most cases of head injury sustained in military conflicts (Dresser *et al.*, 1973; Russell, 1951). During peace-time, the incidence of penetrating head injury is much less common, though in some parts of the United States gunshot wounds (self-inflicted or otherwise) are the most common cause of fatal head injury (Frankowski, 1986). Closed and penetrating head injuries differ not merely in terms of their likely external causes, but also in the patterns of neurological deficit to which they tend to give rise. In particular, penetrating head injuries produced by low-velocity missiles may well give rise to severe focal brain lesions but they often cause little or no disturbance of consciousness (Russell, 1951; Salazar *et al.*, 1986). (The high-velocity bullet wounds produced by modern armaments are much more devastating in their effects, because the pressure gradient that is associated with an object travelling at supersonic speed creates a cavity within the brain; this leads to generalized tissue damage, extensive skull fracturing and a low probability of survival: *see* Allen *et al.*, 1982; Owen-Smith, 1981, pp. 36–7.) In contrast, closed head injuries are much more likely to produce disturbances of consciousness and diffuse cerebral damage. In this book I shall be concerned exclusively with the clinical and neuropsychological aspects of closed head injuries as just defined; that is, *a closed head injury is an injury to the head in which the primary mechanism of damage is one of blunt impact.*

The *International Classification of Diseases* (ICD) has been designed by the World Health Organization for the classification and comparison of morbidity and mortality data and for the indexing of hospital records. In terms of the Ninth Revision, ICD-9 (World Health Organization, 1977, chap. XVII), cases of head injury may be classified as follows (cf. Jennett and Teasdale, 1981, pp. 1–2):

800 Fracture of vault of skull
801 Fracture of base of skull
802 Fracture of face bones
803 Other and unqualified skull fractures
804 Multiple fractures involving skull or face with other bones
850 Concussion
851 Cerebral laceration and contusion
852 Subarachnoid, subdural and extradural haemorrhage, following injury
853 Other and unspecified intracranial haemorrhage following injury
854 Intracranial injury of other and unspecified nature.

Some researchers have excluded ICD category 802 ('Fracture of face bones') from consideration (e.g., Caveness, 1979; Jennett and MacMillan, 1981), apparently on the assumption that such injuries are unlikely to give rise to serious brain damage. To be sure, the facial skeleton consists of compressible, energy-absorbing bones which tend to cushion and protect the intracranial structures in the event of a frontal impact. Nevertheless, many patients with major facial injuries, especially those involving the forehead, show clear deficits on neurological examination, and in such cases computerized tomography (CT) reveals a variety of intracranial lesions (Lee *et al.*, 1987). Following Field (1976, p.1), however, I shall be concerned only with injuries that carry some risk of damage to the brain substance, and I shall therefore exclude from consideration trivial wounds of the face and scalp and direct injuries to the cranial nerves. These would be included in the following ICD categories:

873 Other and unspecified laceration of head
910 Superficial injury of face, neck and scalp except eye
920 Contusion of face, scalp, and neck except eye(s)
950 Injury to optic nerve and pathways
951 Injury to other cranial nerve(s).

The US Department of Health and Human Services has developed a clinical modification of ICD-9 (ICD-9-CM) 'to serve as a useful tool in the area of classification of morbidity data for indexing of medical records, medical care review, and ambulatory and other medical care programs, as well as for basic health statistics' (Public Health Service and Health Care Financing Administration, 1980, p. xvii). The disease classification of the original three-digit categories 800, 801, 803 and 804 (fracture of skull) has been expanded along the following lines (*op. cit.*, chap. 17):

800.0   Closed without mention of intracranial injury
800.1   Closed with cerebral laceration and contusion
800.2   Closed with subarachnoid, subdural, and extradural haemorrhage
800.3   Closed with other and unspecified intracranial haemorrhage
800.4   Closed with intracranial injury of other and unspecified nature
800.5   Open without mention of incracranial injury
800.6   Open with cerebral laceration and contusion
800.7   Open with subarachnoid, subdural, and extradural haemorrhage
800.8   Open with other and unspecified intracranial haemorrhage
800.9   Open with intracranial injury of other and unspecified nature.

The preamble to this section of ICD-9-CM explains that an 'open' fracture subsumes the following descriptions: 'compound', 'infected', 'missile', 'puncture' and 'with foreign body'. All other cases of nonpathological skull fracture (including those described as 'comminuted', 'depressed', 'elevated', 'fissured', 'linear' and 'simple') are classified as 'closed' fractures. A somewhat different subclassification is applied to the original three-digit categories 851–854 (intracranial injury without skull fracture), based on whether there is any mention of an open intracranial wound; this includes both those explicitly specified as open and those where there is mention of infection or a foreign body (*op.cit.*, p. 774).

Concepts and Measures of Severity

Jennett (1976a) pointed out that the *severity* of a head injury can be measured in terms of the occurrence or duration of its initial features, the incidence of complications and its long-term consequences or *sequelae*. To begin with, it is possible to evaluate the severity of head injuries purely in terms of the extent of physical damage to the victim, and this is commonly employed in research into vehicle accidents. For instance, the Abbreviated Injury Scale developed by the Joint Committee on Injury Scaling (1976) of the American Association for Automotive Medicine uses a seven-point scale (from 'no injury' to 'maximal') which can be applied to different body regions as well as to the body as a whole. This was used by Rutherford *et al.* (1985) to classify injuries to vehicle occupants in the 12 months before and after the introduction of legislation in the UK to compel the use of seat belts by drivers and front-seat passengers. It was also used by Gennarelli *et al.* (1989) to evaluate mortality following head injury and extracranial injury of varying degrees of severity.

However, most clinicians attempt to determine the severity of an injury in terms of the degree of neurological or psychological impairment during the immediate post-traumatic period. In particular, closed head injuries tend to produce an immediate loss or impairment of consciousness, and Symonds (1928) suggested that the duration of this impairment could be used as an indication of the degree of cerebral damage. ICD–9–CM incorporates an obligatory fifth digit to identify the manifestations of diseases, and this takes the form of the following subclassification for use with categories 800, 801, 803, 804 and 851–854:

0   Unspecified state of consciousness (e.g., 800.20)
1   With no loss of consciousness
2   With brief [less than one hour] loss of consciousness
3   With moderate [1–24 hours] loss of consciousness
4   With prolonged [more than 24 hours] loss of consciousness and return to pre-existing conscious level
5   With prolonged [more than 24 hours] loss of consciousness, without return to pre-existing conscious level
6   With loss of consciousness of unspecified duration
9   With concussion, unspecified.

A similar subclassification is used as a fourth digit with category 850; for instance, concussion with moderate loss of consciousness is classified as 850.3.

As is implied in the above descriptions, the notion of an immediate loss of consciousness is included in the traditional concept of *cerebral concussion*, but this term has been used in systematically different ways by different authorities. A more rigorous characterization of the onset of cerebral concussion was suggested by Ommaya and Hirsch (1971) for use in experimental research with subhuman primates:

1   loss of coordinated responses to noxious external stimuli;
2   cessation of breathing (apnoea) for more than 3 sec, followed by irregular slow breathing;
3   slowing of the heart rate by 20–30 beats per min (bradycardia);
4   loss of the corneal and eyelid reflexes;
5   loss of voluntary movements;
6   dilation of the pupils for more than 15 sec.

These criteria are supposedly listed in a decreasing order of importance (cf. Ommaya *et al.*, 1966). Symonds (1962) pointed out that in research of this sort the animals were anaesthetized, and he argued that consequently the phenomenon of concussion was 'shorn of its most important clinical symptom, loss of consciousness' (pp.1–2). It is indeed usually assumed that general anaesthesia is an all-or-nothing state that involves a total loss of consciousness. Recent research has nevertheless demonstrated that anaesthesia exhibits varying degrees of 'depth' in terms of the patient's awareness of the external environment (Jones, 1989). (This is to a large extent the crux of the recent ethical controversy concerning the very use of animals in experimental research on head injury.) For example, in one study 44 per cent of patients in whom a general anaesthesia was carefully maintained by means of a commonly used regimen (inhaled nitrous oxide plus increments of intravenous fentanyl) were nevertheless able to respond to verbal commands by making appropriate hand movements, although most were unable to recall such events at a postoperative interview (Russell, 1986).

The clinical usage of the term 'concussion' has been influenced by assumptions about the underlying pathophysiology and the wider effects of closed head injury upon neurological function. To begin with, concussion (or *commotio cerebri*) was traditionally defined as the transient loss of consciousness without permanent damage to the brain (e.g., Denny-Brown and Russell, 1941; Symonds, 1928; Ward, 1966). In this sense, it was to be contrasted with 'contusion' (*contusio cerebri*), the physical bruising of the brain with or without a loss of consciousness (e.g., Eden and Turner, 1941). However, such a distinction has long been recognized to be problematic (Symonds, 1962). As Ommaya and Gennarelli (1974) pointed out, the modern concept of cerebral concussion includes at least the possibility of permanent brain damage (*see* Chapter 2, pp. 39–40). It is still recognized that such damage is not an inevitable consequence of a single concussive blow. Indeed, recent studies using magnetic resonance imaging have shown that lesions to the grey and white matter of the brain itself may well resolve within three months following a minor closed head injury; any residual lesions are likely to be extraparenchymal abnormalities, such as chronic subdural haematomas (Levin *et al.*, 1987a). Nevertheless, there is a narrow range between the force necessary to cause a transient functional impairment and that sufficient to produce irreversible structural change (Shetter and Demekas, 1979).

As a separate issue, it is sometimes assumed that closed head injury gives rise *both* to an impairment of consciousness *and* to an amnesia for episodes immediately preceding the injury, and the latter condition of *retrograde amnesia* has also been incorporated into the concept of cerebral concussion. However, it is important to distinguish carefully between loss of consciousness and retrograde amnesia, since they may be produced by different sorts of cerebral dysfunction. Moreover, research to be discussed in Chapter 3 has suggested that the duration of retrograde amnesia has very little value as an index of the severity of injury (see pp. 71–2).

It is nowadays generally agreed that the duration and extent of the patient's impairment of consciousness is likely to be a characteristic of major importance in evaluating the severity of a closed head injury and in predicting the eventual outcome (e.g., Evans *et al.*, 1976). Brock (1960) even maintained that 'the degree of concussion is measured by the best yardstick presently available, namely, the degree and duration of the unconsciousness and/or abnormalities of consciousness, viz., confusion and dazed states related to it' (p. 20). It has been suggested that a *severe* head injury should be defined as one that produces a state of unconsciousness or *coma* lasting longer than six hours (Jennett *et al.*, 1975a). The duration of coma is however difficult to estimate in the case of less severely injured patients, who have typically recovered consciousness by the time that they are admitted to hospital (Gronwall and Wrightson, 1980). Levin and Eisenberg (1979a) compared the duration of coma with CT findings among 33 children and adolescents with closed head injury. Abnormalities were visualized on CT in six out of 14 patients who had been conscious at the time of their admission to hospital, in all six of the patients who had been unconscious for up to 24 hours, but in only 10 of the 13 patients who had been unconscious for longer than 24 hours. As Levin and Eisenberg concluded, 'persistent coma was clearly not a necessary or sufficient condition for a positive CT scan' (p. 393).

Moreover, even the concept of coma or unconsciousness is not immune to definitional problems. Many definitions that have been offered emphasize the inability to establish intellectual contact with the patient (Bond, 1979; Overgaard *et al.*, 1973; Roberts, 1979, p. 30; Stover and Zeiger, 1976; Thomsen, 1975, 1976): the patient's consciousness is impaired to the extent that he or she cannot be aroused by spoken commands, understand questions, or provide coherent responses. However, other aspects of the patient's behaviour may be important as well. In addition, it may be important to identify states that are intermediate between coma and full consciousness. For instance, Jennett and Plum (1972) noted that certain patients who had recovered from coma (in that they had periods of wakefulness when their eyes were open) nevertheless remained within a 'vegetative state' in which responses were limited to primitive postural and reflex movements of the limbs (see Chapter 7, pp. 221–2). Levin *et al.* (1976a) defined 'coma' as 'a failure of the patient to exhibit vocal responses or carry out purposeful motor activity after verbal or somatic stimulation by the examiner' and 'stupor' as 'an uncommunicative state of the patient from which he could be aroused to vocalisation or purposeful motor activity' (p. 1063; *see also* Plum and Posner, 1980).

The Glasgow Coma Scale

In order to resolve such problems of definition and to facilitate communication among different medical units and different hospital staff, Teasdale and Jennett (1974) developed the Glasgow Coma Scale. This involved the separate assessment of motor responses, verbal responses and eye opening according to an ordered set of criteria indicating the degree of cerebral dysfunction:

Motor responses:
Obeying commands
A localizing response
A flexor response
Extensor posturing
No response

Verbal responses:
    Orientation
    Confused conversation
    Inappropriate speech
    Incomprehensible speech
    No response

Eye opening:
    Spontaneous eye opening
    Eye opening in response to speech
    Eye opening in response to pain
    No response

In the absence of an appropriate motor response to command, this element of the Scale was assessed by observing the responses to painful pressure applied to the fingernail bed with a pencil; if flexion of the relevant limb was observed, stimulation was applied to the head, neck and trunk to test for localization. 'Orientation' referred to awareness of the self and one's environment: 'The patient should know who he is, where he is, and why he is there; know the year, the season, and the month' (p. 82). Preliminary applications of this Scale suggested that it could be readily and routinely used by relatively inexperienced junior doctors or nursing staff to assess a patient's level of consciousness (Teasdale, 1975). High rates of consistency were demonstrated among different raters, whether the Scale was being used by nurses, neurosurgeons or general surgical trainees, and it also seems to be fairly insensitive to linguistic and cultural variations among different observers (*see* Braakman *et al.*, 1977; Teasdale *et al.*, 1974, 1978).

The Glasgow Coma Scale is also useful in monitoring the progress and recovery of individual patients, and for this purpose Teasdale *et al.* (1975) devised a standard chart for recording the results of successive assessments (*see* Figure 1.1). In principle, it is possible to record the patient's best and worst response on each of the three elements of the Scale during a number of time intervals (Jennett *et al.*, 1975a), but it is the best response which has the greater prognostic value (Jennett *et al.*, 1979b) and which is routinely used.

In their original presentation of the Glasgow Coma Scale, Teasdale and Jennett (1974) emphasized that for any particular patient one or other element of the Scale might prove to be untestable. For example, the limbs might be immobilized by splints for fractures, speech might be precluded by intubation or a tracheostomy, and swollen eyelids or bilateral lesions of the third nerve might make eye opening impossible (cf. Marshall *et al.*, 1983a). For this reason, as Jennett (1976a) noted, a patient's state was simply described in terms of his or her place on each individual element, and any attempt to define a series of levels of coma was deliberately avoided. Nevertheless, Jennett *et al.* (1975a, 1975b) suggested that the criteria appropriate to each element of

Figure 1.1   *Glasgow Coma Scale observation record chart*

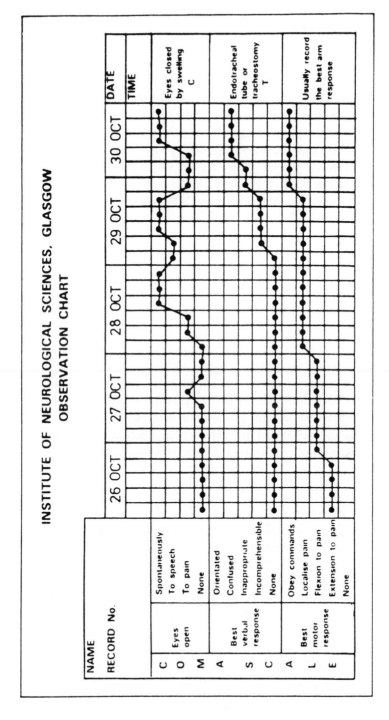

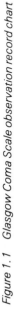

Source: Jennett, B. (1979) 'Defining brain damage after head injury', *Journal of the Royal College of Physicians of London,* 13, pp. 197–200. Reprinted by permission.

the Scale could be rank-ordered from the poorest to the best possible response, and that a patient's overall level of consciousness could be quantified by summing the ranks of the best observed response across the three elements. This yielded a total score between 3 and 14, reflecting various levels of impairment extending from deep coma through mild confusion to normal consciousness. Jennett *et al.* acknowledged that this method of calculating an overall coma score did assume that the intervals between successive criteria on a given element of the Scale were of equal significance. Further research was expected to reveal the relative weights that should be assigned to different intervals in each element of the scale, but no results on this point seem to have been subsequently published. Moreover, Jennett (1979) showed that a full knowledge of the three separate elements of the Scale provided a better prediction of the eventual outcome than the total score, though Teasdale *et al.* (1979a) also showed that the latter was a better prognostic indicator than the score on any individual element alone.

Computing a total score on the Glasgow Coma Scale also assumes that the three different elements of the Scale are strictly commensurable, that they make equivalent contributions to the residual level of consciousness, but that those contributions are additive and independent of one another. Each of these assumptions is certainly false. In the first place, the clinical signs assessed by the different elements of the Glasgow Coma Scale correspond to different levels of damage in the nervous system; as Levy *et al.* (1981) observed:

> Disturbances in the content of speech, recognition of the environment, and response to commands reflect on the integrity of the forebrain. Activities of the eyes other than voluntary gaze . . . primarily express functions regulated by the brain stem. Signs of abnormal limb posturing appear mainly to indicate the extent and severity of deep forebrain injury and do not necessitate brain stem damage. Absent motor responses imply brain stem damage or depression. Deep tendon reflexes are governed largely at the spinal level and bear little correlation with recovery from coma. (p. 299)

In the second place, during the immediate phase of recovery from severe closed head injury the total score on the Glasgow Coma Scale is largely a function of the patient's motor responses (Braakman *et al.*, 1977; Jennett, 1976b, 1979; Levin and Eisenberg, 1979b; Levin *et al.*, 1979a; Teasdale *et al.*, 1979a), whereas during the later phase of recovery from minor closed head injury it is largely a function of the patient's verbal responses (Rimel *et al.*, 1981). Indeed, Jennett and Teasdale (1981, p. 89) suggested that once head-injured patients were speaking the distinction between expletive language, confused conversation and normal orientation provided a useful means of grading their brain dysfunction. In the third place, Levin and Eisenberg (1979a, 1979b) found a highly significant association between the levels of responding on different elements of the Glasgow Coma Scale, and Jennett and Teasdale (1981, p. 89) noted that many patients showed a close correlation between the return of one function and that of another. This is consistent with the idea that the different elements of the Scale are manifestations of some common neurological state, but equally suggests that some other combinatorial procedure than simple addition would be more appropriate for computing an overall score.

Subsequently, Teasdale and Jennett (1976) amended the motor-response element by distinguishing between a normal flexor response (i.e., a rapid withdrawal of the stimulated arm by lateral movement at the shoulder away from the body and often by external rotation of the arm) and abnormal or stereotyped responses (such as the hemiplegic or decorticate posture with the shoulder drawn in towards the body and the elbow and fingers flexed). It has been suggested that this can be a difficult distinction for nurses, nonspecialist doctors and even experienced observers to make (Braakman *et al.*, 1977; Jennett and Teasdale, 1981, p. 78). Nevertheless, this extended version of the Glasgow Coma Scale is the one that is now in general use (*see* Table 1.1). Using the standard scoring method, this version yields a total score between 3 and 15, although Bond (1986) mentioned recent modifications of the Glasgow Coma Scale which rate the poorest performances on each element at zero and which therefore yield a total score between 0 and 12 points. Teasdale and Jennett defined 'coma' clinically as

Table 1.1   Extended Glasgow Coma Scale

Eye opening (E)	
spontaneous	4
to speech	3
to pain	2
nil	1
Best motor response (M)	
obeys	6
localizes	5
withdraws	4
abnormal flexion	3
extensor response	2
nil	1
Verbal response (V)	
orientated	5
confused conversation	4
inappropriate words	3
incomprehensible sounds	2
nil	1

Coma score (E + M + V) = 3 to 15

Source: Jennett, B. and Teasdale, G. (1981) *Management of Head Injuries*, Philadelphia, PA, Davis. Adapted by permission 'a patient who showed no eye opening, who did not obey commands, nor give any comprehensible verbal response' (p. 50); this corresponds to a total score on the original Glasgow Coma Scale of 7 or less (cf. Winogron *et al.*, 1984) and to a total score on the amended Glasgow Coma Scale of 8 or less. The latter has been widely used as an operational definition of 'coma' by researchers in North America, Western Europe and Australia. In particular, the apparent consistency with which the Glasgow Coma Scale could be used by observers in different centres encouraged its use in an international collaborative study, initially between units in Scotland and the Netherlands (Jennett *et al.*, 1976) and subsequently involving also units in the United States (Heiden *et al.*, 1983; Jennett *et al.*, 1977b, 1979b). This eventually encompassed 1000 patients and demonstrated that the total score on the Glasgow Coma Scale was highly predictive of the eventual clinical outcome following head injury. The same conclusion emerged from more recent investigations (*see*, e.g., Alexandre *et al.*, 1983; Bowers and Marshall, 1980; Marshall *et al.*, 1983a; Marshall and Bowers, 1985).

The Glasgow Coma Scale has been supplemented by measurements of systolic blood pressure and respiratory rate to yield an index of the severity of physiological injury, the *Trauma Score*; this is intended to help personnel at the scene of an accident or on admission to hospital to decide whether a patient should be referred for specialized neurosurgical treatment, and can also be used to predict the probability of survival (Champion *et al.*, 1989). The Glasgow Coma Scale has also been found to have both diagnostic and prognostic value in the assessment of coma resulting from nontraumatic causes including cerebrovascular disease, hypoxia-ischaemia and hepatic encephalopathy (Levy *et al.*, 1981). In this study, however, the clinical states demonstrated by 500 patients were classified at various times after their hospitalization into three broad levels of consciousness:

> *Coma* means eyes do not open or open only in response to pain, motor response of withdrawal or poorer, and verbal response no better than incomprehensible sounds. *Vegetative* means eyes open in response to noise or spontaneously, otherwise, like coma. *Conscious* means localizing motor responses, obeying commands, or production of comprehensible words, regardless of eye opening. (p. 295, italics added)

The operational criteria were based upon the work of Plum and Posner (1980) and were slightly different from those that had originally been suggested by Teasdale and Jennett (1976). Moreover, the three levels of consciousness defined above do not seem to be mutually exclusive in terms of the corresponding total scores on the amended Glasgow Coma Scale; in particular, a total score of eight points could in principle be attained by patients in all three clinical states. Nevertheless, all three elements of the Glasgow Coma Scale proved to be useful in predicting outcome on the basis of early clinical signs.

Problems with the Glasgow Coma Scale

Time of administration

There is currently some controversy concerning the appropriate time after injury when the Glasgow Coma Scale should first be administered. Reilly *et al.* (1975) noted that roughly one third of all fatally injured patients were known to have had a 'lucid interval' in which they had talked at some time after their accidents. They suggested that a lucid interval occurred in a similar proportion of severely injured but nonfatal cases, and this was borne out by subsequent research (Jennett *et al.*, 1976, 1977b; cf. Bruce *et al.*, 1978). Teasdale and Jennett (1976) noted that in such patients the development of coma would be delayed. In this situation, they made an initial assessment using the Glasgow Coma Scale after the development of coma, but also noted the patient's clinical state during the interim period. In considering the prognostic value of the Glasgow Coma Scale, they suggested the use of a patient's best level of clinical function during the first 24 hours after the onset of coma, and they restricted their attention just to those patients who remained in coma for at least six hours (*see also* Jennett *et al.*, 1976).

Jennett *et al.* (1977b) sought to justify the latter decision by arguing that a patient's clinical state during the first few hours following a head injury could be contaminated by extracranial injuries and their associated complications (such as shock and respiratory insufficiency). They suggested that other researchers might well have overestimated the extent of brain damage in their patients by taking as a baseline their clinical state during the immediate post-traumatic phase. Bruce *et al.* (1978) considered that such problems were especially likely to arise in studies of the effects of head injury in children. In their study of coma due to nontraumatic causes, Levy *et al.* (1981) also confined their attention to those patients whose coma had lasted at least six hours 'to eliminate from consideration the transient unresponsiveness of syncope (or the unresponsiveness of imminent death)' (p. 293).

Jennett and Teasdale (1977) and Jennett *et al.* (1979b) reinforced these arguments by observing that in adult patients alcohol intoxication would affect brain function during this period. Galbraith *et al.* (1976a) had indeed shown that the influence of alcohol would contaminate the assessment of a head-injured patient's conscious level on admission to hospital and lead to lower scores on the Glasgow Coma Scale (*see also* Rimel *et al.*, 1981). This would in turn mean that impaired consciousness among head-injured patients might be incorrectly attributed to the consumption of alcohol, or that the development of complications such as intracranial haematoma might be disguised. Nevertheless, provided that a head-injured patient's blood alcohol level was less than 200 mg per 100 ml, Galbraith *et al.* recommended that alterations in the patient's conscious state should be ascribed to the head injury itself rather than to intoxication.

Becker (1979) pointed out that delaying the assessment of a patient's level of consciousness for six hours precluded any proper evaluation of the effects of early surgical intervention on outcome. In fact, contemporary clinical practice tends to encourage prompt intervention, thus rendering later neurological assessment invalid (*see* Eisenberg and Weiner, 1987). This is especially true in the United States, where the researchers who instituted a National Traumatic Coma Data Bank involving six urban and regional centres resolved to administer the amended Glasgow Coma Scale following noncranial resuscitation of their patients (that is, after the stabilization of fluid volume and the treatment of hypoxia). Patients were to be included in the Data Bank as cases of acute severe head injury either (a) if they had a total coma score of 8 or less at this point or (b) if they deteriorated to a score of 8 or less during the first 48 hours after injury (Marshall *et al.*, 1983a).

In other studies carried out in North America the investigators have applied the Glasgow Coma Scale retrospectively to the case notes produced by the medical and nursing staff at the time of a patient's admission to hospital. Levin and Eisenberg (1979a, 1979b) found that the best verbal and motor responses of head-injured children could usually be classified in this manner, although the case notes were often equivocal with regard to eye opening. They found that the best verbal response and the best motor response on admission were both closely related to the duration of coma, defined as the period during which the patient failed to respond verbally or motorically to simple verbal commands. Similarly, Winogron *et al.* (1984) classified a head injury as 'severe' if it led to a score of 7 or less on the original Glasgow Coma Scale according to the case notes produced by the staff of the accident department. As a measure of the 'duration of altered consciousness', these researchers employed the time interval that elapsed before a patient attained the maximum score on all three elements of the Glasgow Coma Scale. In their sample of head-injured children this index showed a substantial negative correlation ($r = -0.76$) with a patient's clinical state on admission to hospital according to the Glasgow Coma Scale.

The role of language

A further problem that has only recently come to light concerns the involvement of linguistic skills in the various elements of the Glasgow Coma Scale. In defining consciousness and coma in terms of intellectual contact, Overgaard *et al.* (1973) observed that the latter in most cases meant verbal contact. Similarly, Jennett (1976a) noted that both doctors and relatives tended to characterize the end of coma as the point when a head-injured patient began to talk. Teasdale and Jennett (1974) remarked that intelligible speech had figured in nearly all previous attempts to describe impairments of consciousness, and they explicitly identified the patients' verbal responses as one of the defining elements of the Glasgow Coma Scale. However, they added an important qualification: 'Certainly the return of speech indicates the restoration of a high degree of integration within the nervous system, but continued speechlessness may be due to causes other than depressed consciousness (e.g., tracheostomy or dysphasia)' (p. 82; *see also* Teasdale *et al.*, 1979a). Because the majority of their patients with severe head injuries exhibited problems of communication, Gilchrist and Wilkinson (1979) defined 'unconsciousness' simply as the inability to respond purposefully to the environment.

The role of verbal *comprehension* has received little attention in later applications of the Glasgow Coma Scale, apparently because intelligible speech is totally abolished following severe closed head injury and (as mentioned above) the total coma score is largely determined by the patient's motor reponses. Nevertheless, obeying simple commands is the highest level of response on the latter element of the Scale, and Levin *et al.* (1979a) used this rudimentary level of comprehension as the criterion of termination of coma (*see also* Levin and Eisenberg, 1979a, 1979b). Similarly, Lewin *et al.* (1979) defined 'unconsciousness' as 'persisting until there was comprehension of the spoken word as demonstrated by obeying a verbal request' (p. 1534; *see also* Roberts, 1969, p. 30). Bricolo *et al.* (1980) argued that obeying simple commands was an important 'milestone' in recovery from coma: 'By far the most important step in the evolution of prolonged coma patients is the return of the capacity to execute simple commands: this constitutes unambiguous evidence of resumed mental activity, marks the end of unconsciousness, and is the necessary premise to all further recuperation' (p. 628). Obeying simple commands is also used in surgical practice as a criterion of 'waking up' from general anaesthesia (Russell, 1986).

Research on the sequelae of cerebrovascular accidents has suggested that lesions of the left cerebral hemisphere produce greater disturbances of consciousness than comparable lesions of the right hemisphere (e.g., Albert *et al.*, 1976; Schwartz, 1967). Similar results have been obtained following both penetrating brain wounds (Salazar *et al.*, 1986) and closed head injury (Levin and Eisenberg, 1986). Levin *et al.* (1989) suggested that these latter results might be artefacts due to the verbal demands imposed by the Glasgow Coma Scale. They examined the recovery from coma of 43 severely head-injured patients from the National Traumatic Coma Data Bank who had developed a unilateral intracerebral haematoma. When recovery was defined in terms of the highest level of motor response (obeying simple commands), the patients with lesions of the left hemisphere showed a much longer period of impaired consciousness than those with lesions of the right hemisphere. However, this was no longer true when the criterion of recovery was the next lower motor response (a localizing response to pain). Levin *et al.* concluded that the purported relation between language and consciousness was attributable to the verbal methods used to assess consciousness level, and that it would be necessary to devise alternative, nonverbal indicators of consciousness level in order adequately to assess the recovery of patients with left-hemisphere lesions. Moreover, the implication of these findings is that the side of an intracerebral lesion should be considered in predicting the duration of disturbed consciousness following closed head injury, even in the case of patients who are not clinically aphasic.

Other Measures of Severity

An alternative basis for categorizing cases of closed head injury in terms of the severity of their injuries is the duration of *post-traumatic amnesia* (PTA). The latter expression refers to the characteristic inability of head-injured patients to form new memories for a particular period after they recover consciousness. This concept will be discussed in detail in Chapter 3. Following an original suggestion by Russell and Smith (1961), many clinicians now regard as a 'severe' head injury (as opposed to a 'minor' head injury) one which gives rise to a period of PTA extending for more than 24 hours after the injury. Jennett *et al.* (1975a) mentioned that this corresponded to a period of coma of at least six hours' duration. A more detailed classification based on the duration of PTA was proposed by Jennett and Teasdale (1981, p. 90):

Less than 5 minutes — very mild
5 to 60 minutes — mild
1 to 24 hours — moderate
1 to 7 days — severe
1 to 4 weeks — very severe
More than 4 weeks — extremely severe

A different definition of the severity of a closed head injury might be expressed in terms of the duration of in-patient care. For instance, London (1967) characterized a severe head injury as 'one that either killed the patient or enforced a stay in hospital of at least seven days' (p. 462). Conversely, Rimel *et al.* (1981) defined a minor head injury as 'cranial trauma resulting in a loss of consciousness of 20 minutes or less, an admission Glasgow Coma Scale score of 13 or better, and the need for 48 hours or less of hospitalization' (p. 222). The latter criterion 'excluded patients with severe extracranial associated injuries or medical complications and, in general, reflected the neurosurgeons' assessment that the included patients had sustained minor head injuries not requiring treatment or additional observation' (*loc. cit.*). Gilchrist and Wilkinson (1979) noted that the total length of treatment of 84 patients with severe head injuries in both an acute hospital and a regional rehabilitation unit was directly proportional to the length of time that each patient had been unconscious. Similarly, in their study of 51 head-injured children at a Canadian hospital, Winogron *et al.* (1984) found a substantial negative correlation ($r = -0.67$) between the patient's clinical state on admission according to the Glasgow Coma Scale and the duration of subsequent hospitalization.

Finally, the severity of a head injury can be defined retrospectively in terms of the extent or duration of recovery. Indeed, Jennett (1976a) observed that it was implicit in the traditional concept of cerebral concussion that no structural damage had occurred to the brain and hence that the injury had no persisting sequelae. Nevertheless, as will be explained in Chapter 2, it is nowadays generally recognized that even a brief period of traumatic unconsciousness may well be associated with permanent structural damage, and indeed that a 'concussional' head injury is not necessarily a 'minor' one with regard to its consequences. The idea that severity might be defined with regard to the quality of the eventual outcome is however well motivated, and is especially relevant to those concerned with the social and economic impact of head injuries and with the provision and evaluation of rehabilitation services. Because of their dissatisfaction with earlier schemes, Jennett and Bond (1975) proposed a classification of patients with severe brain damage that was based on the degree of residual disability among the survivors and their consequent need for continuing social support: death; persistent vegetative state; severe disability (conscious but disabled); moderate disability (disabled but independent); and good recovery. This will be discussed in more detail in chapter 7 (pp. 226–9).

Epidemiology

England and Wales

Until very recently, the most convenient source of information on the epidemiology of closed head injuries in England and Wales was the Hospital In-patient Enquiry (Office of Population Censuses and Surveys, 1976–1987). This provided an annual analysis based upon a one-in-ten sample of all nonmaternity in-patient records from hospitals in the National Health Service, excluding hospitals and beds designated for the treatment of mental illness and mental handicap. Estimates of the corresponding national figures in any calender year can be obtained by dividing the statistics in the published tables by the exact sampling ratio.

Although information was provided for both England and Wales until 1981, subsequently the published findings covered only the English health authorities. Moreover, after 1985 the Hospital In-patient Enquiry was discontinued, and at the time of writing no statistics for subsequent years have been published. The year 1985 will therefore be taken as the baseline for discussing the epidemiology of closed head injuries in Great Britain. (The Hospital In-patient Enquiry has been replaced by a new system of Hospital Episode Statistics, which is intended to provide more detailed information based on a broader, 25 per cent sample of patients, but which is based on financial years rather than calendar years. Initial results from the first year of operation with effect from April 1987 were due to be published towards the end of 1989, but these are not likely to include information on detailed diagnostic categories. The results from subsequent years should be more useful for epidemiological purposes.)

As Field (1976) noted, hospital activity data 'will exclude mild cases not admitted to hospital, as well as the most severe who die before admission. Admission will depend not only on the severity of the injury, but also the admission policy of the hospital, which in turn will reflect the facilities and skills available in that hospital' (p. 3; *see also* Kraus, 1980). Jennett (1976a) observed that 'about a third of patients admitted to hospital with head injury have another injury, and it may be this rather than the head injury which leads to hospital admission, or which determines the length of stay' (p. 648). Subsequently, Jennett and MacMillan (1981) reported that patients with a minor head injury but a major extracranial injury accounted for 11 per cent of admissions but for one-third of all occupied bed days attributed to head injuries. Moreover, one recent study carried out in the United States found that 41 per cent of patients who had been admitted to hospital following traumatic spinal cord injuries provided histories that were consistent with a concomitant closed head injury (Davidoff *et al.*, 1986). Jennett also suggested that there were differences among hospital personnel in their use of the rubrics in the International Classification of Diseases. (This certainly seems to be true of personnel in England and in the United States, as will be seen below.) Nevertheless, the Hospital In-patient Enquiry data can be used to obtain an approximate estimate of the numbers of patients who in any one year received a head injury sufficiently serious to warrant their admission to hospital.

For 1985, the estimated incidence of the ten diagnostic categories described in the previous section is shown in Table 1.2. (Because of rounding errors the individual entries do not necessarily produce the totals shown.) This indicates that over 127 500 people out of a total national population of 47 111 700 were admitted to hospital that year with a diagnosis reflecting a head injury. This corresponds to an annual incidence rate of 2.71 cases of head injury per 1000 population, though this standardized admission rate shows pronounced regional variation, as Jennett and MacMillan (1981) pointed out. In addition, Jennett (1975b) suggested that 'probably four or five times as many patients attend casualty departments as are admitted' (p. 267). Rather more specifically, Jennett and MacMillan (1981) reported an annual rate of attendance during 1974 at accident and emergency departments in an area in the North-East of England of 16.20 cases of head injury per 1000 population, corresponding to 11 per cent of all new patients attending such departments. Out of the cases of head injury seen by the accident and emergency departments in the area in question, 22 per cent were subsequently admitted to hospital for treatment. When taken together with the figures shown in Table 1.2, these estimates would imply that in England rather more than 600 000 individuals receive a head injury each year that is sufficiently serious to lead them to seek medical treatment at a hospital. However, fewer than 5 per cent of these patients have received head injuries that are serious enough for them to be transferred to specialist neurosurgical units for investigation or treatment (Jennett *et al.*, 1979a).

Table 1.2   Estimated total number of discharges and deaths following head injury from hospitals in England in 1985 by nature of injury and gender of patient

Nature of injury (with ICD code)	Males	Females
Fracture of vault of skull (800)	2173	942
Fracture of base of skull (801)	1718	1004
Fracture of face bones (802)	12364	3559
Other and unqualified skull fractures (803)	1242	341
Multiple fractures involving skull or face with other bones (804)	93	0
Concussion (850)	9540	4532
Cerebral laceration and contusion (851)	331	93
Subarachnoid, subdural and extradural haemorrhage, following injury (852)	631	497
Other and unspecified intracranial haemorrhage following injury (853)	207	124
Intracranial injury of other and unspecified nature (854)	57134	31050
Totals	85432	42142

Source: Office of Population Censuses and Surveys (1987) *Hospital In-patient Enquiry 1985* (Series MB4, No. 27), London, Her Majestry's Stationery Office.

United States

In the United States, national epidemiological data were until recently available only from the household interviews of the civilian, noninstitutionalized population conducted annually by the National Health Interview Survey (National Center for Health Statistics, 1988a), in which respondents are asked to report any injuries received during the previous two weeks. Head injuries are unfortunately not differentiated from other sorts of injuries in the published results of these interviews. However, Caveness (1979) presented unpublished findings on head injuries reported during the period from 1970 to 1976, and a similar analysis was carried out in the case of the 1977 Survey. The results identify those head injuries associated with 'skull fracture and intracranial injury' (i.e. ICD–8 codes N800, N801, N803, and N850–854, which are identical to the corresponding ICD–9 codes). The findings suggest that in 1977 roughly 2 211 000 persons suffered an injury of this sort which either required medical attention or restricted their activity for at least one day. Of these, 226 000 were under six years of age, 516 000 were between 6 and 16 years of age, 1 123 000 were between 17 and 44 years of age, 213 000 were between 45 and 64 years of age, and 133 000 were 65 years of age or more. The total national population was approximately 212 153 000, yielding an annual incidence rate of 10.42 cases per 1000 population.

As Frankowski (1986) noted, these data 'are subject to a number of limitations. The data on injuries are self-reported and thus lack clinical confirmation. The data include self-treated injuries as well as medically-treated injuries; new injuries are not distinguished from previous injuries, and the extent of recall bias is unknown' (p. 154). Such criticisms do not apply to the National Head and Spinal Cord Injury Survey, which was a multistage probability survey of relevant hospital discharges in the United States between 1970 and 1974 (Anderson *et al.*, 1980). For the year 1974, it was estimated that 422 000 persons were hospitalized following head injuries, corresponding to an incidence rate of 2.00 cases per 1000 population (Kalsbeek *et al.*, 1980). Similar figures for hospitalization following head injury have been reported in several local surveys within the United States (e.g., Annegers *et al.*, 1980; Cooper *et al.*, 1983; Jagger *et al.*, 1984; Klauber *et al.*, 1978; Kraus *et al.*, 1984; cf. Whitman *et al.*, 1984). Finally, it is interesting to note that a retrospective questionnaire survey conducted by Crovitz *et al.* (1983) found that roughly 20 per cent of college students in the United States claimed to have been 'knocked out by a head injury' at some time in their lives, usually during childhood. (This latter is of course a measure of the *prevalence* of head injury, rather than its *incidence*.)

More recently, however, information about detailed diagnoses among hospital inpatients in the United States has been available from the National Hospital Discharge Survey. This covers an annual multistage sample of patients discharged from civilian, noninstitutional hospitals, and provides estimates of the annual incidence of all diseases according to the ICD–9–CM classification. Table 1.3 shows the estimated incidence during 1987 of the ten diagnostic categories described in the previous section. This

Table 1.3   Estimated total number of discharges and deaths (in thousands) following head injury from hospitals in the United States in 1987 by nature of injury and gender of patient

Nature of injury (with ICD code)	Males	Females
Fracture of vault of skull (800)	10	5
Fracture of base of skull (801)	22	12
Fracture of face bones (802)	90	48
Other and unqualified skull fractures (803)	10	4
Multiple fractures involving skull or face with other bones (804)	0	0
Concussion (850)	103	61
Cerebral laceration and contusion (851)	17	7
Subarachnoid, subdural and extradural haemorrhage, following injury (852)	15	7
Other and unspecified intracranial haemorrhage following injury (853)	7	5
Intracranial injury of other and unspecified nature (854)	67	39
Totals	341	188

Source: Graves, E. J. (1989) 'Detailed diagnoses and procedures, National Hospital Discharge Survey, 1987' *Vital and Health Statistics*, Series 13, No. 100, DHHS Pub. No. (PHS) 89–1761, Hyattsville, MD, Public Health Service.

indicates that approximately 530 000 people were admitted to hospital in the United States that year with a diagnosis reflecting a head injury. Since the total national population was 241 661 000, this figure corresponds to an incidence rate of 2.20 cases per 1000 population. A comparison between these figures and those produced by the National Health Interview Survey implies that, in line with the experience of the United Kingdom, only 20 per cent of all individuals who sustain head injuries are actually admitted to hospital in the United States (cf. Jennett, 1975b).

The most obvious difference between Table 1.2 and Table 1.3 is the predominant use in England of the diagnostic category 854 ('Intracranial injury of other and unspecified nature') as opposed to diagnostic category 850 ('Concussion'). Moreover, compared with the corresponding figures for England, roughly twice as many patients admitted to hospitals in the United States with a diagnosis reflecting head injury had a skull fracture (800–804). This probably reflects different admission policies in the two countries, as does the overall discrepancy in their annual incidence rates for hospitalization following head injury (i.e., 2.71 versus 2.21 cases per 1000 population: cf. Jennett and MacMillan, 1981). In both countries, patients with minor head injuries may be admitted to hospital purely for observation in case of the development of complications such as intracranial haematoma, intracranial infection, or post-traumatic epilepsy (*see* chapter 2, pp. 56–66). In fact, comparatively few go on to develop such complications, and most are discharged within a few days (Jennett and MacMillan, 1981). However, given the difficulty of predicting exactly *which* patients might develop complications, the criteria for their admission remain vague and vast numbers are apparently admitted unnecessarily and at considerable cost to the health services (Jennett, 1975b, 1976b; Jennett *et al.*, 1975a).

Analysis of the fourth-figure classifications applied to the patients who are shown in Table 1.3 suggests that fewer than one per cent of the head injuries sustained by the civilian population of the United States during 1987 were open head injuries. Moreover, although in many cases the post-traumatic state of consciousness was not adequately specified, and although many of the relevant estimates are based upon relatively few records and hence are of doubtful reliability, further analysis of the fifth-figure classification suggests that in the overwhelming majority of head injuries the duration of post-traumatic unconsciousness was less than one hour (data from Graves, 1989, Table 3). As Langfitt and Gennarelli (1982) commented, the 10–20 per cent of all hospitalized patients who have sustained severe head injuries may constitute only the tip of the iceberg.

Scotland

Comparable data are not always available from other countries. The Scottish Health Service (1987) publishes annual analyses of all patients discharged from Scottish hospitals using a short list of diagnoses which collapses together the categories contained in the full ICD–9. For 1985, the actual incidence of relevant diagnostic categories is shown in Table 1.4. This indicates that nearly 19 000 people were admitted to hospital that year with a diagnosis reflecting head injury out of a total national population of 5 136 500. This corresponds to an annual incidence rate of 3.68 cases per 1000 population; the latter is somewhat higher than the corresponding figure for England, but it does include the additional ICD categories 950 (injury to the optic nerve and pathways) and 951 (injury to other cranial nerves). In 1974 a survey was carried out of all patients who had been admitted to primary surgical wards in Scotland in two 2-week periods with a diagnosis that reflected head injury (Jennett *et al.*, 1977a). This yielded a total of 820 males and 361 females, which corresponds to an estimated annual incidence of 15 000 cases of head injury or 3.13 cases per 1000 population (Jennett and MacMillan, 1981). As in the case of patients in England and Wales, fewer than 5 per cent of these patients had sustained head injuries that were sufficiently serious to warrant their transfer to a regional neurosurgical unit for specialized investigation or treatment (Jennett *et al.*, 1979a).

The 1974 study also surveyed all new attendances at accident and emergency departments in Scotland during two separate weeks (Strang *et al.*, 1978). This yielded 3558 patients with a diagnosis reflecting head injury, of whom roughly 70 per cent were male. This corresponded to an estimated annual incidence of 84 000 or 17.78 cases per 1000 population (Jennett and MacMillan, 1981; Jennett *et al.*, 1977a). It was noted that cases of head injury represented about 11 per cent of all new attendances at accident and emergency departments and about 15 per cent of those attending after recent trauma. The estimated annual incidence rate is rather higher than the corresponding figure which was mentioned earlier for an English health authority. Nevertheless, the proportion of all patients attending such departments who had a head injury was essentially identical in these two regions, as was the proportion of all attenders with a head injury who were subsequently admitted to hospital (Jennett and MacMillan, 1981). Moreover, a comparison of Tables 1.2 and 1.4 shows that the

Table 1.4   Total number of discharges and deaths following head injury from hospitals in Scotland in 1985 by nature of injury and gender of patient

Nature of injury (with ICD codes)	Males	Females	Total
Fracture of skull (800, 801, 803, 804)	1013	333	1346
Fracture of face bones (802)	2149	547	2696
Concussion (850)	538	212	750
Other intracranial injuries (851–854, 950, 951)	9767	4357	14124
Totals	13467	5449	18916

Source: Scottish Health Service (1987) *Scottish Hospital In-Patient Statistics 1985*, Edinburgh, ISD Publications.

proportion of head-injured patients admitted to Scottish hospitals who had sustained a skull fracture is quite similar to that in England.

Changes over Recent Years

Table 1.5 shows the estimated incidence of the dignostic categories described in the previous section in England between the introduction of ICD–9 in 1979 and 1985. This indicates that the incidence of closed head injury has been relatively constant during the last few years. Indeed, the annual incidence rate of 2.71 cases per 1000 population that was cited above is almost identical to the corresponding figure for England and Wales in 1974 that was calculated by Jennett and MacMillan (1981). In contrast, several commentators noted that there had been a steady rise in hospital admissions during the 1960s and early 1970s. Epidemiological variations of this sort might have been produced by changes in environmental conditions, and some concern was expressed that the existing hospital resources were inadequate to accommodate the apparently increasing numbers of survivors (e.g., Jennett, 1976d; London, 1967).

However, Field (1976, pp.18–21) argued that the steady rise in hospital admissions during this period was largely the result of more liberal admission policies and the increased availability of resources (*see also* Jennett and MacMillan, 1981). He presented three sets of data to support this conclusion. First, the increase in hospital admissions was largely attributable to the less serious ICD categories 802, 850 and 854, and especially to the last of these, 'intracranial injury of other and unspecified nature'.

Table 1.5 Estimated total number of discharges and deaths following head injury from hospitals in England in 1979–1985 by nature of injury

ICD code	1979	1980	1981	1982	1983	1984	1985
800	2978	3322	2957	3130	3458	3089	3114
801	2876	3250	3070	2967	2611	2935	2721
802	13844	14178	14660	15435	14976	15364	15923
803	1469	1645	1848	1703	1961	1720	1583
804	185	248	216	204	248	196	93
850	18455	17044	17801	15608	15007	16456	14071
851	555	693	482	469	475	566	424
852	935	942	1027	1325	1115	1246	1128
853	339	207	267	326	279	350	331
854	89145	89134	88728	89561	88513	87766	88184
Totals	130780	130663	131054	130727	128641	129688	127574

Source: Office of Population Censuses and Surveys (1983–87) *Hospital In-patient Enquiry 1974–1985* (Series MB4, Nos. 14–27), London, Her Majesty's Stationery Office.

Second, the increase was largely attributable to patients whose stay in hospital was of seven days or less. Third, there was no sign of any corresponding increase in the number of deaths caused by head injury. Indeed, Jennett and MacMillan (1981) suggested that there had actually been a fall in the number of fatal and serious head injuries in Britain during the relevant period. Similarly, Caveness (1979) reported a decline in the number of head injuries associated with skull fracture or intracranial injury in the United States between 1970 and 1976, which he attributed to advances in occupational safety.

Age and Gender

Table 1.6 shows the estimated incidence of head injury in England during 1985 with the total number of patients classified separately by age and gender. (Once again, because of rounding errors the individual entries do not always produce the totals and subtotals shown.) It is apparent that there were roughly twice as many male patients as females overall (*see also* Tables 1.3 and 1.4), and that this discrepancy was most pronounced in the case of young adults. Not only are men more likely to suffer closed head injuries than women, but they are also likely to sustain more severe injuries, as evidenced by their scores on the Glasgow Coma Scale on admission and by the subsequent duration of coma (Levin *et al.*, 1979a). The age distribution for cases of head injury in the United States in 1987 was as follows: 0–14 years, 17.0 per cent; 15–44 years, 60.2 per cent; 45–64 years, 10.7 per cent; 65 years and over, 12.1 per cent (Graves, 1989, Table 3). Similar proportions have been obtained in previous investigations of the incidence of closed head injury both in the United Kingdom (Jennett *et al.*, 1977a; Rowbotham *et al.*, 1954; Steadman and Graham, 1970) and in the United States (Annegers *et al.*, 1980; Cooper *et al.*, 1983; Kalsbeek *et al.*, 1980;

Table 1.6   *Estimated total number of discharges and deaths following head injury from hospitals in England in 1985 by age and gender of patient*

Age	Males	Females	Total
0–4 years	8608	6487	15096
5–14 years	18324	8339	26663
15–44 years	45142	14051	59193
45–64 years	8215	4221	12437
65–74 years	2732	2680	5411
75–84 years	1718	4170	5887
85 years and over	693	2193	2887
Totals	85432	42142	127574

Source: Office of Population Censuses and Surveys (1987) *Hospital In-patient Enquiry 1985* (Series MB4, No. 27), London, Her Majesty's Stationery Office.

Kraus *et al.*, 1984; Marshall *et al.*, 1983a). These investigations have also indicated that in males the incidence of closed head injury increases progressively during childhood and early adulthood, reaching a peak around 20 years of age; in females, it tends to decline gradually with age (Annegers *et al.*, 1980; Jennett and MacMillan, 1981; Kraus *et al.*, 1984). The net result of these trends is that more than half of all head-injured patients seen in accident and emergency departments and more than half of all head-injured patients subsequently admitted to hospital are children or young adults (Field, 1976, p. 8; Jennett *et al.*, 1977a; Kalsbeek *et al.*, 1980). Klonoff (1971) found that a particularly high proportion of patients seen in a Canadian general hospital but not admitted were young children.

Social Class

Another personal characteristic which might be expected to influence the likelihood of closed head injury is the patient's social class. While Steadman and Graham (1970) found no clear differences between a sample of 390 head-injured patients and the general population in the distribution of social class, subsequent studies have found a higher incidence of closed head injury both among the lower social classes (Kerr *et al.*, 1971; Rimel *et al.*, 1981; Selecki *et al.*, 1968) and among their children (Klonoff, 1971; Rutter, 1980). Field (1976, pp. 10–1) presented unpublished material which suggested that male patients in unskilled manual occupations were overrepresented among the total number of admissions to hospital, especially those between 35 and 54 years of age. Similarly, there is a negative correlation between the incidence of head injury and the number of years of full-time education (Kraus, 1978). The effect of social class is presumably also responsible (at least in part) for the increased incidence of closed head injuries among the inner-city population (Whitman *et al.*, 1984).

Alcohol Consumption

It is generally assumed that a major predisposing factor in cases of traumatic injury is the use and abuse of alcohol (e.g., Reilly *et al.*, 1986), although as Fields (1976, p. 12) pointed out comparable data are not available as to the proportion of the population at risk who have consumed alcohol but not had accidents. In cases of head injury, in particular, alcohol intake is frequently recorded as a contributory factor (Jennett *et al.*, 1977b, 1979b). As O'Shanick (1986) noted, 'The typical scenario is one in which drunk driving young men hit drunk old pedestrians resulting in head trauma to both' (p. 174). Moreover, chronic alcoholism may be endemic in certain urban areas; in one study, it was suggested that approximately 20 per cent of the entire patient population of the hospital in question were known alcoholics, and that amongst head-injured patients the proportion was even higher (Heilman *et al.*, 1971). In another study, two-thirds of the patients were said to have had a history of heavy drinking (Livingston, 1986).

It would appear that between 20 and 40 per cent of all head-injured patients have consumed alcohol shortly before their accidents (Jennett *et al.*, 1977a; Kerr *et al.*, 1971; Selecki *et al.*, 1968). However, research carried out in Scotland has suggested that this proportion may be as high as 50 per cent among the patients attending the accident departments of inner-city hospitals (Strang *et al.*, 1978; Swann *et al.*, 1981) and among the patients subsequently admitted to such hospitals (Galbraith *et al.*, 1976a). The latter studies also found that the recent consumption of alcohol was related to a number of different factors:

1   Male patients who had sustained a head injury were more than twice as likely to have consumed alcohol as female patients, and the mean level of blood alcohol that resulted was higher in men (193 mg per 100 ml) than in women (165 mg per 100 ml). Nevertheless, since the national legal limit for driving was 80 mg per 100 ml, both of these figures represent a significant degree of intoxication.

2   More than 40 per cent of all head-injured patients are seen between 5.00 p.m. and midnight. Over one-third of all head-injured patients attending accident departments and nearly a half of all such patients who are admitted to hospital arise from injuries on a Friday or Saturday. The proportion of patients with detectable levels of blood alcohol is much higher on these two days of the week (62 per cent) than on other days (43 per cent).

3   The proportion of all head-injured patients in these samples, the proportion of such patients with detectable levels of blood alcohol, and the mean levels of blood alcohol that result are higher following assaults and falls than following traffic accidents or other causes.

The importance of alcohol as a contributory cause of head injuries was confirmed in a subsequent study by Rimel *et al.* (1981) which involved 538 patients with minor head injury (defined by a Glasgow Coma Scale score on admission of 13–15) and 260 patients with severe head injury (defined by a Glasgow Coma Scale score on admission of 8 or less). In this study, alcohol was detected on admission in the blood of 43 per cent of the former and 84 per cent of the latter; the mean level of blood alcohol across all patients tested was 80 mg per 100 ml in those with minor head injuries and 190 mg per 100 ml in those with severe head injuries (Rimel *et al.*, 1981). As noted earlier (p. 13), this obviously makes it more difficult to assess the patient's clinical state. Moreover, as McMillan and Glucksman (1987) pointed out, excessive alcohol consumption can mimic PTA and can therefore make estimations of the duration of PTA inaccurate, especially in the case of patients who have sustained minor head injuries.

Other Predisposing Factors

There has been somewhat less investigation of other predisposing or constituional factors in the incidence of closed head injuries. There have been some suggestions that certain victims are 'accident-prone' because of being psychiatrically disturbed or socially maladjusted (Ruesch *et al.*, 1945; Sims, 1985), and Dencker (1958) concluded a study of closed head injuries in twins by commenting that 'the head injured persons seemed to differ in pretraumatic mental make-up from the average subject' (p. 119). On the basis of their enquiries into the family backgrounds of 162 children admitted to hospital following head injury, Hjern and Nylander (1964) concluded as follows:

> A remarkably large number came from homes with mentally ill or asocial parents, a remarkably large number had parents with anxious and grossly exaggerated fears of the sequelae of head injuries, a remarkably large number had already had head injuries previously or had been involved in other accidents and a remarkably large number had already manifested pronounced symptoms of mental illness before the head injury. (p. 35)

The absence of any comparison group in this study makes it difficult to evaluate how 'remarkable' the findings really were, but Jennett (1972) concurred that 'socially deprived and mildly backward children are more frequently encountered than in the general population' (p. 143). There is some evidence that this is especially true of those children who sustain only moderately severe head injuries (Rutter *et al.*, 1980; although cf. Klonoff, 1971).

Moreover, one recent study in the United States found a history of poor premorbid academic performance in 42 per cent of a sample of adult patients with severe closed head injuries, and in 50 per cent of those who had been born after the concept of learning disability had been legally recognized (Haas *et al.*, 1987). It is interesting in this context to note that figures of 33–35 per cent have been reported in the case of patients suffering from spinal injuries (Hall *et al.*, 1987; Wilmot *et al.*, 1985). The role of constitutional 'risk' factors is also shown by the relatively high incidence of subsequent accidents in those who have received an initial head injury (Klonoff, 1971; and cf. Rimel *et al.*, 1981). Among adults the single most important characteristic mediating this effect is probably persistent alcohol abuse (Annegers *et al.*, 1980). Some writers have sought to characterize those most at risk in particular contexts, such as those drivers who are likely to be involved in traffic accidents (Jamieson, 1971b). However, it is not really feasible at present to attempt to give a general or systematic account of the constitutional factors determining the incidence of head injury.

Mortality

Information on mortality following closed head injury in England and Wales is available from the Registrar General's annual review of deaths which is published by the Office of Population Censuses and Surveys (1980–88). The number of deaths in each of the ten diagnostic categories described earlier during 1985 is shown in Table 1.7. This indicates that there were 4065 fatal head injuries in England and Wales that year, corresponding to a figure of 8.14 deaths per 100 000 population. Such injuries represented 0.96 per cent of all deaths among males, 0.42 per cent of all deaths among females, and 0.69 per cent of all deaths across the population as a whole. Skull fractures appear to be especially related to a high mortality after head injury.

Unpublished figures supplied by the Office of Population Censuses and Surveys show that there were 3747 cases of fatal head injury during 1985 in England alone. According to the Hospital In-patient Enquiry for the same year, approximately 1645 deaths of patients who had been admitted to English hospitals fell under the ten diagnostic categories concerned. It follows that the remaining 2102 or 56 per cent of all deaths ascribed to head injury occurred before admission to hospital. This is very much in line with previous estimates of the proportion of patients with fatal head injuries who are dead on arrival in hospital that have been offered both in Britain (W. B. Jennett, quoted by Henry, 1979; but cf. Jennett and MacMillan, 1981) and in the United States (Frankowski, 1986). In the case of the US National Head and Spinal Cord Injury Survey, the proportion of fatally injured cases who received no hospital in-

Table 1.7   Total number of deaths following head injury in England and Wales in 1985 by nature of injury and gender of patient

Nature of injury (with ICD code)	Males	Females
Fracture of vault of skull (800)	29	4
Fracture of base of skull (801)	184	84
Fracture of face bones (802)	18	11
Other and unqualified skull fractures (803)	1407	550
Multiple fractures involving skull or face with other bones (804)	330	121
Concussion (850)	10	1
Cerebral laceration and contusion (851)	211	118
Subarachnoid, subdural and extradural haemorrhage, following injury (852)	166	164
Other and unspecified intracranial haemorrhage following injury (853)	56	40
Intracranial injury of other and unspecified nature (854)	387	174
Totals	2798	1267

Source: Office of Population Censuses and Surveys (1987) *Mortality Statistics 1985: Cause* (Series DH2, No. 12), London, Her Majesty's Stationery Office.

patient care seems to have been even greater (Anderson and Kalsbeek, 1980). However, Jennett (1976a) suggested that 'a number of pre-hospital deaths ascribed to head injury are due to other causes, such as fracture-dislocation of the cervical spine or multiple injuries' (p. 648).

The World Health Organization (1977, p. xvi) recommends that deaths due to injury should be classified according to the external cause of the injury rather than according to its nature. As a result, in the mortality statistics of certain countries, deaths caused by closed head injury are subsumed with other accidents and are not shown as a distinct category. This is true, for example, of the Annual Reports produced by the Registrar General for Scotland (1987) and also of the annual mortality data published by the United States National Center for Health Statistics (1988b). Goldsmith (1972) suggested that the total number of deaths due to head injury in the United States might be as many as 100 000 per year, corresponding to a mortality rate of more than 40 per 100 000 population. However, Jennett and MacMillan (1981) suggested that the annual mortality rate in the United States following closed head injury was roughly 22–25 per 100 000 population, although this is still more than twice the rate found in Britain. The US National Center for Health Statistics (1984) reported an analysis of the ascribed causes of all resident deaths which occurred during 1978. Summary data were not reported separately for cases of skull fracture, but 49 797 out of the 210 942 deaths due to injury fell within the ICD–8 categories corresponding to intracranial injury without skull fracture, N850–N854. Finally, Gennarelli *et al.* (1989) described the results of a survey of 49 143 patients admitted to trauma centres in the US over a 4-year period, of whom 4982 subsequently died. Those with head injuries (defined as injuries to the brain or skull according to the Abbreviated Injury Scale: *see* p. 4) accounted for 34 per cent of all admissions but for 60 per cent of all deaths. More than 80 per cent of all patients with head injuries also had extracranial injuries (which in nearly half of such cases were judged as severe). The mortality rate was if anything lower in these patients (17 per cent) than in those with pure head injuries (23 per cent), but this was because the latter included a disproportionate number of highly lethal penetrating gunshot wounds. In other respects, the presence of extracranial injury had little impact on the mortality of head-injured patients unless it was of maximal severity.

Table 1.8 shows the number of deaths in England and Wales in each of the ten diagnostic categories since the introduction of ICD–9 in 1979. In his own analysis, Field (1976, pp. 29–31 and Fig. 10) elegantly showed how fluctuations in the annual mortality rate associated with closed head injuries were attributable almost entirely to variations in the number of such deaths caused by motor vehicle accidents (though cf. Kalsbeek *et al.*, 1980). In this context it is interesting that the total number of deaths following closed head injury in England and Wales was consistently around 4500 per year throughout the 1960s and 1970s (corresponding to a rate of 9–10 deaths per 100 000 population) and reached a peak of 5053 in 1978. However, it then fell to

Table 1.8   Total number of deaths following head injury in England and Wales in 1979–1986 by nature of injury

ICD code	1979	1980	1981	1982	1983	1984	1985	1986
800	46	29	29	36	28	38	33	24
801	415	429	300	379	373	311	268	313
802	36	31	27	31	40	29	29	25
803	2297	2223	1953	1992	1959	2063	1957	1973
804	527	542	334	467	540	508	451	419
850	26	29	13	20	16	19	11	14
851	418	322	357	337	325	353	329	282
852	343	301	328	315	348	332	330	331
853	111	118	119	92	101	87	96	95
854	287	361	450	395	399	432	561	546
Totals	4506	4385	3910	4064	4129	4172	4065	4022

Source: Office of Population Censuses and Surveys (1980–88), *Mortality Statistics 1979–1986: Cause* (Series DH2, Nos. 6–13), London, Her Majesty's Stationery Office.

around 4000 per year, apparently in response to official Government campaigns to promote the wearing of seat belts by the drivers and front-seat passengers in road vehicles. The latter was made compulsory on 31 January 1983, and Rutherford *et al.* (1985) demonstrated that the total number of fatal head injuries among front-seat occupants declined by one-third between the 12 months before and after this date. In the United States the introduction of laws to compel the use of seat belts in cars and the use of helmets by motorcyclists has had a similar beneficial effect (Cooper, 1982a; Frazee, 1986).

During the early 1970s, researchers in several European countries consistently found that the mortality rate following severe head injury (defined in terms of a period of coma of six hours or more) was about 50 per cent (*see* Teasdale and Jennett, 1976), and similar rates were yielded by the international collaborative study involving patients in Scotland, the Netherlands and the United States (Heiden *et al.*, 1983; Jennett *et al.*, 1977b, 1979b). However, Jennett and his colleagues (Jennett and Carlin, 1978; Rose *et al.*, 1977) identified a number of avoidable factors in the management of head-injured patients which might contribute to mortality, of which the most common was delayed treatment of intracranial haematoma in primary surgical wards. They suggested that 50 per cent of deaths in neurosurgical units exhibited one or more of these factors, and that the development of more effective policies for the early management of head-injured patients would make a significant impact upon both mortality and morbidity.

Indeed, in a study of 53 head-injured children which used precisely the same selection criteria as the international collaborative study, Bruce *et al.* (1978) recorded a mortality rate of just 6 per cent. These researchers acknowledged that there were probably differences in the pathophysiology of head injury in children and adults (*see* chapter 7, pp. 260–1), but they suggested that the particularly good outcome obtained in their study resulted also from the introduction of computerized tomography as a routine diagnostic tool permitting early surgical intervention and from the aggressive control of intracranial hypertension. Similarly, Bowers and Marshall (1980) suggested that mortality rates could be markedly improved by 'the skilful management of patients at the scene of the accident by well-trained paramedical and police personnel, the availability of rapid diagnostic scanning techniques, and the rapid response and aggressive treatment by the community's neurosurgeons' (p. 241). In accordance with this notion, Clifton *et al*. (1980) achieved a mortality rate of 29 per cent with a consecutive series of 124 severely injured patients, which they ascribed to early evacuation of haematomas and efficient control of intracranial pressure. Subsequent studies carried out during the 1980s have certainly produced lower mortality rates (*see* Eisenberg and Weiner, 1987), but to what extent these were due to improvements in clinical management rather than to changes in public behaviour on the roads and elsewhere is not clear.

Table 1.9 shows the mortality statistics in England and Wales for 1985 with regard to both the age and the gender of the victim. There are three major features of interest here. First, the overall proportion of males to females is comparable with that contained in the statistics of the estimated incidence of closed head injury in Table 1.5. Second, the prognosis appears to be rather poorer in the case of older patients. Thus, over half of all deaths following head injury occur in victims over the age of 40. Carlsson *et al* (1968) also observed a marked increase in mortality among patients over 40 years old, but they demonstrated that this was solely the result of extracranial

Table 1.9 Total number of deaths following head injury in England and Wales in 1985 by age and gender of patient

Age	Males	Females	Total
0–4 years	63	38	101
5–14 years	199	76	275
15–24 years	739	181	920
25–34 years	384	85	469
35–44 years	333	82	415
45–54 years	265	85	350
55–64 years	271	127	398
65–74 years	237	190	427
75–84 years	244	289	533
85 years and over	63	114	117
Totals	2798	1267	4065

Source: Office of Population Censuses and Surveys (1987) *Mortality Statistics 1985: Cause* (Series DH2, No. 12), London, Her Majesty's Stationery Office.

complications such as pneumonia, thromboembolism, or myocardial infarction: as complications of fatal head injuries, these occurred almost exclusively and increasingly among the higher age groups, and the likelihood of mortality due to primary cerebral injury was found to be essentially constant across all age groups over 10 years. Third, however, there is also a marked increase in the number of deaths amongst adolescent and young adult males. Indeed, among young people aged between 15 and 19, closed head injury accounts for 26 per cent of all deaths in males and 17 per cent of all deaths in females. Similar trends have been noted in other studies (Annegers *et al.*, 1980; Jennett and MacMillan, 1981; Kraus *et al.*, 1984; National Center for Health Statistics, 1984). With regard to social class, there is a tendency for mortality for most causes of death to be higher in patients from the lower social classes; however, Field (1976, p. 26) noted that this tendency was especially pronounced in deaths following closed head injury.

Causes

Detailed information concerning the circumstances in which closed head injury occurs is not routinely collected. In England (and formerly in Wales), the Hospital In-patient Enquiry analysed accidental injuries by their place of occurrence into four broad categories: road traffic accidents; accidents occurring at home; accidents occurring at work; and other and unspecified places of occurrence. Of those patients who had suffered head injuries during 1985, the proportions in these four categories were 19.4 per cent, 13.5 per cent, 2.0 per cent and 65.1 per cent, respectively. The latter figure is inflated by instances where the relevant information was simply not specified, but the first three figures give a good indication of the relative contribution of traffic, domestic and occupational accidents to the hospitalization of patients with closed head injuries. In Table 1.10, the relevant figures are analysed further by age and gender.

In the United States, the National Head and Spinal Cord Injury Survey used three broad categories of external cause of injury taken from ICD–8: motor vehicle accidents, falls and all other causes. The proportions of cases falling into these three categories who had received head injuries during 1974 were 49 per cent, 28 per cent and 23 per cent, respectively (Kalsbeek *et al.*, 1980). The National Health Interview Survey classifies all incidents into motor vehicle injuries, work injuries, home injuries and injuries at play, in school, or in the public domain. In the analysis of head injuries in the 1977 survey, the estimated numbers of cases in these categories were: motor vehicle, 536 000; work, 301 000; home, 1 058 000; and other, 472 000. The corresponding proportions are 24 per cent, 14 per cent, 48 per cent and 21 per cent, respectively (the four categories are not mutually exclusive).

On the basis of the limited number of special studies which had then been carried out on the circumstances of closed head injury, Field (1976, pp. 13–7, 26) concluded that road traffic accidents were the major cause of injuries amongst adults, that falls

Table 1.10   *Estimated total number of discharges and deaths following head injury from hospitals in England in 1985 by cause of injury and gender and age of patient*

Age	RTA*	At home	At work	Other causes
	(a) Male patients			
0–4 years	621	3549	0	4439
5–14 years	3104	1180	207	13833
15–44 years	10957	1459	1449	31278
45–64 years	1655	641	476	5442
65–74 years	445	579	41	1666
75–85 years	269	414	0	1035
85 years and over	62	300	0	331
All ages	17113	8122	2173	58024
	(b) Female patients			
0–4 years	341	2711	10	3425
5–14 years	1314	1086	41	5898
15–44 years	4014	1649	186	8381
45–64 years	1045	745	62	2369
65–74 years	507	673	21	1480
75–84 years	331	1511	0	2328
85 years and over	93	962	0	1138
All ages	7646	9157	321	25018

*Road traffic accidents.
Source: Office of Population Censuses and Surveys (1987) *Hospital In-patient Enquiry 1985* (Series MB4, No. 27), London, Her Majesty's Stationery Office.

were the major cause of injuries amongst children, and that domestic accidents and falls were the major cause of injuries amongst the elderly. Subsequent research has confirmed and elaborated Field's conclusions.

Road Traffic Accidents

As a general point, it is quite clear that road traffic accidents represent the major cause of closed head injuries amongst adults up to the age of 65 (Annegers *et al.*, 1980; Frankowski, 1986; Gennarelli *et al.*, 1989; Hawthorne, 1978; Jennett *et al.*, 1977a; Kalsbeek *et al.*, 1980; Kerr *et al.*, 1971; Klonoff and Thompson, 1969; Kraus *et al.*, 1984; Rowbotham *et al.*, 1954). In more precise terms, Jennett and MacMillan (1981) noted that road accidents accounted for only a small minority of patients attending accident and emergency departments who were not subsequently admitted to hospital, but that they accounted for more than one-half of all fatal and severe head injuries. Bowers and Marshall (1980), Jennett *et al.* (1979b), Kalsbeek *et al.* (1980), Marshall *et al.* (1983a), and Rutter *et al.* (1980) all found that vehicular accidents were responsible for over 70 per cent of severe closed head injuries. Such accidents also seem to be chiefly responsible for the rise in the incidence of head injuries between the ages of 15 and 24 years among males (Annegers *et al.*, 1980; Kalsbeek *et al.*, 1980; Marshall *et al.*, 1983a). Nevertheless, road traffic accidents are also the second most likely cause of closed head injuries among both children and the elderly (Annegers *et al.*, 1980; Hjern and Nylander, 1964; Kalsbeek *et al.*, 1980; Klonoff, 1971; Marshall *et al.*, 1983a; Rowbotham *et al.*, 1954; Rune, 1970). The converse relationship also holds: closed head injuries are the most common cause of death and serious permanent disability following road traffic accidents (Gennarelli *et al.*, 1989; Grattan and Hobbs, 1980; Jennett and MacMillan, 1981; Perrone, 1972). In particular, injuries to the head and face are the most likely outcome of accidents among the occupants of cars (Elia, 1974; Hobbs, 1981; Perrone, 1972; Rutherford *et al.*, 1985, p. 48). They are somewhat less likely in the case of occupants of larger vehicles but are still a frequent outcome of serious accidents (Grattan and Hobbs, 1978).

The circumstances of accidents occurring on the roads often have direct implications for the design of motor vehicles. As a result, the biomechanics of road traffic accidents are fairly well understood (Hobbs, 1978; Perrone, 1972; Sims *et al.*, 1976). First, those drivers and passengers who are not restrained by seat belts may come into violent contact with the windscreen, its frame, or the side of the vehicle compartment, or they may be thrown from the vehicle and collide with the exterior of another vehicle, a roadside obstacle, or the road surface. In particular, unrestrained children sitting on the laps of front-seat passengers are liable to be thrown against or through the windscreen and to suffer severe frontofacial injuries as a result (Jennett, 1972). The risk of head injury to front-seat occupants who are restrained by seat belts is increased by the presence of unrestrained rear-seat passengers; the latter may themselves sustain injury by coming into violent contact either with the vehicle roof or with the front-seat occupants (Roberts, 1983; Rutherford *et al.*, 1985, p. 54).

Rutherford *et al.* (1985) found that the introduction of legislation in the UK to compel the wearing of three-point lap-diagonal belts among front-seat occupants of cars produced a decline in the incidence of brain injury of 30 per cent in the case of drivers and 57 per cent in the case of front-seat passengers; similar reductions were evident in the overall frequency of injuries to the head and neck (pp. 40–1, 48–9). However, this masked an *increase* of 44 per cent in the incidence of major brain injury among car drivers (but not among front-seat passengers). There was also a substantial decline in the number of fatally injured drivers with skull and facial fractures and in the number of fatally injured front-seat passengers, but little change in the number of fatally injured drivers who had suffered intracranial injuries (p. 97). Previous research, together with the pattern of other injuries, led Rutherford *et al.* to conclude that the inertial reel belts then in use permitted contact between the driver's head and the steering wheel in a frontal collision. *A fortiori*, vehicle occupants who are restrained only by lap belts may sustain head injury by coming into contact either with the steering wheel or with the dashboard. Even those occupants who are restrained by lap-diagonal belts may suffer a 'whiplash' injury caused by rapid movement of the head about a restrained torso; two such cases were described by Ommaya and Yarnell (1969).

Closed head injury is also the most common form of life-threatening injury involving pedestrians and users of two-wheeled vehicles (Grattan *et al.*, 1976). Indeed, motorcycle accidents tend to be the cause of the most severe closed head injuries (Annegers *et al.*, 1980; Grattan and Hobbs, 1980). Conversely, closed head injuries account for approximately one-third of all moderate and for most fatal injuries following motorcycle accidents. These injuries are usually caused by the rider's head coming into violent contact with the road or an obstacle such as another vehicle (Whitaker, 1976, 1980). Among pedestrians, closed head injury is a common outcome of severe accidents, as well as the most frequent cause of accidental death, often as the result of the patient's colliding with the windscreen, the windscreen frame, or (in the case of children) the bonnet of the vehicle involved (Ashton *et al.*, 1977). Among pedal cyclists, closed head injury is once again a common outcome of both falls and collisions with other vehicles, and it is a frequent cause of death following such accidents (Thorson, 1974). Most bicycle accidents seem to occur in the 5–14 age group (Kraus *et al.*, 1984; Steadman and Graham, 1970). However, Field (1976, p. 13) commented that it was as pedestrians that children were mainly at risk of being involved in road accidents leading to closed head injuries rather than as cyclists or as passengers in vehicles. The same seems to be generally true of head-injured patients in European countries (Jennett *et al.*, 1977b).

Domestic Accidents

Domestic accidents and especially falls represent another significant cause of closed head injuries. Steadman and Graham (1970) found that more than half of their cases of head injury resulted from falls, but they had included falls from bicycles, motorcycles and other vehicles which together constituted roughly one half of these cases. A more realistic impression was given by Kerr *et al.* (1971), who found that domestic accidents accounted for 16 per cent of admissions following head injury (*see also* Gennarelli *et al.*, 1989); these tended to be falls from a height (usually down stairs) or onto a level surface. Such falls appear to be the major cause of head injuries among children under 15 years and among the elderly (Annegers *et al.*, 1980; Hjern and Nylander, 1964; Kalsbeek *et al.*, 1980; Klonoff, 1971; Kraus *et al.*, 1984; Marshall *et al.*, 1983a; Strang *et al.*, 1978). Falls among adults up to the age of 65 are relatively uncommon and tend to give rise to relatively milder forms of injury (Annegers *et al.*, 1980), although they may be encountered more often at inner-city hospitals (Swann *et al.*, 1981).

Assault

Cases of assault account for up to 20 per cent of adult head injuries (Bowers and Marshall, 1980; Gennarelli *et al.*, 1989; Hawthorne, 1978; Jennett *et al.*, 1977a, 1979b; Kerr *et al.*, 1971; Klonoff and Thompson, 1969; Kraus *et al.*, 1984; Marshall *et al.*, 1983a; Steadman and Graham, 1970). In their multinational study, Jennett *et al.* (1977b) noted that 'assaults and "falls under the influence of alcohol" were common in Glasgow and Los Angeles, accounting between them for almost a third of all injuries over the age of 10 years; these kinds of accident were rare in the Netherlands' (p.293). In general, the proportion of head injuries due to assault is increased and may be as high as 40 per cent in depressed urban areas such as inner-city Glasgow (Swann *et al.*, 1981), the Bronx (Cooper *et al.*, 1983) and inner-city Chicago (Whitman *et al.*, 1984). However, in the United States these are often penetrating head injuries resulting from gunshot wounds (Frankowski, 1986); Gennarelli *et al.* (1989) found that such injuries accounted for 25 per cent of all head injuries by assault and were associated with a mortality rate of 68 per cent. There seems to be an increased incidence of head injuries by assault among 15–24 year old males, but not in females (Annegers *et al.*, 1980; Kraus *et al.*, 1984). Indeed, Jennett and MacMillan (1981) stated that assaults were twice as common as road accidents as causes of head injuries among men of between 15 and 24 years of age who were treated in Scottish accident and emergency departments. However, Marshall *et al.* (1983a) found a relatively high incidence of closed head injuries resulting from assaults in all adult age-groups, and they noted that in patients aged 60 and over falls and assaults caused more than half as many head injuries again than motor-vehicle accidents.

Klonoff (1971) found that cases of assault accounted for 4 per cent of head injuries among children, in whom they were frequently associated with battering by a parent. It has even been suggested that child abuse is the most common cause of severe head injuries during the first year of life (Chadwick, 1985). Jennett (1972) advised that the possibility of head injury should be considered whenever child abuse was suspected, regardless of whether there was any direct evidence of head trauma. One potential source of injury among so-called battered children is concussion induced by repeated severe shaking. Caffey (1972, 1974) observed that infants were highly vulnerable to many kinds of whiplash stresses because their heads were relatively heavier and their neck muscles relatively weaker than at any other age. He described children who had suffered subdural haematomas in the absence of obvious external signs of head impact and concluded that many so-called 'battered babies' were really cases of a 'whiplash shaken infant syndrome'. However, he also noted that whiplash shaking was considered to be a socially acceptable means of disciplining young children in the UK and the USA, and that it was involved in a number of activities habitually engaged in by adults playing with young children.

One problem in interpreting such findings, however, as Leventhal and Midelfort

(1986) pointed out, is that neurological problems may have preceded (and perhaps even precipitated) child abuse rather than being caused by it. Moreover, Duhaime *et al.* (1987) pointed out that any history of documented occurrences of shaking was typically lacking in such children. These researchers noted that evidence of blunt head impact had been apparent in only seven out of 13 fatal cases of the syndrome, but was found in every single case at post mortem; in particular, all had cerebral contusions as well as diffuse and usually massive brain swelling. Duhaime *et al.* then demonstrated that the measurements of angular acceleration and velocity obtained in shaking inanimate models of infants were considerably below the range associated with significant brain injury in experiments on primates, whereas similar measurements obtained with impact against a hard object or surface fell well within that range. They inferred that shaking alone in an otherwise normal baby was unlikely to cause the syndrome.

Occupational Accidents

Kerr *et al.* (1971) found that industrial accidents reflected 14 per cent of admissions following head injury; one-half of these were caused by falls at work, one-quarter were caused by falling objects, while one-fifth were the result of mining accidents. In the survey of Scottish hospitals during 1974, Jennett *et al.* (1977a) found that 10 per cent of all patients with head injury who attended accident and emergency departments and 8 per cent of all those who were admitted to hospital had sustained their head injuries at work. However, more recent research (e.g., Annegers *et al.*, 1980) has tended to confirm the implication of the Hospital In-patient Enquiry findings that occupation-related head injuries are relatively infrequent and relatively constant between the ages of 15 and 64; they occur predominantly among men in manual occupations such as farming and the construction industry.

Recreational Accidents

Accidents relating to recreational activities also account for up to 14 per cent of head injuries (Annegers *et al.*, 1980; Jennett *et al.*, 1977a; Kraus *et al.*, 1984; Whitman *et al.*, 1984), especially among patients in middle-class occupations (Kerr *et al.*, 1971). However, they constitute only 7 per cent of serious cases admitted for treatment to neurosurgical units (Lindsay *et al.*, 1980). Contact sports such as football are often implicated in such injuries, and Gurdjian and Gurdjian (1978) pointed to subdural haematomas as an important cause of deaths in American college football, even among players wearing protective helmets. The most common sort of injury is helmet-to-helmet collision in the course of tackling or blocking manoeuvres (Barth *et al.*, 1989).

In children, Kraus *et al.* (1984) emphasized the importance of accidents involving pedal cycles, roller skates and skateboards. Barber (1973) observed that head injuries were also a common outcome of horse-riding accidents; he concluded that such injuries were more common and more severe than was generally appreciated and comparable with those sustained by motorcyclists. Foster *et al.* (1976) found that professional National Hunt jockeys in particular were exposed to frequent and often severe concussive head injuries; these could lead to permanent brain damage and intellectual deterioration but often went unreported. Finally, although it is perhaps not strictly a recreational activity, closed head injuries obviously arise in the course of boxing. There are some serious methodological problems involved in the neuropsychological assessment of boxers (*see* Stewart *et al.*, 1989). However, these injuries seem to be the cause of significant neurological damage, not only in the case of professionals (Roberts, 1969), but even among amateurs (McLatchie *et al.*, 1987).

Concluding Summary

For the purposes of this book, a 'closed head injury' is an injury to the head in which the primary mechanism of damage is one of blunt impact. Such injuries are a major cause of deaths following accidents, especially those that involve children and young people, and they are also a major cause of handicap and morbidity among the survivors.

The severity of a head injury can be measured in terms of its initial effects, the incidence of complications, or its long-term consequences. In particular, the duration and extent of the patient's impairment of consciousness is of major importance in evaluating the severity of a closed head injury. The Glasgow Coma Scale provides a standard set of criteria for quantifying the depth of unconsciousness in terms of motor responses, verbal responses and eye opening. However, there are certain problems in its use concerning the time after injury when it should be administered and the involvement of linguistic skills in the different elements of the Scale.

The number of individuals who receive a head injury each year that is sufficiently serious to lead them to seek treatment at a hospital is roughly 600 000 in England, 84 000 in Scotland and 2 200 000 in the USA. However, only 20 per cent of these patients are subsequently admitted to hospital as patients, and in the UK fewer than 5 per cent are transferred to specialist neurosurgical units for investigation and treatment. The incidence of head injury is higher in males than in females, in young adults than in children or the elderly, and in the working classes than in the middle classes, and it is higher following the consumption of alcohol. Each year, roughly 4000 individuals die following head injury in England and Wales; comparable figures are not available for Scotland or the USA. The major causes of head injury are road traffic accidents, domestic falls, assaults, occupational injuries and recreational accidents.

Chapter 2

Mechanisms of Structural Pathology

To obtain a proper understanding of the clinical and neuropsychological effects of a closed head injury, it is vitally important to appreciate the physical and physiological mechanisms by which these effects have come about. This chapter describes the different types of damage which occur at the time of injury and are directly attributable to the trauma itself, as well as the various complications that may result.

In the previous chapter, it was noted that the notion of concussion, as traditionally conceived, represented a transient disturbance of cerebral function without any associated permanent structural damage to the brain. However, an early investigation by English (1904) suggested that bruising (or *contusions*) and tearing (or *lacerations*) might be identified even in patients who sustained a relatively slight head trauma but who then died of unrelated causes, such as thoracic or abdominal injuries. He found macroscopic damage in the brains of eight out of ten such patients for whom there was an unambiguous history of loss of consciousness lasting less than 5 min. In addition, an examination of the brains of a number of patients who had died a substantial time after sustaining a minor closed head injury revealed in most cases residual structural changes such as meningeal thickening and a discolouration of the cerebral cortex from old extravasated blood.

Microscopic changes to the brain as the result of minor closed head injury were demonstrated by Windle *et al.* (1944) in the course of an experimental investigation using both anaesthetized and unanaesthetized guinea-pigs. Progressive degeneration of nerve cells was observed over the course of one week following a closed head injury sufficient to induce concussion (defined as the abolition of the corneal reflex). However, subtle intraneuronal disorganization was observed in animals killed by vascular perfusion with formalin within 30 sec. of the injury. These changes were confined (in this species, at least) to interneurones within the brainstem and spinal cord, and they occurred despite the absence of any significant intracranial bleeding or brain swelling (*see below*, pp. 56–62). It was concluded that concussive injury gave rise to immediate cell changes within the brain. Degeneration of nerve cells was also shown in a more recent study by Jane *et al.* (1982) of just two monkeys killed seven days after sustaining a minor head injury. In research on fatal injuries amongst human patients,

Oppenheimer (1968) reported abnormal clusters of microglial cells even in the brains of patients who had sustained mild concussion but had subsequently died from other causes. As he himself concluded, 'permanent damage, in the form of microscopic destructive foci, can be inflicted on the brain by what are regarded as trivial head injuries' (p. 306).

It has subsequently been shown that minor head injuries give rise to persistent changes in cerebral blood flow (Taylor, 1969), in physiological activity according to electroencephalographic indices and evoked potential (Binder, 1986; MacFlynn *et al.*, 1984; Montgomery *et al.*, 1984; Noseworthy *et al.*, 1981), and (as will be described at length in later chapters) in performance in neuropsychological tests. Moreover, the cumulative effects in both pathological and neurological terms of repeated mild head injuries in boxers are well recognized (Roberts, 1969). The contemporary position as summarized for example by Jennett and Galbraith (1983, p. 216) is that a blow to the head which is sufficient to cause even a brief disturbance of consciousness may produce detectable structural damage. This is also the implication of studies using computerized tomography (*see* Hardman, 1979) and magnetic resonance imaging (e.g., Jenkins *et al.*, 1986; Levin *et al.*, 1987a). In considering neuropathological evidence obtained from patients who have sustained severe or even fatal head injuries, therefore, it should be born in mind that nowadays the difference between these patients and those who have sustained relatively mild or minor closed head injuries is conceived of as a quantitative rather than a qualitative one.

Cerebral Contusions

As explained above, closed head injuries typically give rise to contusions and lacerations on or within the surface of the brain. Strictly speaking, lacerations are lesions that breach the membrane which encloses the brain itself (the pia mater), whereas contusions leave the latter intact. This distinction is however difficult to make in practice and the distributions of the two sorts of damage are essentially identical (Adams, 1988). These lesions are usually found on the crests of the convolutions (or *gyri*) on the surfaces of the cerebral hemispheres, but they may penetrate the whole thickness of the cortex and extend into the subcortical white matter (*see* Adams *et al.*, 1980, 1985b). They are haemorrhagic lesions (that is, they involve the loss of blood) and lead to the accumulation of fluid (*oedema*) and the death of nerve cells (*necrosis*) within the brain. They usually heal within a few weeks and leave yellow-brown atrophic scars that are easily recognized at *post mortem*.

Clinicians have traditionally distinguished among several different potential sites of cerebral contusions following closed head injury (e.g., Jamieson, 1971a, pp. 32–3). First, contusions and lacerations may arise at the site of impact; this is normally referred to as the 'coup' injury. Second, local changes in intracranial pressure may give rise to damage in cerebral regions which are diametrically opposite to the site of impact; this is usually described as the 'contrecoup' injury. Third, movement of the brain within the skull gives rise to lacerations and contusions in the region of the sphenoidal ridge, which produces damage to both the frontal and temporal lobes. Finally, movement of the brain is also likely to produce a variety of surface lesions, especially by causing tearing (or *avulsion*) of the veins that leave the upper borders of the cerebral hemispheres. These four possible types of physical damage are illustrated in Figure 2.1.

Coup Injury

It would be intuitively reasonable to expect contusions and lacerations to occur beneath the site of impact following a closed head injury. In most cases, the latter will obviously be marked by contusions and lacerations on the scalp. Indeed, 40 per cent of all head-injured patients who attend an accident and emergency department have scalp

Figure 2.1   Mechanisms of injury to the brain surface in closed head injury

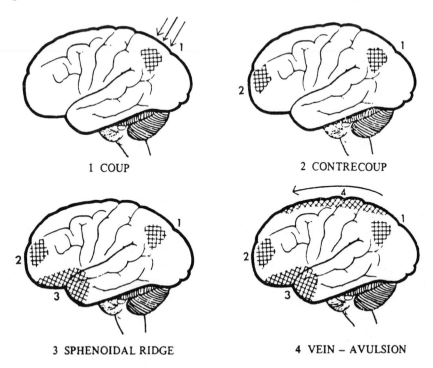

1 COUP   2 CONTRECOUP

3 SPHENOIDAL RIDGE   4 VEIN – AVULSION

Source: Jamieson, K. G. (1971) *A First Notebook of Head Injury*, 2nd ed., London, Butterworths. Reprinted with permission.

lacerations that require closure by suture or other means (Jennett *et al.*, 1977a). Nevertheless, provided that the skull remains intact, only a superficial bruising occurs in the region of the point of application of the blow as a result of local deformation of the skull (Holbourn, 1943, 1945). Of course, as Adams and Graham (1972) noted, a fatal brain injury may occur without discernible damage to the scalp or the skull, but it follows that in such cases the critical lesions are to be found elsewhere in the brain (*see below*). In contrast to the sorts of head injuries that are associated with missile wounds, where the principal damage occurs beneath the point of impact even when the skull has been left intact (Russell, 1951), serious neurological damage at the site of impact tends to arise in cases of closed head injury only when the skull has been fractured.

Tables 1.2–1.4 indicate that the proportion of patients admitted to hospital with a diagnosis reflecting closed head injury who have sustained a fractured skull is roughly 18 per cent in the United Kingdom and roughly 38 per cent in the United States. Nevertheless, at least two-thirds of all *severe* head injuries are associated with a fractured skull (Jennett *et al.*, 1977a, 1977b, 1979b), and Table 1.7 shows that the same proportion of all *fatal* head injuries is associated with a fractured skull. The likelihood of a skull fracture obviously depends on the mass, the velocity and the shape of the object that causes the head injury. Courville (1942) suggested that the location of a fracture tended to indicate the point at which the blow was applied, and that its direction tended to indicated the direction of the relevant force. However, Adams *et al.* (1980a) found that in 69 out of 120 cases of fatal head injury with skull fracture the latter was centred on the midline of the vault of the skull or restricted to the base of the skull, and hence gave no indication as to the site of the injury. Only 30 of these cases exhibited a predominantly unilateral fracture with a corresponding laceration or bruising of the scalp.

The presence of a fracture indicates that the skull has absorbed some of the kinetic energy of the object causing the head injury, but it also increases the probability of complications both because of damage to the underlying tissue and because of the possibility of infection. *Linear* fractures constitute roughly 70–80 per cent of all skull fractures, and result from the deformation of the skull inwards at the point of impact and outwards further away. Fractures of the base of the skull are of particular significance: they are associated with a major physical impact to the head and are common among the most severely injured patients who do not survive to reach hospital. Such fractures carry an appreciable risk of intracranial infection derived from the sinuses or the middle ear, and they may lead to a leakage of cerebrospinal fluid from either the nose (rhinorrhoea) or the ear (otorrhoea). A *depressed* fracture is one where a piece of bone is displaced by at least the thickness of the skull; this is of prognostic importance because damage to the underlying cerebral cortex may lead to post-traumatic epilepsy (*see below*, pp. 65–6). In a *closed* or *simple* fracture, the scalp is intact; in an *open* or *compound* fracture, the overlying scalp is lacerated or torn, and this carries the risk of intracranial infection. In a *comminuted* depressed fracture, the fractured portion of bone is broken into several fragments, and these may lacerate the brain surface. In roughly half of all depressed fractures, the scalp is lacerated and the dura mater is penetrated, which allows infection to enter the subdural space.

The important characteristic of most cases of closed head injury is that substantial pressure gradients are temporarily set up within the brain as a result of its motion relative to the skull. This inertial loading within the brain is the major cause of neurological damage following closed head injury (Ommaya and Gennarelli, 1976). Obviously, the extent of the damage depends once again upon the mass, the velocity, and the shape of the object which produces the injury. (Consequently, in the specific case of traffic accidents, adequate clinical treatment of the victims may depend upon detailed knowledge of the characteristics of the vehicle or vehicles involved: Sims *et al.*, 1976). However, animal experiments have shown that even subconcussive blows to the head may lead to clear gliding movements of the brain relative to the skull, chiefly in the sagittal (that is, dorsoventral) and horizontal planes (e.g., Gosch *et al.*, 1970; Pudenz and Shelden, 1946); and blunt, heavy weapons may produce massive neurological damage with only slight contusions to the scalp.

There are two important corollaries to the idea that neurological damage following closed head injury is produced by inertial loading of the cerebral tissues. First, significant widespread damage depends upon the free acceleration or deceleration of the cranium. Therefore, if the cranial vault is fixed at the time of impact, or if the injurious forces are applied in a static, compressive manner (as in crushing), diffuse injuries are less likely and consciousness may even be unimpaired (Adams, 1969; Ommaya and Gennarelli, 1976; Pudenz and Shelden, 1946). Second, and conversely, injuries which produce inertial loading within the skull without actual head impact (such as 'whiplash' injuries in road accidents or falling onto the buttocks) may nevertheless give rise to concussion and gross cerebral contusions (Ommaya and Gennarelli, 1976). This has been repeatedly demonstrated in experiments with infrahuman primates in which inertial angular acceleration has been administered without head impact (Adams *et al.*, 1983; Gennarelli, 1983; Gennarelli *et al.*, 1982, Graham *et al.*, 1988a; Jane *et al.*, 1985). In this connection, it is interesting that 15 per cent of patients admitted to a regional spinal injury centre had neurological signs of significant brainstem or cortical damage (Hall *et al.*, 1987). It is also worth noting that closed head injuries may be associated with blast injury as the result of explosions transmitted through water (Hirsch and Ommaya, 1972) or through air (Hill, 1979), although injuries of this sort are fairly rare in peace-time.

Contrecoup Injury

Following a closed head injury, the dynamic impact produces an inertial stress propagation in the direction of the force applied (Gurdjian and Gurdjian, 1975), which may give rise to lesions and contusions at points within the skull that are roughly opposite the original site of impact. Such 'contrecoup' damage has been discussed for more than 200 years, but it was first described in detail by Russell (1932) and Courville (1942). Unlike the superficial bruising which occurs at the point of impact, these lesions and contusions are not caused by local deformation of the skull, nor by local changes in cerebral circulation (Pudenz and Shelden, 1946). Rather, contrecoup injury results from the movement of the brain against the interior surfaces of the skull.

In his original analysis, Courville claimed that the combination of coup and contrecoup damage was only found in deceleration injuries, when a moving head undergoes a rapid decrease in velocity by coming into contact with a fixed or stationary object. In these injuries, he argued, the propagation of inertial stress was predominantly in the direction of the force applied, and typically along a diameter of the cranial cavity. On the other hand, in acceleration injuries, when a stationary head undergoes a rapid increase in velocity by being struck by a moving object, Courville claimed that the propagation of inertial stress radiated from the point of impact and that the resultant forces were quickly diffused. While it has been suggested that deceleration injuries are usually associated with a greater compression of cerebral tissue (Gurdjian and Gurdjian, 1978), Pudenz and Shelden (1946) appear to have had no difficulty in producing contrecoup damage in primates by acceleration injury, and nowadays most authorities seem to assume that acceleration and deceleration injuries are likely to be essentially equivalent in terms of their neuropathological mechanisms and consequences (e.g., Gurdjian, 1971).

In the past, the results of *post mortem* investigations tended to encourage the idea that contrecoup lesions were typically more serious than those arising under the site of impact itself, though Russell (1932) commented that this impression was merely the result of the fact that the contrecoup injury was often marked by subarachnoid haemorrhage. However, recently this notion has been brought into question by more rigorous work on fatal head injuries. Adams *et al.* (1980b) devised a 'contusion index' in order to quantify the depth and extent of contusions in various parts of the brain in a systematic manner. In cases of fatal head injury where the principal site of skull impact could be established with a reasonable level of confidence, these researchers concluded that there was no real tendency for contusions to be more severe in contrecoup locations than elsewhere. In particular, among 30 patients who had suffered a unilateral fracture of the vault of the skull and an overlying scalp injury, there was no sign of any difference in the severity of contusions between the hemisphere contralateral to the fracture and the ipsilateral hemisphere. Moreover, there was no sign of any difference in the relative severity of frontal and occipital contusions between 23 patients with predominantly frontal fractures and 44 patients with predominantly occipital fractures. The former result was confirmed by Adams *et al.* (1985) in a much larger series of patients with fatal head injuries.

Sphenoidal Injury

Closed head injuries characteristically produce movements of the brain relative to the skull. Courville (1942) observed that the vault of the skull is relatively smooth, whereas the base of the skull contains major irregularities which restrict the movement of the cerebral tissues after a sudden impact: namely, the three cranial fossae on each side, separated by the sphenoidal and petrosal ridges. The latter bony projections tend to induce substantial shearing forces and give rise to contusions of the orbital surfaces of the frontal lobes, the areas of cortex above and below the Sylvian fissures, the temporal poles and the inferior aspect of the temporal lobes. Most of this damage seems to occur in the vicinity of the sphenoidal ridge (*see* Figure 2.2).

Courville's analysis was unequivocal in identifying frontotemporal contusions as the major source of contrecoup injury. Although chains of haemorrhages may occur along the line of maximal propagation of inertial stress, he argued that the most serious lesions were not necessarily produced along this line of force at all, but were dependent upon 'local bony relations' (p. 34). In fact, Courville showed that damage to both the frontal and temporal lobes was a likely outcome of all closed head injuries. This damage might reflect ipsilateral, coup lesions following frontal or temporal impact; or

Figure 2.2   Composite drawing showing the size and location of contusions found in a series of forty consecutive cases of closed head injury

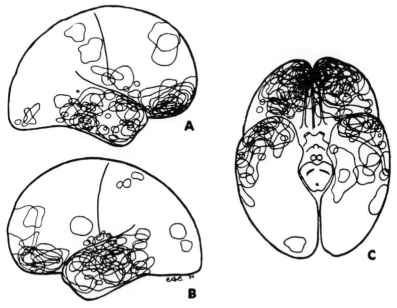

Source: Courville, C. B. (1950) *Pathology of the Central Nervous System*, 3rd ed., Mountain View, CA, Pacific Press Publishing Association. Reprinted with permission.

it might reflect contralateral, contrecoup lesions following parietal or occipital impact. Coup lesions of the occipital regions only followed injuries which gave rise to depressed fractures, and contrecoup lesions of those areas were never found. Similar results have been produced by many other autopsy studies of the relation between the site of head impact and the location of brain contusions in human beings and also by experimental investigations using infrahuman primates (*see* Ommaya *et al.*, 1971b).

In particular, Adams *et al.* (1985) applied their contusion index to a series of 434 fatal cases of head injury. The typical patient exhibited *no* contusions in the occipital lobes, the parietal lobes, the Sylvian fissures, or the cerebellum, but bilateral contusions of either moderate extent or moderate depth in the frontal and temporal lobes. Patients with fractured skulls exhibited contusions of greater severity, but those with unilateral fractures and a corresponding scalp injury showed essentially the same pattern regardless of the presumed side of impact. Moreover, a broadly similar distribution of contusions across the different cerebral regions was obtained in infrahuman primates subjected to inertial angular acceleration of the head which did not involve any actual impact. There was, in short, no evidence that cerebral contusions were produced by any 'contrecoup' mechanism in the sense that they were systematically more severe diametrically opposite to the point of impact, nor even that they were dependent upon the occurrence of any 'coup' at all.

Research using computerized tomography (CT) and magnetic resonance imaging (MRI) has confirmed this distribution of cerebral lesions among the survivors of closed head injuries, and has also demonstrated that it generalizes to patients who have sustained less severe brain damage. For instance, Levin *et al.* (1987a) reported findings from CT and MRI carried out upon 20 cases of mild or moderate head injury. MRI disclosed nearly five times as many lesions as CT, and in the case of lesions detected by both techniques MRI generally indicated that they were larger in volume than CT; these disparities were especially pronounced in lesions within the grey and white matter of the brain (*parenchymal* lesions). (Similar assessments of the relative sensitivity of CT and MRI in cases of closed head injury have been given by other researchers: *see* Gandy *et al.*, 1984; Han *et al.*, 1984; Jenkins *et al.*, 1986; Kalisky *et al.*, 1987.) Lesions were detected in 17 out of 20 patients, and the vast majority of these were situated in the frontal and temporal lobes (*see also* Jenkins *et al.*, 1986). However, none of the additional lesions disclosed by MRI required surgical intervention, and most resolved within a period of three months.

In short, the findings of autopsy studies following severe, fatal head injury and those of brain imaging research following minor or mild head injury are totally consistent with each other in implying that the notion of sphenoidal damage is rather more useful than that of contrecoup damage in evaluating the neurological damage consequent upon closed head injury. *A fortiori*, since the frontotemporal region is a primary location of surface contusions, irrespective of the point of impact (Ommaya *et al.*, 1971b), it follows that the locus of impact is relatively uninformative in establishing a likely prognosis unless the injury has produced a depressed fracture. Moreover, even though patients with a fractured skull reveal a much wider incidence of cerebral contusions, these are usually distributed across the surface of the brain and are not particularly associated with the principal site of skull impact (Adams *et al.*, 1980b, 1985).

Gliding Contusions

The free movement of the brain within the skull is also constrained by the falx cerebri, which is a sickle-shaped process of dura mater that descends vertically into the longitudinal fissure that divides the two cerebral hemispheres. This restricts any rotation of the brain within the coronal plane and thus gives rise to contusions of the medial surfaces of the cerebral hemispheres and also along the upper surface of the corpus callosum. Conversely, the falx cerebri also ensures that movement of the brain is mostly within the sagittal and horizontal planes (Pudenz and Shelden, 1946). Indeed, precisely because there is relatively little restraint to this movement between the superior surfaces of the cerebral hemispheres and the vault of the skull, there may be considerable avulsion of nerve fibres and blood vessels, with the consequent risk of subdural haematoma (*see* pp. 58–9 *below*).

In recent work, attention has been directed towards the phenomenon of 'gliding contusions', which are haemorrhagic lesions located in the dorsal paramedial regions of the cerebral hemispheres (Lindenberg and Freytag, 1960). Microscopic investigation often reveals that they extend into the deeper layers of the cerebral cortex and the adjacent white matter. Adams *et al.* (1986b) identified gliding contusions in over 30 per cent of cases of fatal head injury, although they were less likely in patients who had sustained a fractured skull, more likely in the victims of road traffic accidents, and more likely in patients who exhibited evidence of diffuse brain damage. Adams *et al.* noted that similar lesions had been produced in experimental animals using inertial angular acceleration of the head, and they suggested that these contusions might result from the relative movement of the skull, the cortical surface, and subcortical structures. More specifically, they pointed out that the parasagittal bridging veins tethered the cortical surface to the superior sagittal sinus (which runs along the upper margin of the falx cerebri). They noted that the failure of a bridging vein itself would produce an acute subdural haematoma, and they hypothesized that gliding contusions were caused by a failure of the branching vessels of these veins that penetrate into the brain substance.

As was mentioned in Chapter 1 (p. 6), cerebral contusions (or *contusio cerebri*) have been traditionally regarded as the hallmark of a clinically significant closed head injury. Nevertheless, it is clear from recent research on the neuropathology of fatal head injury that patients may die as a result of such an injury without having any contusions or lacerations of the brain (Adams, 1988). For instance, Adams *et al.* (1985) identified 27 cases of fatal head injury in whom cerebral contusions were entirely absent, plus another 28 cases in whom such lesions were minimal. Graham *et al.* (1988a) added that cases had also occurred in experimental research with primates where fatal brain damage had arisen in the absence of cerebral contusions. Conversely, Adams *et al.* (1980a) identified only three out of 151 cases of fatal head injury where severe contusions seemed to be the principal cause of death insofar as they were the only evidence of severe brain damage. Indeed, Jennett and Teasdale (1981, p. 25) stated that a head injury could give rise to extensive cerebral contusions in the absence of any prolonged disturbance of consciousness. As they explained, the clinical significance of cerebral contusions usually lies in the fact that they can initiate brain swelling and intracranial haemorrhage, and that such processes can themselves result in turn in the deterioration of the patient's level of consciousness or the prolongation of a coma that was caused initially by other mechanisms (*see also* Teasdale and Mendelow, 1984).

Diffuse Axonal Injury

Linear and Rotatory Components

Earlier in this chapter, it was emphasized that the neurological damage which is produced by a closed head injury is critically dependent upon whether or not the head is restrained at the time of impact. In addition experimental research using inanimate models and laboratory animals has shown that the dynamic effects of a head injury upon the movement of the brain relative to an unconstrained skull should be analysed in terms of an axial, linear translation together with a rotatory component (Holbourn, 1943, 1945; Ommaya and Gennarelli, 1974, 1976). These physical components produce quite different patterns of neurological damage.

The linear component of the head injury produces a translational acceleration or deceleration of the skull, and this gives rise to pressure gradients within the brain. However, the effects of these forces are both focal and relatively minor. There may be contusions at the site of impact and possibly also at points which are diametrically opposite to that site; but an axial translation by itself does not produce diffuse lesions throughout the brain. In particular, while linear blows which are severe or which are applied repeatedly may interfere with consciousness by producing profound circulatory disturbances, they rarely give rise to cerebral concussion.

The nonlinear component of a closed head injury produces a rotational acceleration of the skull, and this gives rise to a rotation of the skull relative to the brain. As was pointed out earlier in this chapter, such movement may well produce contusions and lacerations at points where the cerebral tissues come into contact with major bony irregularities. Thus, the rotation of the skull will cause major damage in the region of the sphenoidal ridge and possibly also at the vertex, with consequent risk of intra-cranial haemorrhage. In short, as Holbourn (1943, 1945) argued, the so-called 'contrecoup' injuries are really neurological damage that is caused by the rotation of the frontal and temporal lobes against the sphenoidal ridge.

However, the rotation of the brain within the skull does not simply give rise to contusions at the point of contact between the cerebral hemispheres and the bony projections of the cranium. Depending upon the inertial loading to which the head is subjected, it also produces damaging shearing strains within the brain which decrease in magnitude from the surface of the brain to its centre. As Holbourn (1943) explained using a somewhat helpful analogy, this is 'the type of deformation which occurs in a pack of cards, when it is deformed from a neat rectangular pile into an oblique-angled pile' (p. 438). In the absence of any complications, these forces seem to be the major cause of the brain damage that follows closed head injury. In particular, the rotational component of a head injury is usually necessary for consciousness to be impaired and for diffuse damage to occur throughout the brain. Thus, the rotation of the brain following a closed head injury may give rise to both focal and diffuse lesions which are relatively independent of the original site of impact.

Ommaya and Gennarelli (1974) integrated the results of experimental research into a formal hypothesis which defined cerebral concussion as

> a graded set of clinical syndromes following head injury wherein increasing severity of disturbance in level and content of consciousness is caused by mechanically induced strains affecting the brain in a centripetal sequence of disruptive effect on function and structure. The effects of this sequence always begin at the surfaces of the brain in the mild cases and extend inwards to affect the diencephalic-mesencephalic core at the most severe levels of trauma. (pp. 637–8)

This hypothesis was in turn elaborated into a proposed classification of the possible grades of cerebral concussion (*see* Figure 2.3). According to this 'centripetal' conception of the biomechanics of brain injury, the distribution of damaging strains induced by inertial loading decreases in magnitude from the surface of the brain to its centre. It follows that in less severe cases (Grades I to III in the model) the patient's conscious awareness is only partially impaired and damage is confined to the cortex, subcortex, and diencephalon. However, more severe shearing forces disrupt the rostral brainstem and in particular the reticular activating system, thus producing traumatic unconsciousness or even death (Grades IV to VI).

This sort of analysis predicts the occurrence of specific functional disconnections, depending upon the amount of inertial loading to which the brain is subjected (*see* Ommaya and Gennarelli, 1974, 1976). First, linear translation of the brain in the absence of a rotatory component should lead only to focal damage at the site of impact. Second, low levels of inertial loading should produce cortical damage at the site of

Figure 2.3 Diagrammatic description of Ommaya and Gennarelli's (1974, 1976) hypothesis for the syndromes of cerebral concussion

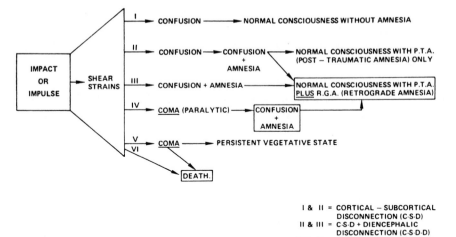

Source: Ommaya, A. K. and Gennarelli, T. A. (1974) 'Cerebral concussion and traumatic unconsciousness', *Brain*, 97, pp. 633–54. Reprinted with permission.

impact and at the sphenoidal ridge, but may well not lead to impaired consciousness. Third, high levels of inertial loading may produce loss of consciousness, as well as significant lesions of the frontal and temporal lobes. Thus, focal damage to cortical structures may result from a closed head injury without loss of consciousness; and, in addition, neurological signs of fronto-temporal damage may result from a closed head injury without loss of consciousness. Nevertheless, cerebral concussion only follows large rotational strains, and will be largely independent of the site of injury and the direction of the blow, although it will always be associated with frontaltemporal signs and possibly with other major cortical effects (cf. Holbourn, 1945).

Of course, in real life most closed head injuries will have both linear and rotatory components, and relatively pure linear or pure rotatory forces are rarely seen (Gurdjian and Gurdjian, 1978). Indeed, accidental closed head injuries may involve multiple blows and it may prove very hard to disentangle their linear and rotatory components after the event. The clinical value of this distinction may thus be limited; as Teasdale and Jennett (1976) emphasized, 'a complete description of the severity of brain injury requires the assessment of impaired consciousness to be complemented by eliciting signs of focal brain dysfunction' (p. 48). Moreover, it certainly cannot be assumed that the patterns of impaired consciousness obtained in anaesthetized animals in the laboratory will inevitably mirror those observed following accidental injury in humans (Gurdjian and Gurdjian, 1975; Symonds, 1962).

Nevertheless, 'whiplash' injuries in traffic accidents (Ommaya and Yarnell, 1969) and perhaps also in cases of child abuse (Caffey, 1974; but cf. Duhaime *et al.*, 1987) constitute examples of fairly pure rotatory movements of the brain within the cranial cavity in the absence of linear translation. Falls onto the buttocks have already been mentioned as examples of inertial loading without actual head impact. Finally, it is well known in boxing that an axial blow to the head is the least damaging, whereas the most devastating blow in effecting the opponent's loss of consciousness is one which induces major rotational forces within the brain (Lampert and Hardman, 1984; Parkinson, 1977). In other words, it is probably true, as Ommaya and Yarnell (1969) commented, that 'rotation of the head is the common denominator to the cerebral trauma of both head injury and whiplash injury' (p. 239).

Diffuse Damage in Fatal Head Injury

It is now generally recognized that diffuse cerebral damage produced by shearing forces within the brain is the primary mechanism of brain lesions following closed head injury. However, the damage in question would not have been evident in the early work of Courville and others for at least two different reasons. First, the lesions in question are typically not visible to the naked eye and their identification depends on comprehensive histological analysis using microscopic inspection of carefully preserved brain tissue (Jennett and Teasdale, 1981, p. 26). This is often precluded in forensic examinations of the sort on which much of this early work was based (*op. cit.*, p. 19). As Adams *et al.* (1980a) pointed out, this led to an inevitable tendency for pathologists in determining the cause of death to lay particular stress on readily identifiable macroscopic abnormalities such as skull fractures, intracranial haematomas, and cerebral contusions. Second, these lesions take about 12–18 hours to develop and are difficult to diagnose in patients who survive for less time than this (Adams *et al.*, 1989a). Whilst more than half of all patients with fatal head injury die before they reach hospital (*see* Chapter 1, p. 28), *post mortem* findings in such cases reflect the overwhelming nature of their injuries, including severe basal skull fracture, brainstem laceration, or even disruption of the whole brain, as well as fracture or dislocation of the cervical spine or serious chest injury (Jennett and Carlin, 1978). Lesions of this kind are quite different from the injuries found in those patients who survive long enough to reach a specialist neurosurgical unit and this is reflected in differences between the reports of forensic pathologists and those of neuropathologists (W. B. Jennett, personal communication). As a result, our current understanding of structural pathology in survivors of closed head injury has been immeasurably enhanced by careful histological analysis of patients who have died in specialist units.

For instance, Strich (1956) originally described extensive degeneration in the white matter of five patients who had suffered apparently uncomplicated head injuries, but who had remained in a profoundly demented state with gross neurological deficits until their deaths some months later. Strich (1961) reported similar results in a larger series of cases whose survival had extended from as little as two days to as much as two years after trauma. A number of subsequent *post mortem* investigations confirmed the existence of diffuse white-matter damage following closed head injuries (*see* Strich, 1969, for a review). To the naked eye, the brain may often have a rather shrunken appearance and the ventricular system may be enlarged because of the reduction in the bulk of the white matter. This is especially likely in patients who have survived for many months or even years in a persistent vegetative state (Adams *et al.*, 1989a; *see* Chapter 7, pp. 212–2). Among young infants, grossly visible tears in the cerebral white matter are a characteristic finding following a closed head injury (Lindenberg and Freytag, 1969). Among adult patients, the extent of the underlying damage may not be immediately obvious. Microscopically, however, there may well be axonal damage to the corpus callosum, the internal capsule, and the subcortical mechanisms of both cerebral hemispheres, to the cerebellum, and to a number of sites within the brainstem, including the pyramidal tracts, the medial lemnisci, the medial longitudinal bundles, and the superior cerebellar penduncles (e.g., Nevin, 1967).

As implied earlier, clinical signs of brainstem dysfunction are commonly seen at an early stage after major closed head injury. This has led to the notion of 'primary brainstem damage': that is, of severe focal damage to the brainstem. Over 80 per cent of patients demonstrating such signs following closed head injury will not recover (Turazzi *et al.*, 1975). Neuropathological and electrophysiological studies have however challenged the notion that this clinical picture is specifically associated with isolated damage to the brainstem (e.g., Mitchell and Adams, 1973), and it would seem that selective 'primary brainstem damage' does not, in fact, occur. In one major study, for instance, not one of the patients who fitted this clinical syndrome was found at *post mortem* to have lesions confined to the brainstem (Adams *et al.*, 1977). On the contrary, as is indeed predicted by Ommaya and Gennarelli's (1974, 1976) 'centipetal' conception of the biomechanics of head injury, primary damage to the rostral brainstem represents just one aspect of the widespread and diffuse damage that occurs to the white matter (though cf. Jane *et al.*, 1982).

Adams *et al.* (1980a) identified a total of 19 patients with diffuse lesions of the cerebral white matter in a consecutive series of 151 cases of fatal nonmissile head injury. Adams *et al.* (1982b) added another 26 patients with diffuse white-matter damage to this series. Every one of these 45 patients displayed a characteristic pattern of focal lesions in the corpus callosum and in the dorsolateral quadrant or quadrants of the rostral brain stem, together with diffuse damage to axons. Although the latter could only be determined by microscopic scrutiny of appropriately stained neural tissue, Adams *et al.* described this condition as one of *diffuse axonal injury*. All the patients had been unconscious from the time of impact and had remained in a coma or a persistent vegetative state with no lucid interval until they died. Adams *et al.* found that they were more likely to have been involved in road traffic accidents and less likely to have been involved in falls than other cases of fatal head injury. They suggested that rotational movements necessary to induce primary brain-stem damage would be more likely to ensue from road traffic accidents than from falls. Subsequently, Adams *et al.* (1984) found that this pattern of brain damage only arose in head injuries caused by falls when the patient had fallen a considerable distance (that is, one greater than his or her own height).

Adams *et al.* (1982b) also demonstrated that the patients with diffuse axonal injury had a much lower incidence of skull fracture, cerebral contusions, intracranial haematoma, and raised intracranial pressure than the other head-injured patients, although the two groups showed no difference in the incidence of brain swelling or hypoxic damage. From these observations they argued that the degeneration of white matter seen in diffuse axonal injury did not occur secondary to hypoxia, brain swelling, or raised intracranial pressure. Instead, they supported the contention of Strich (1961, 1969) that the degeneration of white matter was a direct result of physical damage to nerve fibres at the moment of impact, and they inferred from this that such lesions could be neither prevented nor remedied. They concluded that diffuse axonal damage was probably the single most important factor influencing the outcome in cases of closed head injury.

Adams *et al.* (1989a) confirmed these basic observations with a much larger sample of patients with fatal head injuries, except that in this series 14 per cent of the patients with diffuse axonal injury had in fact exhibited a lucid interval. Moreover, there was an increased incidence of both gliding contusions and deep intracerebral haematomas among patients with diffuse axonal injury. On the basis of their experience with these patients, Adams *et al.* suggested that the basic clinicopathological entity of diffuse axonal injury could be differentiated into three broad types, reflecting various grades of severity. Grade 1 could be identified only on the basis of histological evidence of axonal injury in the white matter of the cerebral hemispheres, the corpus callosum, the brain stem, and also occasionally in the cerebellum. Grade 2 was identified by an additional focal lesion in the corpus callosum; this was typically haemorrhagic and tended to lie to one side of the midline, although it might also extend to the midline and involve the interventricular septum and the pillars of the fornix. Finally, Grade 3 was defined by focal lesions in both the corpus callosum and the dorsolateral quadrant of the rostral brain stem. In many cases these focal lesions could only be identified microscopically.

Diffuse Axonal Injury in Survivors of Head Injury

Gennarelli *et al.* (1982) showed that precisely the same lesions could be produced in infrahuman primates that were subjected to concussion through inertial angular acceleration of the head, although only when motion was in the coronal plane (that is, at right angles to the body midline). The extent of such damage was directly proportional to the duration of coma. Gennarelli *et al.* concluded that diffuse axonal injury produced by coronal head acceleration was a major cause of prolonged traumatic coma, and that in the absence of complications the outcome of head injury depends on the amount and distribution of axonal damage. It is also pertinent to remark that once again these lesions had been induced without actual head impact (*see* Adams *et al.*, 1983). The precise mechanism of diffuse axonal injury in such cases has yet to be established, but recent research suggests that it involves subtle structural changes within the cell membrane enclosing the axon (the axolemma) and within the myelin sheath, rather than actual tearing of the axon itself (Maxwell *et al.*, 1988).

In the case of survivors from head trauma, CT scans usually fail to provide direct evidence of damage to the cerebral white matter (Zimmerman *et al.*, 1978b). Indeed, Snoek *et al.* (1979) found normal CT scans in 23 (or 38 per cent) out of 60 severely injured patients who did not have an acute intracranial haematoma, and in five (or 26 per cent) out of the 19 of these patients who subsequently died. In 15 of the latter cases *post mortem* examinations were carried out; diffuse damage to the cerebral white matter was identified in six of these cases, despite the fact that no parenchymal lesions had been identified in their CT scans. Snoek *et al.* pointed out that the pathological lesions typical of diffuse white matter damage are either small or only recognizable at a microscopic level; it is therefore not particularly surprising that such lesions are not evident on CT scans, although there may be circumstantial evidence from CT scans to suspect their presence. Bruce *et al.* (1981) used this sort of evidence obtained from head-injured children to confirm the idea of a link between diffuse damage to the cerebral white matter and the absence of a lucid interval. However, the main point emphasized by Snoek *et al.* was that caution was called for in drawing conclusions based solely on CT scans, expecially in regarding a normal or near normal scan as excluding severe brain damage. Indeed, Gennarelli (1983) used as an indicator of diffuse axonal injury prolonged traumatic coma in the absence of any mass lesions (intracranial haematomas) on CT scans.

Intracerebral lesions can be readily detected in patients with either severe or minor closed head injury using MRI (Kalisky *et al.*, 1987; Levin *et al.*, 1985a, 1985c, 1987a). In agreement with Ommaya and Gennarelli's (1974, 1976) 'centripetal' conception of the biomechanics of head injury, the depth of lesions visualized in this way is inversely related to the patient's total score on the Glasgow Coma Scale and positively related to the duration of impaired consciousness, and they are typically smaller in volume than lesions to the brain surface (Jenkins *et al.*, 1986; Levin *et al.*, 1988b). Unfortunately, it is not at present entirely clear whether these lesions reflect regional variations specifically in the extent of diffuse axonal injury, as opposed to subsequent complications such as a transient elevation of intracranial pressure or to degenerative changes during the post-injury interval. Nevertheless, Levin *et al.* (1988b) found that the exclusion of patients who exhibited neurological deterioration and raised intracranial pressure did not affect the overall relationship between the depth of the lesion and the level of consciousness. Two additional problems are that MRI is known to be sensitive to pre-existing demyelinating conditions such as multiple sclerosis (Levin *et al.*, 1987a), but that it is unable to visualize compact bone (Han *et al.*, 1984).

A fairly common outcome of severe closed head injury is an enlargement of the Sylvian aqueduct and of the lateral ventricles despite the absence of communicating hydrocephalus. On the basis of pneumoencephalographic studies Boller *et al.* (1972) argued that this clinical condition was the result of degeneration of the periventricular white matter, a notion that is entirely consistent with the results of the *post mortem* investigations cited above. Levin *et al.* (1981b) showed that the extent of ventricular enlargement according to CT was significantly related to the duration of coma, though only among patients who had been involved in motor vehicle accidents. More recently, Levin *et al.* (1988b) found that the extent of ventricular enlargement was correlated with the depth of lesions that had been visualized by means of MRI.

Nevertheless, shearing forces at the time of impact may give rise to lesions in a variety of other intracranial structures. For instance, the possibility of damage to the corpus callosum was mentioned earlier. Adams and Graham (1972) found some damage of this sort amongst 80 per cent of a consecutive series of 400 fatal head injuries. In particular, there were gross lesions within the corpus callosum in every patient who demonstrated diffuse degeneration of the white matter or evidence of primary injury to the brain stem. These lesions may sometimes be visualized by means of CT (Zimmerman *et al.*, 1978b) or more readily by means of MRI (Jenkins *et al.*, 1986), and can even lead to a hemispheric disconnection syndrome (Rubens *et al.*, 1977). There may also be damage to the cranial nerves, and the resulting sensory impairment can affect the quality of subsequent recovery. Neurological deficits of this sort are seen in between 2 and 8 per cent of survivors of severe head injuries. The olfactory, optic, and auditory nerves seem to be the most vulnerable. A detailed though now rather dated account of cranial nerve problems after closed head injuries was given by Russell (1960), who attributed these to small vascular lesions within the brain stem, while Sumner (1964) provided an early but authoritative analysis of post-traumatic anosmia (loss of the sense of smell). A review chapter by Rovit and Murali (1982) is somewhat more up-to-date. Damage to the hypothalamo-pituitary system is also well recognized. More than 40 per cent of patients who die as the result of head injuries show some evidence of haemorrhagic or ischaemic damage to the hypo-thalamus (Crompton, 1971), and complete or partial necrosis of the anterior lobe of the pituitary gland and haemorrhage into the posterior lobe are common findings at *post mortem*. Among patients who survive severe head injury, disordered hypothalamic or pituitary function may be evident: for instance, diabetes insipidus, which involves the excretion of large volumes of urine of low concentration and thus reflects a failure of secretion of antidiuretic hormone, is sometimes seen after head injury.

Secondary Brain Damage

Jennett and Teasdale (1981, p. 23) pointed out that a crucial distinction needs to be drawn between immediate impact damage after closed head injury (that is, skull fractures, cerebral contusions and diffuse axonal injury), and subsequent complications or secondary brain damage. The complications of closed head injury are the only treatable aspects of closed head injury and it follows that the main objective of medical management is to prevent or at least to minimize the various forms of secondary brain damage. The primary complications are *intracranial haematomas* and *brain swelling* (*see* Adams *et al.*, 1980a). These changes can usually be identified by means of CT (Clifton *et al.*, 1980; Tarlov, 1976; Weisberg, 1979), although they may only be evident on close inspection of relevant images (Zimmerman *et al.*, 1978), and they can also be detected by means of MRI (Snow *et al.*, 1986).

Intracranial Haematomas

Intracranial haemorrhage tends to occur in all but the most minor head injuries, but it is only of clinical significance if it gives rise to a space-occupying clot or intracranial haematoma. This occurs in almost 50 per cent of severely injured patients, more commonly in older patients, and it often accounts for the delayed development of coma after a lucid interval or for the deterioration of patients already in coma (Jennett *et al.*, 1976, 1977b, 1979a, 1979b; Reilly *et al.*, 1975; Teasdale *et al.*, 1979b). Jennett and Teasdale (1981, pp. 100–1) stated that the diagnosis of a skull fracture increased the likelihood of an intracranial haematoma by about 20 times in comatose patients and by about 400 times in conscious patients. Prompt surgical intervention is necessary to deal with this condition (Marshall *et al.*, 1983b). Nevertheless, Bowers and Marshall (1980) suggested that the occurrence of an intracranial haematoma did not itself have any adverse effect upon prognosis once it had been surgically treated. These researchers as well as others (e.g., Gennarelli, 1983) have also noted that intracranial haematomas are about half as common in head injuries resulting from motor accidents as in those resulting from other causes. Intracranial bleeding may be categorized in terms of its anatomical location with respect to the brain and the three membranes or *meninges* by which it is enveloped. These are illustrated schematically in Figure 2.4. It should however be noted that the dura mater normally adheres to the inner surfaces of the cranial bones and is separated from the arachnoid mater just by a film of serous fluid. In contrast, the arachnoid and the pia mater are separated by a layer of cerebrospinal fluid and are in close contact only on the crests of the cerebral gyri (Williams and Warwick, 1975, pp. 986–92). This means that in normal individuals the extradural and subdural spaces are merely 'potential' spaces, and that the subarachnoid space is the only true space. Intracranial haemorrhage can be classified as extradural, subdural, subarachnoid, intracerebral, or intraventricular, although more than one of these forms may be involved in the same patient.

Extradural haematoma

An extradural haematoma (sometimes described as an *epidural* haematoma) forms when blood from torn meningeal vessels strips the dura away from the skull and produces a lens-shaped bulging mass within the extradural space. This mass of blood is well-defined, because the dura at the edges of the haematoma remains firmly attached to the inner table of the skull. Extradural haematomas are found in 1–2 per cent of patients admitted to hospital with closed head injuries, and they are most common over the temporal and parietal regions, since it is the branches of the middle meningeal vessels that are most frequently damaged in cases of closed head injury (Jennett and Teasdale, 1981, p. 153). Although haematomas at this site are not uncommonly seen after what clinically seems to have been only a slight trauma, a skull fracture is present in 85 per cent of patients (Jamieson and Yelland, 1968). Indeed, Adams *et al.* (1983) concluded that extradural haematomas were essentially a complication of skull fracture, because neither extradural haematomas nor skull fractures were induced as the result of inertial angular acceleration of the head in experiments on infrahuman primates. The subsequent mortality rate may be high (between 15 and 30 per cent in different series), despite the fact that there may often be no discernible brain damage other than that which is attributable to the space-occupying effects of the haematoma

Figure 2.4   Schematic anatomical representation of the cerebral meninges

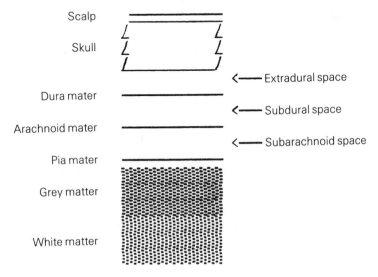

itself. Nevertheless, it is just these effects which make an extradural haematoma such a dangerous complication and death may supervene without prompt surgical intervention.

Subdural haematoma

A subdural haematoma is a collection of blood lying between the dura and the arachnoid. It most commonly results from the tearing of the bridging veins which run across the subdural space to the dural venous sinuses, but the cause may also be direct injury to the sinuses themselves or bleeding from arteries and veins in areas of damaged cerebral cortex. Whereas the spread of extradural haematomas is circumscribed by dural attachments to the skull, subdural haematomas tend to be much more widespread and often extend beneath and between the cerebral hemispheres (Adams, 1988, p. 11): indeed, they are commonly found over the convexities of the hemispheres, against the falx cerebri in the longitudinal fissure, or in the floor of the anterior, middle, or posterior cranial fossae. Subdural haematomas of the same density as brain tissue are difficult to detect on CT images, but can be readily identified using MRI (Han *et al.*, 1984).

The expression 'acute subdural haematoma' is often used to refer to those occurring within 48 hours of injury. A thin film of subdural blood is in fact commonly seen in cases of closed head injury and need not have any great clinical significance. However, in about 5 per cent of cases the collection of blood is large, often as a result of haemorrhages from the capillaries in the outer membrane. In this situation prompt surgical intervention is certainly warranted, although the resulting mortality may still be relatively high (Bowers and Marshall, 1980; Gennarelli, 1983). Some authors describe as 'subacute' a haematoma that occurs between three days and two to three weeks following a head injury, but Jennett and Teasdale (1981, p. 156) doubted whether this constituted a distinct diagnostic category. They suggested that any haematoma occurring within the first two weeks after injury should be described as 'acute', while a haematoma diagnosed later than this should be described as 'chronic' (*see* Cooper, 1982b).

In experimental research using infrahuman primates, Ommaya *et al.* (1968) demonstrated that rapid rotation of the head without direct impact could produce cerebral concussion, superficial cortical contusions, and subdural haematomas (*see also* Ommaya *et al.*, 1971b). It has subsequently been extensively confirmed that inertial angular acceleration of the head can induce subdural haematomas, but only when the acceleration is rapid and within the sagittal (that is, dorsoventral) plane (Adams *et al.*, 1983; Gennarelli, 1983). Similarly, Ommaya and Yarnell (1969) described two cases of subdural haematoma in human patients which had apparently been produced by whiplash injury alone. Moreover, in his account of the 'whiplash shaken infant syndrome', Caffey (1974) specifically noted the occurrence of bilateral subdural haematoma in the absence of external signs of trauma to the head and neck. Cortical atrophy and ventricular enlargement are now well documented as sequelae of subdural haematomas (Cullum and Bigler, 1985).

Subarachnoid haemorrhage

A subarachnoid haemorrhage occurs when blood is released into the space between the arachnoid and the pia. Some degree of subarachnoid bleeding is almost universal after a closed head injury, particularly if there is an occipital fracture of the skull. A more substantial haematoma within the subarachnoid space is however somewhat rare, because the collection of blood tends to rupture into the brain or the subdural space. The presence of blood in the subarachnoid space seems to be involved in the genesis of arterial spasm, which may give rise to ischaemic brain damage (Macpherson and Graham, 1978). Moreover, the presence of blood and, in the longer term, the development of fibrous adhesions in the subarachnoid space may obstruct the flow of cerebrospinal fluid. This results in communicating high pressure hydrocephalus, which may arise even following a minor head injury in a patient with congenital narrowing (stenosis) of the Sylvian aqueduct (Jennett and Teasdale, 1981, p. 40; Teasdale and Mendelow, 1984).

Intracerebral haematomas

Intracerebral haematomas are characteristically associated with cerebral contusions, and therefore tend to occur most frequently within the frontal and temporal lobes (*see* Figure 2.5). They can also arise in other regions of the cerebral hemispheres and within the cerebellum and brainstem. They have been variously reported as occurring in 5–20 per cent of serious head injuries (e.g., Levin *et al.*, 1989), and in over 50 per cent of the latter cases are associated with a fractured skull (Jamieson and Yelland, 1972). Nevertheless, they have also been reported in experimental research where inertial angular acceleration has been used to induce closed head injury in infrahuman primates without actual head impact, although like subdural haematomas they tend to arise only with rapid acceleration in the sagittal plane (Adams *et al.*, 1983).

Three forms of intracerebral haematoma are associated with particularly severe head injuries. First, there may sometimes be a gross disruption of one lobe of the brain (usually the frontal or temporal pole) where severe contusions and lacerations are combined with an intracerebral haematoma in continuity with a related subdural haematoma at the same location. Such a phenomenon is described as a 'burst lobe' (Jennett and Teasdale, 1981, p. 155). Second, an intracerebral haematoma may extend

Figure 2.5   Composite drawing showing the size and location of intracerebral haemorrhages found in a series of twenty-seven cases of closed head injury

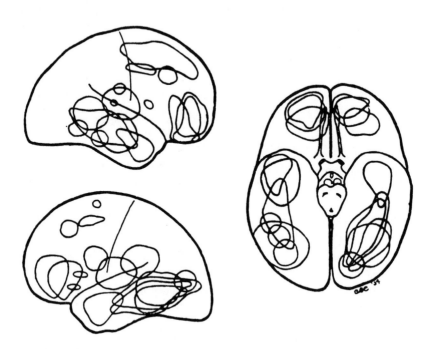

Source: Courville, C. B. (1950) *Pathology of the Central Nervous System*, 3rd ed., Mountain View, CA, Pacific Press Publishing Association. Reprinted with permission.

into the ventricular system and thus generate an *intraventricular haemorrhage*. This was formerly regarded as having an extremely poor prognosis, but the advent of CT has led to this view being revised. Third, intracerebral haematomas may also arise deep within the brain from vessels which have been torn by shearing forces at impact. Adams *et al.* (1986a) found such deep intracerebral haematomas (or 'basal ganglia' haematomas) in the brains of 10 per cent of patients with fatal head injuries. These patients showed more severe contusions and an increased incidence of diffuse axonal injury, and this led Adams *et al.* to conclude that a deep intracerebral haematoma was a primary event occurring at the moment of injury and not merely a form of secondary brain damage.

Brain Swelling

This type of brain damage may arise from the accumulation of excess water in brain tissue (i.e., cerebral oedema), but it can also arise following closed head injury as the result of the leakage of plasma from cerebral blood vessels because of vasodilation (*see* e.g., Adams *et al.*, 1980a). Some local swelling is an almost invariable consequence of contusions and lacerations, from which plasma can spread to the underlying white matter by passing between the myelin sheaths. It may also occur in the vicinity of intracerebral haematomas, as well as beneath extradural and subdural haematomas. However, Adams (1988) argued that the term 'brain swelling' should be restricted to cases of diffuse swelling of one or both cerebral hemispheres. Diffuse swelling of an entire cerebral hemisphere arises in about 10 per cent of patients with severe head injury, and often follows the evacuation of an overlying acute subdural haematoma, although it is much more common in children (Adams *et al.*, 1989b). Adams *et al.* (1983) found that diffuse swelling was also a frequent occurrence in infrahuman primates who had developed an acute subdural haematoma as the result of inertial angular acceleration of the head. However, they also noted that a generalized brain swelling affecting both cerebral hemispheres was rare in human adults and could not be produced in infrahuman primates.

Nevertheless, this latter condition of generalized swelling is seen in children and adolescents, in whom it may develop after apparently minor head injuries and in the absence of significant primary impact damage such as marked contusions or lacerations (*see* Bruce *et al.*, 1981). Indeed, an early study by Hendrick *et al.* (1964) suggested that up to 50 per cent of children who died following head injury had been conscious on admission to hospital but had deteriorated dramatically over the subsequent 48 hours. However, a recent study by Graham *et al.* (1989a) reported that only 16 per cent of children with fatal head injuries had had a lucid interval of any kind, which was taken to mean that children died most often as a result of brain damage sustained at the moment of injury. In the latter series, 18 per cent showed unilateral brain swelling and 52 per cent showed bilateral swelling. The findings that are typical of diffuse cerebral swelling from autopsy or CT are 'slit-like' compressed ventricles and venous congestion (Bruce *et al.*, 1978; Snoek *et al.*, 1979; Zimmerman *et al.*, 1978a). In a study of 60 patients with severe head injury, Snoek *et al.* (1979) recorded findings of this sort in the CT scans of 15 cases and in the autopsies of six out of the 15 fatally injured cases, all of whom were under 20 years of age. Similarly, Levin and Eisenberg (1979a) reported that compressed ventricles were visualized in eight out of 33 children and adolescents who had been referred for CT following closed head injury; four of these eight patients had been awake and responsive to commands at the time of their admission to hospital. The pathophysiology of this phenomenon is probably cerebral vasodilation and increased cerebral blood volume secondary to disturbance of vasomotor tone (Adams, 1988; Bruce *et al.*, 1981).

Finally, a similar though transient condition may be responsible for the so-called 'fall-asleep syndrome' (*Einschlafsyndrom*), in which a child with a relatively mild head injury shows a delayed impairment of consciousness after a lucid interval, but improves within a matter of hours and exhibits little or no residual neurological impairment (Todorow and Heiss, 1978; cf. Bruce *et al.*, 1981; Levin *et al.*, 1982a, pp. 195–96).

Raised Intracranial Pressure

The cranial cavity is a relatively rigid container, but increases in the volume of blood (due to haematoma) or tissue (due to brain swelling) can be readily compensated for within certain limits by the displacement of cerebrospinal fluid. Nevertheless, there comes a point at which this buffering is exhausted, and the patient is then at risk from brain damage secondary to raised intracranial pressure. Although many of the classical features may even occur in patients whose intracranial pressure has never been significantly elevated, the neuropathology of this condition includes some or all of the following features: a compression and flattening of the cerebral convolutions; a herniation of the cingulate gyrus, the parahippocampal gyrus and uncus, and the cerebellar tonsils and medulla; infarction in the territory of the posterior cerebral artery; haemorrhage or infarction of the brain stem; and a shift in the interventricular septum across the midline, with a consequent distortion of the ventricles. More than 80 per cent of fatally injured cases show evidence of elevated intracranial pressure, usually as the result of diffuse brain swelling or an intracranial haematoma (Adams and Graham, 1976; Graham *et al.*, 1987; Jennett and Teasdale, 1981, pp. 31–4). Conversely, in fatally injured cases with no evidence of raised intracranial pressure, brain swelling is rare, intracranial haematomas are typically not found at all, and death usually results from extracranial complications such as bronchopneumonia, pulmonary embolism, sepsis and renal failure (Graham *et al.*, 1988).

Adams and Graham (1976) established that the most common and consistent pathological marker of raised intracranial pressure between head injury and death was the presence of a wedge of pressure necrosis as the result of downward herniation within one or both parahippocampal gyri where they impinge against the free anterior border of the tentorium cerebelli (the arched layer of dura mater that separates the occipital lobes of the cerebral hemispheres from the cerebellum). In neuropathological studies of fatal head injury, the incidence of this phenomenon has proved to be consistently around 85–90 per cent (*see* Graham *et al.*, 1989b). Results presented by Adams *et al.* (1983) showed that on this criterion raised intracranial pressure was a common outcome of head injury induced in infrahuman primates without head impact, but once again only when there was rapid acceleration within the sagittal plane. Graham *et al.* (1987) identified pressure necrosis of either one or both parahippocampal gyri in 324 out of 434 cases of fatal nonmissile head injury, and in 42 of these patients there was no other brain damage attributable to raised intracranial pressure. However, they pointed out that a rapid increase in intracranial pressure might well prove fatal before internal herniation could appear, and this largely explained the apparently anomalous occurrence of other forms of brain damage conventionally ascribed to raised intracranial pressure among 16 patients with no evidence of pressure necrosis in the parahippocampal gyri.

Reilly *et al.* (1975) noted that raised intracranial pressure was a feature of 17 out of 22 head-injured patients who had died after a lucid interval but who had no intracranial haematoma. They suggested that the monitoring and treatment of elevated intracranial pressure would have a significant impact on mortality following severe head injury, and subsequent research has tended to confirm this (Bowers and Marshall, 1980). However, Graham *et al.* (1987) found no support at all for the specific proposition that death in head-injured patients after a lucid interval was associated with raised intracranial pressure as indicated by pressure necrosis in either one or both parahippocampal gyri.

Ischaemic Brain Damage

Uncontrolled intracranial pressure is an important factor determining mortality after severe closed head injury because it leads to vascular complications and is especially associated with ischaemic brain damage (that is, damage caused by an inadequate flow of blood). This tends to take the form of the death of nerve cells as the result of an inadequate blood supply (*infarction*) leading to a deficiency of oxygen in the brain tissues (*hypoxia*). For instance, tentorial herniation leads to infarction in the brainstem and in the territory supplied by the posterior cerebral artery, especially in the medial occipital cortex. The latter occurs in 30 per cent of all cases of fatal head injury (Graham *et al.*, 1978) and in 36 per cent of those cases that show evidence of pressure necrosis (Graham *et al.*, 1987). It was not identified by Adams *et al.* (1983) in infrahuman primates following inertial angular acceleration of the head, but this was attributed to the short period of survival before they were sacrificed.

Ischaemic brain damage can also take the form of focal infarction and necrosis in the vicinity of cerebral contusions as well as more widespread lesions associated with cardiorespiratory arrest, status epilepticus, and fat embolism (Graham *et al.*, 1978). Hypoxic damage is particularly common in the boundary zones between the major cerebral arterial territories, and especially in the parasagittal cortex between the regions supplied by the anterior and middle cerebral arteries (Adams, 1988); this occurs in up to 50 per cent of patients with fatal head injuries, regardless of whether or not they have suffered diffuse axonal injury, but it occurs only rarely in infrahuman primates that are subjected to inertial angular acceleration and monitored for systemic hypoxia and hypotension (Adams *et al.*, 1983). Adams *et al.* (1980a) noted that hypoxic brain damage had previously not been emphasized as a consequence of severe head injury, perhaps because it could often only be identified microscopically. For the same reason, the pathological lesions that are typical of recent hypoxic brain damage are unfortunately often not evident on CT scans (Snoek *et al.*, 1979), although they are associated with angiographic evidence of post-traumatic arterial spasm (Macpherson and Graham, 1978).

Diffuse cortical damage of the sort seen after cardiac arrest or status epilepticus occurs in 30–40 per cent of fatally injured patients (Graham *et al.*, 1989b). Lesions associated with fat embolism are more common in patients who have sustained multiple injuries. When there is a fracture of a long bone (or sometimes following the internal fixation of such a fracture), emboli of fat may be released into the circulation and be transported to the lungs and brain. This condition is heralded by an abrupt onset of confusion, drowsiness, and, in the more severely affected cases, coma. The characteristic features are fever, an increase in heart rate (tachycardia), and deficiency of oxygen in brain tissues (hypoxia); small haemorrhages may develop on the skin and conjunctivae, and epileptic seizures may occur. Cerebral fat embolism carries a high mortality risk, but it is fortunately a rare complication that normally does not produce additional deficits in those who survive. Emboli of brain tissue may also produce pulmonary insufficiency, and are found at autopsy in the lungs of 2 per cent of patients with fatal head injuries (Wacks and Bird, 1970).

Nevertheless, a more important mechanism of ischaemic brain damage is widespread cerebral infarction resulting from a generalized reduction in blood flow. Cerebral blood flow depends upon the pressure difference between the arteries and the veins (the cerebral perfusion pressure), and the latter is essentially the difference between the systematic arterial pressure and the intracranial pressure. In principle, then, either lower systemic arterial pressure or elevated intracranial pressure would reduce the cerebral perfusion pressure, resulting in reduced cerebral blood flow and therefore in diffuse ischaemic hypoxia (*see* Graham, 1985). Studies of fatal head injury have produced good evidence of small localized areas of dead tissue (infarcts) or widespread foci of ischaemic necrosis throughout the brain, and especially in the areas that are known to be differentially sensitive to hypoxia, such as the hippocampus and the thalamus (Teasdale and Mendelow, 1984; cf. Brierley, 1976). In particular, ischaemic damage to the hippocampus has been reported in roughly 80 per cent of all cases of fatal head injury (e.g., Graham *et al.*, 1987, 1989b). There is a high incidence of such lesions among infrahuman primates subjected to inertial angular acceleration of the head (Adams *et al.*, 1983).

This type of ischaemic damage is more common in patients with a history of hypertension or hypoxia, as well as in those whose head injuries lead to an elevation of intracranial pressure (Graham *et al.*, 1978; Price and Murray, 1972). Nevertheless, Adams and Graham (1976) found no correlation between pressure necrosis in the para-hippocampal gyri and hypoxic necrosis in the hippocampus, and they concluded that high intracranial pressure was not an important factor in the pathogenesis of hypoxic necrosis following severe head injury. The effective causal mechanism might instead involve low arterial pressure (Graham *et al.*, 1978) or else poor oxygen saturation (arterial hypoxaemia) as the result of obstruction of the airways (Adams, 1988), but at present the exact pathogenesis of diffuse hypoxic damage in head-injured patients has yet to be established. It might be added that the findings of Graham *et al.* (1978) led many centres to attach more importance to the treatment of hypoxia and hypotension in head-injured patients at the accident scene, during transfer to and between hospitals, and during intensive care, and also to the detection and treatment of intracranial haematoma. However, there is no evidence that such endeavours in management and organization of patient care have had any effect on the incidence of ischaemic damage following closed head injury, perhaps because they have been outweighed by the increasing numbers of very severely injured patients who are referred for specialist neurosurgical treatment that might otherwise have died in accident departments or primary surgical wards (Graham *et al.*, 1989b).

Infection

Another source of complications following closed head injury is that of intracranial infection (*see* Landesman and Cooper, 1982, for a detailed review of this topic). Post-traumatic infection is seen especially in patients who have suffered skull fracture; conversely, it is not seen in infrahuman primates subjected to inertial angular acceleration of the head (Adams *et al.*, 1982a). *Meningitis* is a well recognized problem that occurs in 2–3 per cent of severely injured patients. The most common causative organism is pneumococcus. If the dura has been penetrated, then infection may enter, leading to the formation of a collection of pus in the subdural space (a *subdural empyema*). This is most frequently located over the convexity of the cerebral hemispheres or in the interhemispheric fissure. The condition of *extradural empyema* may also occur. A serious complication which characteristically develops in the subacute phase after head injury is that of *cerebral abscess*. Despite the introduction of antibiotics, this is still associated with a 10 per cent mortality. Among the survivors there may be additional residual neurological deficits, and epilepsy is especially frequent.

Post-traumatic Epilepsy

This is a condition that has received considerable discussion, although it is less common following closed head injury than following penetrating missile wounds. Indeed one study of 117 individuals with closed head injuries found just one instance where seizures had clearly started after the injury in question (Dencker, 1960). Jennett and Lewin (1960) identified a specific condition of *early* post-traumatic epilepsy which occurred during the first week after a closed head injury. Jennett (1969, 1974) subsequently elaborated the logical basis for distinguishing a separate diagnostic entity thus: (a) that the first epileptic fit occurred many times more often in the first week after injury than in subsequent weeks; (b) that focal motor attacks were far more likely in the first week than in subsequent weeks; and (c) that fewer than one-third of the patients who had any seizures in the first week after injury had any further epileptic fits during the next four years (*see* Jennett, 1973). This condition appears to affect at most 5 per cent of all patients admitted to hospital with closed head injuries, although it is more common in patients who have experienced severe head injuries and in children (*see also* Kollevold, 1976). Early epilepsy may indicate certain complications such as intracranial haematoma or infection, but it is not in itself a clinical hazard unless status epilepticus develops.

The prognostic importance of early epilepsy is that it increases the probability of *late* epilepsy, in which seizures begin at any time after the first week (and possibly not for many years after the original closed head injury). The incidence of this condition is also about 5 per cent of all admissions, and it is related to the occurrence of early epilepsy, a depressed fracture of the skull, or an intracranial (and more especially an intradural) haematoma (Jennett, 1973, 1975a; Jennett and Lewin, 1960; Roberts, 1979, chap. 10; cf. Kollevold, 1978, 1979). Nevertheless these predisposing factors do not contribute additively to the incidence of late epilepsy. In particular, Jennett (1973) showed that after early epilepsy the incidence of late epilepsy was over 20 per cent even following trivial injuries (with no post-traumatic amnesia, no depressed skull fracture, and no intracranial haematoma) and regardless of the patient's age. However, in patients who have sustained a compound depressed fracture of the skull, the incidence of both forms of epilepsy is increased overall, and that of late epilepsy can exceed 70 per cent, depending upon the occurrence of early epilepsy, the duration of post-traumatic amnesia, and whether the dura was torn (Jennett *et al.*, 1973, 1974). Late epilepsy tends to be focal in nature, often implicating the temporal lobe, and, unlike early epilepsy, can be a recurrent debilitating condition. Nevertheless, in most cases epileptic convulsions become progressively less frequent over a period of ten years or so, and nearly half of all patients with late post-traumatic epilepsy eventually achieve complete remission (Lewin *et al.*, 1979; Roberts, 1979, p. 123).

Concluding Summary

Any discussion of the effects of closed head injury must begin with the obvious but fundamental observation that the damage which is sustained by the brain is the most important factor determining the eventual outcome (Adams *et al.*. 1980a, 1983). Even a blow to the head which causes merely a brief disturbance of consciousness may produce detectable structural damage to the brain. Some of this damage occurs at the moment of head injury (the primary brain damage), but some may be caused by subsequent complications (the secondary brain damage), of which the most important are intracranial haematoma, brain swelling, raised intracranial pressure, ischaemic brain damage, infection and post-traumatic epilepsy.

The principal mechanism of brain damage following closed head injury is diffuse axonal injury as the result of shearing forces which decrease in magnitude from the surface of the brain to its centre. Nowadays, indeed, it is generally recognized that diffuse axonal injury is the single most important mechanism governing the outcome from closed head injury (Adams, 1988; Adams *et al.*, 1980a). Closed head injury also gives rise to contusions and lacerations on the surface of the brain which may extend into the subcortical white matter. Such lesions are themselves neither necessary nor sufficient for a head injury to prove fatal; their clinical significance lies rather in the fact thay they initiate brain swelling and intracranial haemorrhage. Contusions are predominantly the result of the rotational movement of the frontal and temporal lobes against the bony projections within the base of the skull. They do not occur principally at the site of original impact ('coup' injury), unless the skull has been fractured. Nor do they occur specifically at the point which is diametrically opposite the site of head impact ('contrecoup' injury). In fact, a similar distribution of cerebral contusions can be induced in infrahuman primates as a result of inertial angular acceleration that involves no impact at all (Adams *et al.*, 1985).

The distinction between primary and secondary brain damage is obviously fundamental in the clinical management of head-injured patients, because in principle the complications are the only treatable aspects of a closed head injury. Nevertheless, a final point to be made is that in terms of understanding the consequences of head injury it may be more important to consider the resulting brain damage as being either *focal* or *diffuse*. As Adams *et al.* (1983, 1986a, 1986b) explained, the focal brain damage which results from closed head injury includes cerebral contusions, intracranial haematomas, and the damage that is characteristic of raised intracranial pressure and brain herniation. This can often be visualized by means of CT during life, and is readily identified by the naked eye at *post mortem*. Although all of the broad types of brain damage that occur in human beings as the result of closed head injury can be induced in infrahuman primates by means of inertial angular acceleration (Adams *et al.*, 1982a, 1983; Gennarelli, 1983; Graham *et al.*, 1988a), the amount of focal brain damage is increased substantially by the occurrence of skull fracture and to that extent it is associated with actual head impact of the sort encountered in assaults and falls (Adams *et al.*, 1989b; Gennarelli, 1983).

The diffuse brain damage which results from closed head injury unless the patient fails to survive more than a few hours includes diffuse axonal injury, hypoxic damage and brain swelling. At present the precise form which this damage takes in any particular patient is rarely identifiable during life. However, the incidence of diffuse axonal injury is significantly increased among those patients who have sustained either deep intracerebral haematomas (Adams *et al.*, 1986a) or gliding contusions (Adams *et al.*, 1986b), and it has been suggested that the visualization of either of these lesions on a CT scan shortly after a head injury could be taken as evidence of diffuse axonal injury (Adams *et al.*, 1989b). The amount of diffuse brain damage is primarily dependent upon the rate of acceleration and deceleration and to that extent it is associated with high inertial loading of the head of the sort which is encountered in vehicular accidents (Adams *et al.*, 1989b; Gennarelli, 1983).

Chapter 3

Retrograde Amnesia and Post-Traumatic Amnesia

In the previous chapter, it was noted that a closed head injury tends to produce shearing forces within the brain that give rise to diffuse lesions and disturbance of function, and the most common effect of these forces is the immediate loss of consciousness known as coma or concussion. Russell (1971) gave a vivid account of the process of recovery from this state:

> The immediate effects of concussion are usually that the individual drops to the ground motionless, often with an arrest of respiration, and at this stage basic reflexes such as the corneal response may be abolished. After respiration returns, restless movements appear and by very gradual stages the patient begins to speak, resist interference, make a noise, and becomes restless, talkative, abusive, and irritable in one way or another. Slowly his speech becomes more intelligible and then as the effect of the trauma wears off he looks around wondering where he is: the period of traumatic confusion is at an end, but he has no recollection of any event that occurred since the injury.
> (p. 1)

To facilitate the observation and categorization of behavioural responses during this early phase of recovery, Hagen *et al.* (1979) devised a formal 'Levels of Cognitive Functioning' scale that described the relevant aspects of behavioural change in terms of a sequence of distinct stages, although the latter can be conveniently grouped within four basic recovery phases covering decreased responding, agitated responding, confused responding and automatic responding (Malkmus, 1983).

It was also pointed out in the previous chapter that the rotational motion of the brain within the skull gives rise to lacerations and contusions in the region of the sphenoidal ridge, producing damage to both the frontal and the temporal lobes. These frontotemporal lesions are not only a frequent outcome of closed head injury; they are also likely to constitute the area of greatest cortical damage wherever the site of impact. It is well established that the physiological integrity of the temporal lobes is a prerequisite for many of the important higher cognitive functions and especially for the normal functioning of human memory (*see* e.g., Walsh, 1978, chap. 5). It is therefore not surprising that disturbances of learning and remembering are a reliable outcome of closed head injury. Specifically, post-traumatic memory impairment seems to be associated with lesions of the hippocampal gyri of the temporal lobes (Ommaya and Gennarelli, 1976).

These characteristic disturbances of human memory are of considerable interest, both to the clinician and to the neuropsychologist. From the clinical point of view, the length of time over which remembering is impaired is broadly proportional to the duration of coma or concussion, and is relevant to both diagnosis and prognosis. It appears to be a reliable measure of the severity of the injury and a sensitive predictor of the eventual outcome. From the neuropsychological point of view, the study of head-injured patients offers a quasi-experimental model for testing theories of normal memory function. A variety of psychological theories of learning and remembering have been used in trying to give a useful analysis of the disorders manifested by these patients, and the more important frameworks will be discussed in this chapter and the next.

The impairment of memory function which is characteristic of closed head injury takes three different forms. First, head-injured patients manifest a reliable inability to recall events experienced during a short period immediately prior to their injury. Second, head-injured patients manifest a reliable inability to recall events experienced during a certain period immediately following the cessation of coma. Third, head-injured patients also manifest a measurable disturbance of memory function that persists beyond the latter period. The first and second type of memory deficit will be considered in this chapter; the third type will be considered in Chapter 4.

Retrograde Amnesia

Retrograde amnesia (RA) is a specific impairment of memory for events that were experienced immediately before a closed head injury. The duration of the period before the injury that is affected in this way normally varies with the severity of the head injury, judged according to the duration of unconsciousness (Russell, 1932), and by implication with the later prognosis. Consequently, as Symonds (1940) noted, a long period of RA is generally an indication of severe or extensive brain damage. However, occasionally a rather mild head injury may trigger an amnesic attack that is grossly disproportionate to the degree of trauma, with the RA extending over days or even weeks (Haas and Ross, 1986). It is thought that a loss of consciousness inevitably gives rise to RA, although the latter may certainly occur without the former. More specifically, Yarnell and Lynch (1970) described four subjects who had received head injuries while playing American college football that resulted in transient confusion or motor incoordination; in three out of the four cases there seemed to have been no loss of consciousness. When these subjects were examined immediately following their injuries, they all showed good recall of the events leading up to the relevant incidents. Nevertheless, on repeated questioning between 3 and 20 min later, all of this information had been lost. Subsequently, Lynch and Yarnell (1973) increased their sample to six subjects, all of whom showed this pattern of findings (*see also* Yarnell and Lynch, 1973). These results suggest that RA is a condition which may develop within a few minutes of a closed head injury even when the victim has not lost consciousness.

Nevertheless, the measurement of RA in individual clinical cases presents a number of serious problems (Blomert and Sisler, 1974; Schacter and Crovitz, 1977). First, the precise timing of the most recent event which can be remembered before the head injury can often be determined only from the patients' own reconstructions of their previous activities; it may therefore be highly unreliable, especially in severely injured cases. Second, the period in question is not always characterized by a continuous amnesia; rather, patients may still be able to recollect isolated events or, as Russell and Nathan (1946) described them, 'islands' of accessible memories. However, these are not necessarily memories of personally significant episodes or events; indeed, Williams (1969) claimed that RA 'tends to take little account of emotional bias ... When islands of memory are retained, they are typically of trivial visual images' (p. 75). Third, RA does not seem to affect a fixed period immediately prior to the accident, but typically varies on repeated testing (Sisler and Penner, 1975). More specifically, a closed head injury often results in a retrograde amnesia which seems to 'shrink' or gradually shorten during the course of the patient's recovery (Russell, 1935; Russell and Nathan, 1946), though this may leave persistent amnesic gaps or haziness within the otherwise continuous sequence of memories for events preceding the injury (Williams and Zangwill, 1952).

The latter process of shrinkage affects both the absolute interval of time over which the impairment extends and also the number of 'islands' of memories occurring within that period. Much of this process occurs during the period of post-traumatic amnesia (Schilder, 1934), and it has been suggested that after that period any retrograde impairment of biographical memory is relatively permanent (Teuber, 1969). However, Symonds (1940) stated that 'shrinkage of the retrograde amnesia may continue for some time after the patient has regained his orientation and memory for recent events, and may be taken as evidence of continued recovery of cerebral function' (p. 87). Similarly, Russell and Nathan (1946) claimed that in cases of shrinking RA 'the P.T.A. [post-traumatic amnesia] terminates long before the R.A. shrinks to its final duration' (p. 292), and Benson and Geschwind (1967) described a patient whose RA continued to shrink well beyond the end of the period of post-traumatic amnesia. Nevertheless, even at this point, more than half of all head-injured patients report a period of RA extending for less than a minute before their accidents, and a complete amnesia extending for more than two days is somewhat rare (Eden and Turner, 1941; Russell, 1932, 1935; Russell and Nathan, 1946). In general, the duration of persistent retrograde amnesia is normally too brief for it to be of any practical value as a reliable indication of the severity of injury or of the prognosis for recovery (Long and Webb, 1983).

Symonds (1962) likened the RA observed in cases of head injury to the memory disorders that result from bilateral temporal lobectomy and herpes simplex encephalitis (which also produces damage to the temporal lobes). He argued that post-traumatic RA resulted from bilateral and symmetrical damage to the cerebral white matter, although he suggested that it could also result from lesions elsewhere in the cerebral hemispheres than in the temporal lobes. A more recent account by Goldberg *et al.* (1981) described a patient with a dense and persistent RA that extended back over nearly 20 years. On the basis of detailed investigations using computerized tomography, this was attributed to a lesion in the ventral tegmental region, and Goldberg *et al.* concluded that the selective activation of limbic structures by the mesencephalic reticular formation was important in the retrieval of long-term memories.

Encoding, Storage and Retrieval

From a logical point of view, remembering can be characterized with reference to three consecutive processes or stages: an original event is witnessed or experienced; it is retained in memory over a period of time; and finally the relevant information is retrieved or otherwise put to use. The identification of these three distinct stages of *input* (or *encoding* or *acquisition*), of *storage* (or *retention*), and of *retrieval* goes back to the time of Plato and Aristotle. It is a purely conceptual device which in itself tells us very little about the structure and function of the cognitive system that makes learning and remembering possible. It has nevertheless formed the basis of theoretical discussions about the nature of RA following closed head injury. As Levin *et al.* (1985b) summarized these discussions, 'Brief RA confined to immediate preinjury events has been attributed to disruption of memory consolidation, that is, encoding and storage, whereas impaired retention of events from the distant past has been interpreted as retrieval failure' (p. 561).

The metaphorical notion of *consolidation* as a process whereby memory traces or representation are somehow rendered with a cerebral substance has an exceedingly long history in thought and discussion on the nature of remembering. It has a natural application to cases of disordered memory, according to which patients are assumed to lack the ability to develop consolidated memory traces. Various specific suggestions have been made as to why a closed head injury might disrupt such a consolidation process. One is that recent events are erased from memory by the interruption of protein synthesis (Dixon, 1962); another is that a concussive head injury stimulates the nervous system in a manner analogous to electroconvulsive shock, thus leading to the extinction of recent neural activity (Ommaya *et al.*, 1971). However, accounts of the initial duration of RA that are grounded upon deficits of storage or consolidation are inherently implausible, because it can extend over as much as a year or more into the past. In such cases, as Russell and Nathan observed, 'there is clear inability to recall important events which must previously have been well registered, retained and recalled before the injury' (p. 294; *see also* Symonds, 1966). Moreover, Benson and Geschwind (1967) argued that the phenomenon of shrinking RA was wholly incompatible with the idea that a closed head injury disrupted the process of memory consolidation, because remote memories that are not recalled in the early stages of recovery may well prove to be accessible when patients are retested at a later date. They inferred that 'the disturbance is therefore a failure of retrieval rather than a loss of established memories' (p. 542), although Schilder (1934) pointed out that some apparent shrinkage of RA may be partially based on information provided by other people. Nevertheless, Benson and Geschwind did concede that a permanent, residual RA of only a few seconds' or a few minutes' duration might well reflect the true abolition of memories which had not yet been consolidated.

Wasterlain (1971) described 24 patients with closed head injury among whom the duration of RA had been confirmed by eyewitness testimony. Four patients showed electroencephalographic abnormalities, skull fractures and persistent neurological sequelae; their RA, which originally extended over periods of up to six months, was subject to progressive shrinking over subsequent months. In keeping with previous ideas, Wasterlain suggested that this pattern of forgetting was incompatible with any failure of storage or consolidation, but was strongly indicative of a failure of memory retrieval. In the remaining patients, however, the RA was of less than a minute's duration, was relatively constant on repeated testing, and showed no preserved 'islands' within this period; Wasterlain considered this pattern of forgetting to be entirely consistent with an account of RA expressed in terms of a failure of memory consolidation.

Short-term Memory and Long-term Memory

Such an account implies that experiences remain available in memory for a relatively brief period of time, but that they leave no permanent record. Contemporary thinking in psychology would regard such a pattern of results as manifesting a distinction between *short-term memory* and *long-term memory* as different structural components of the human memory system. During the 1950s and 1960s, these expressions were introduced to refer to different types of research paradigm: experiments in which the subjects were required to remember a relatively small amount of material for a relatively short period of time (of the order of several seconds) on the basis of a single presentation were characterized as investigations of short-term memory; experiments where the subjects were required to learn a relatively large amount of material over several trials or presentations and to retain that material for a longer period of time were characterized as investigations of long-term memory. This dichotomy bears no relation to the common clinical distinction between 'recent' and 'remote' memory, both of which would count as 'long-term' memory in this sense. Moreover, it is in itself a purely operational description that carries no necessary theoretical implications. Nevertheless, it came to be used quite quickly by many researchers to demarcate different hypothetical components of the total memory system. Fortunately a large amount of subsequent evidence tended to support this notion of two separate components of human memory (*see* Baddeley, 1976, chap. 6), and nowadays some such distinction between short-term and long-term storage is broadly accepted, if only as a useful first approximation, in discussing the architecture of human memory.

Yarnell and Lynch (1970) noted that in the case of their head-injured football players information about events which had immediately preceded the injury was intact when the patients were examined shortly afterwards. It had therefore clearly been stored by some short-term memory process, contrary to the view put forward, for example, by Williams and Zangwill (1952), that RA was the result of a failure of initial registration. The fact that this information was subsequently lost suggested instead that the injury had damaged 'the fixation into long-term traces' (p. 864). As Lynch and Yarnell (1973) elaborated this account, RA is best interpreted as the preserved storage of information within some relatively transient, short-term memory system, combined with the disruption of the consolidation or transformation of information into a relatively permanent, long-term memory system. Nevertheless, they also acknowledged that their findings could be handled equally well by the assumption of a single time-dependent and continuous consolidation process (*see also* Yarnell and Lynch, 1973).

A common finding in research into any retrograde memory disorder is that recently acquired information is impaired while remote memories are spared (Ribot, 1882). The fact that head-injured patients seem to have little or no difficulty in remembering events experienced in the remote past creates problems for the idea that RA results from defective retrieval processes. However, this temporal gradient might be caused by a number of confounded factors. First, biographical events from the remote past whose retention is assessed by clinicians may well have special personal significance for patients themselves. Second, because questions about the remote past tend to cover a broader time scale, they may well be cast in more general terms than questions about the more recent past (Squire *et al.*, 1975). Third, as Ribot (1882) himself noted, significant personal events from the remote past will have had more opportunity to be retrieved and rehearsed during the intervening years. When 28 patients with neurological damage of a variety of aetiologies (including 12 patients with closed head injury) were tested on objective events that had little personal salience (the titles of old television programmes), Levin *et al.* (1977a) found that there was no selective sparing of the oldest memories. Levin *et al.* (1985b) used a similar task extended across a longer chronological interval with a sample consisting exclusively of head-injured patients. They also showed a persistent, partial RA extending back over more than a decade, which was entirely consistent with an explanation of RA as a dysfunction of the retrieval of established memories. When the patients were tested on personally salient life events, there was a significant temporal gradient indicating the relative preservation of older memories, but only among patients who were still exhibiting post-traumatic amnesia.

This relates to a feature of RA that has been relatively neglected by researchers: that memory for personal experiences is severely impaired, whereas general world knowledge is only partially disrupted and skilled behaviour seems not to be affected at all. In particular, Russell (1971) emphasized the fact that 'training experiences during the RA period may be preserved as a learned skill although the learning cannot be recalled' (p. 48). Current discussions of the functional architecture of long-term memory differentiate between *declarative memory* and *procedural memory*: the former contains knowledge about events and objects which can be consciously retrieved and described, while the latter is responsible for skills or capabilities that can only be manifested in overt behaviour. Within the domain of declarative memory, Tulving (1972) distinguished between *episodic memory* and *semantic memory*: episodic memory was concerned with the retention of particular events and episodes in a person's life, whereas semantic memory was concerned with general knowledge about language and the world. Like the demonstration of skills or capacities held in procedural memory, the retrieval of declarative knowledge from semantic memory is an *implicit* expression of memory, insofar as it is not accompanied by the conscious recollection of a biographical episode; the retrieval of information from episodic memory is in contrast an *explicit* expression of memory that is characterized by just this sort of conscious recollection (Schacter, 1987a). Graf and Schacter (1985) made the specific claim that the amnesic syndrome was predominantly a disorder in the explicit expression of memory, and the same appears to be true of RA following closed head injury.

The hypothesis that RA extending back beyond the immediate preinjury events is predominantly a problem of the retrieval of information from memory also seems to be supported by evidence that it can be alleviated by the application of barbiturates (Russell and Nathan, 1946), neuropeptides such as vasopressin (Oliveros *et al.*, 1978), or lithium (Kline, 1979). To some clinicians it even implies that extensive RA is an hysterical dissociative reaction (Russell, 1935; cf. Kline, 1979), although others have disputed whether this is always so (Symonds, 1966). Recent experimental research suggests that at least some of these preparations influence memory performance by enhancing a person's general level of arousal rather than by affecting specific aspects of retention (*see* Sahgal, 1984; Wolkowitz *et al.*, 1985). Experience with other clinical groups indicates that vasopressin may have some clinical potential, although severely impaired patients tend to be less likely to show any benefit from such treatment (e.g., Strupp and Levitsky, 1985; Van Ree *et al.*, 1985). A retrieval interpretation of RA is also consistent with suggestions that it can be alleviated by hypnosis (Milos, 1975; cf. Raginsky, 1969). In principle, this ought to be of considerable forensic importance, but there are grave methodological reservations about much of the research that has been carried out to date. The safest conclusion at present, according to one authoritative evaluation, is that 'hypnotically induced testimony is not reliable and ought not be permitted to form the basis of testimony in court' (Orne *et al.*, 1984, p. 211).

Post-traumatic Amnesia

Following concussion (that is, following the return of normal somatic mobility and normal responsiveness to external stimuli), head-injured patients manifest a characteristic impairment of cognitive function. Symonds (1928) emphasized that 'it is important to distinguish between complete unconsciousness or coma and the condition of stupor or clouded consciousness' (p. 829), and he argued that the persistence of the latter state more than 24 hours after a head injury was the hallmark of 'major cerebral contusion' rather than simple concussion. Symonds also noted of the head-injured patient that 'on regaining his senses he is found to have an amnesia for the period of clouded consciousness' (*loc. cit.*). Russell (1932) subsequently gave a similar account of this state as the 'loss of full consciousness' (p. 552), and he suggested that the return of normal consiousness was best estimated from the patient's subsequent memory of when he or she 'woke up' (p. 554). Elsewhere, Russell (1934) summarized this analysis:

> A fair indication of the severity of the cerebral injury can be obtained from the duration of the loss of full consciousness. This is a useful indication from the practical point of view, as it can be estimated at an interval after the injury from the duration of amnesia following the injury. This may be calculated by comparing the time of the injury with the time or date at which the patient again became fully orientated with regard to time and place. (p. 135)

Symonds (1937) made a similar proposal:

> The outstanding feature of mental disorder after head injury is loss of consciousness in some degree ... For purposes of description in head injuries, if a man has no memory of what he has done, we assume that he was not at that time fully conscious. Therefore, the duration of unconsciousness may be measured by that of the traumatic amnesia following the accident. (p. 1081)

Symonds (1940) subsequently used the phrase 'post-traumatic amnesia' (PTA) to refer to this state, which he took to indicate 'a general defect of cerebral function after consciousness has been regained' (p. 77). Symonds and Russell (1943) added that it was 'taken to end at the time from which the patient can give a clear and consecutive account of what was happening around him', and that it could be estimated 'by careful questioning after recovery of full consciousness and normal orientation' (p. 7).

In short, although the post-traumatic phase is at the time marked by a mental state of *disorientation* (i.e., an inability to locate oneself with regard to one's time, place and situation), it can subsequently be regarded as a state of *anterograde amnesia* (i.e., an inability to remember the continuous flow of new experiences). Russell and Nathan (1946) were explicit that the period of PTA terminated with the return of continuous memory for experienced events, as determined from the patient's own retrospective reports. Russell and Smith (1961) in a similar manner described PTA as 'the interval during which current events have not been stored' (p. 16). As Russell (1971) remarked, 'the retrospective assessment of the duration of the amnesic period after the injury is a remarkably good guide to the duration of loss of full consciousness' (p. 12). There are therefore two important points to note about the contemporary concept of PTA:

1   As was indicated in the passage by Russell (1971, p. 1) which was quoted at the beginning of this chapter, this phase of recovery following closed head injury is dominated by two forms of mental dysfunction: (a) an anterograde memory disorder; and (b) a state of disorientation. The duration of the anterograde amnesia appears to be closely related to the duration of post-traumatic disorientation, and after the recovery of full consciousness the former is used as a retrospective estimate of the latter (Moore and Ruesch, 1944).

2   PTA terminates with the return of full consciousness as measured retrospectively by the return of continuous memory. However, contemporary practice follows Russell and his colleagues in measuring PTA from the time of the original head injury. In other words, the duration of PTA includes not only the period of anterograde amnesia as strictly understood but also the period of coma (Levin *et al.*, 1982a, p. 74).

PTA and Severity of Closed Head Injury

The duration of PTA tends to vary directly with the duration of coma, though this relationship is by no means a perfect one (Evans *et al.*, 1976; Guthkelch, 1980; Levin and Eisenberg, 1986; Moore and Ruesch, 1944; Norrman and Svahn, 1961) and it is to some extent an artefact since (as has just been pointed out) the latter is contained within the former. Nevertheless, the relationship tends to be weaker in the case of older patients, where relatively short periods of coma may be followed by disproportionately long periods of PTA (von Wowern, 1966). The duration of PTA also tends to be directly related to the duration of RA, although the former is typically much longer than the latter (Russell, 1932; Russell and Nathan, 1946; Russell and Smith, 1961). Parkinson (1977) suggested that the total duration of PTA was about nine times that of the residual extent of RA, but other researchers have proposed more complex relationships (Crovitz *et al.*, 1983). Symonds (1940) suggested that a permanent period of RA longer than a few hours would always be associated 'with a story of severe injury, with a long post-traumatic amnesia, and with some permanent defects of mental function other than the amnesia' (p. 87). Exceptions to this general pattern can certainly arise, however, with cases of both disproportionately long RA (Symonds, 1962) or of PTA in the absence of any persistent RA (Crovitz *et al.*, 1983).

Moreover, PTA can also occur without the patient losing consciousness at all. On the basis of one such case, Fisher (1966) suggested that PTA and coma might result from damage to distinct neural mechanisms. Yarnell and Lynch (1973) described a further four American football players who demonstrated a marked post-traumatic memory impairment with no apparent alteration in their levels of consciousness. When tested immediately after their injuries, they had intact orientation and good memory for the episodes in question. They rejoined their games, but within a few minutes had great difficulty remembering the course of play, and they subsequently showed little or no recollection of the original neurological examination. A similar though more anecdotal example was quoted by Strauss and Savitsky (1934) of the boxer Gene Tunney who after colliding with his opponent's head proceeded to knock him out and then boxed three rounds with another sparring partner, and yet had no subsequent recollection of these events. In addition, Haas and Ross (1986) described several cases of transient global amnesia which had apparently been triggered by relatively mild head injuries that failed to induce any loss of consciousness. These attacks involved some degree of disorientation as well as a severe anterograde memory impairment that lasted for several hours after the injury itself, but no other symptoms. Haas and Ross argued that such episodes were a form of traumatic migraine.

PTA was described by Miller (1966) as 'the signature of significant closed head injury' (p. 257), and the duration of PTA is usually regarded by clinicians as an excellent indicator of the severity of a closed head injury (e.g., Smith, 1961). Indeed, in 1961 an anonymous annotation in *The Lancet* described the duration of PTA as 'the best yardstick we have' in the absence of any definitive evidence of structural damage, although this was in fact an inaccurate paraphrase of the comment by Brock (1960) quoted in Chapter 1 (p. 00) which actually concerned coma and not PTA. Moore and Ruesch (1944) demonstrated that the duration of post-traumatic disorientation increased with the incidence of several clinical features, including raised intracranial pressure, skull fracture and intracranial haemorrhage. Similarly, Russell and Smith (1961) showed that duration of PTA tended to increase systematically with a number of 'organic' signs such as skull fracture, anosmia, dysphasia and motor disorders, although not with 'nonorganic' symptoms such as headache, anxiety, depression and dizziness. They did however note that the duration of PTA had much greater prognostic value in the case of closed head injuries than in the case of crushing injuries or missile wounds, in which the duration of both coma and PTA can often be remarkably short (*see also* von Wowern, 1966).

For Symonds (1928) the criterion for a diagnosis of 'major contusion' was that 'the patient should have been in a state of unconsciousness, or partial unconsciousness, for more than twenty-four hours following the injury' (p. 832). Similarly, it is nowadays common for both clinicians and researchers to distinguish between cases of 'severe' closed head injury and 'minor' closed head injury according to whether the period of PTA has exceeded 24 hours. This is roughly concordant with a dichotomy between 'severe' and 'minor' cases of head injury determined by whether or not the patients have spent more than six hours in coma (Jennett *et al.*, 1975a), although a lucid interval or complications such as an intracranial haematoma may lead to disproportion-ately long periods of disorientation. Patients in whom PTA extends beyond 24 hours are much more likely to have open fractures and intracranial haemorrhages, and they are therefore more likely to need surgical intervention. Nevertheless, this probably applies to fewer than 10 per cent of all patients admitted to hospital with closed head injuries (Artiola i Fortuny *et al.*, 1980). Finer gradations of severity based upon both the duration of coma and the duration of PTA have been proposed. Russell and Smith (1961) themselves suggested a four-fold classification of patients with closed head injury as follows: 'slight concussion', PTA lasting less than one hour; 'moderate concussion', PTA lasting between one and 24 hours; 'severe concussion', PTA lasting between one and seven days; and 'very severe concussion', PTA lasting more than seven days. Nowadays, however, these categories would be referred to simply as cases of 'mild', 'moderate', 'severe' and 'very severe' closed head injury.

There is considerable evidence that the duration of PTA is of value in determining the eventual prognosis. It is known to predict the extent of the patient's physical recovery (Evans *et al.*, 1976), the patient's long-term neurological, psychological and social assessment (Bond, 1975, 1976), and the patient's eventual occupational outcome (Russell and Nathan, 1946; Russell and Smith, 1961; Symonds and Russell, 1943). Evidence on this point will be discussed in more detail in Chapter 7. Nevertheless, this relationship is qualified by the effect of the patient's age. Older patients tend to have longer periods of PTA and a poorer prognosis, but they also show a more pronounced relationship between these two variables than younger patients. Thus, a more reliable assessment of the severity of a closed head injury may be obtained by taking both the patient's age and the duration of PTA into account (Russell and Smith, 1961).

Measuring Post-traumatic Amnesia

In seeking to define and measure the duration of PTA, however, problems arise that are similar to those already discussed in connection with RA (*see* e.g., Schacter and Crovitz, 1977; Sisler and Penner, 1975). First, the period in question need not be characterized by a continuous memory loss. In other words, as Symonds (1942) emphasized, the patient's first memory after a closed head injury may not coincide with the return of continuous awareness, but may sometimes amount to an 'island' of accessible memory that is then followed by a further period of amnesia (*see also* Symonds and Russell, 1943). Russell and Nathan (1946) mentioned just 13 cases who had shown such an 'island', which they likened to the phenomenon of the lucid interval (*see* Chapter 1, p. 13). They implied that these 'islands' occurred fairly early during the period of PTA and were often concerned with events of personal significance, such as the visit of a relative. Gronwall and Wrightson (1980) carried out a detailed investigation of PTA in the case of 67 patients with minor head injuries. They found that 26 (or 39 per cent) of their sample reported a total of 39 events as 'islands' of memory during the period of PTA. Almost 80 per cent of these events were apparently recalled from the first quarter of the period in question, and over 70 per cent fell within the first 15 minutes after their accidents. Typically, the events in question were specific and personally significant, such as having their wounds sutured or the arrival of their relatives at the hospital. In contrast, the patients who reported no 'islands' of memory tended to give as their first recollections marking the return of continuous memory mundane or nonspecific events such as being in a hospital bed or cubicle.

A second point, related to the first, is that many practitioners and researchers follow Russell and Nathan (1946) in identifying the end-point of PTA with the return of continuous normal memory, while others identify it with the earliest (or perhaps the earliest authenticated) memory after the closed head injury (e.g., Sisler and Penner, 1975). As Symonds (1942; Symonds and Russell, 1943) pointed out, the latter step does not of course exclude the isolated 'islands' of memory which have just been described. The inclusion of these 'islands' may well make a significant difference to the estimated duration of PTA. Symonds and Russell concluded that careful questioning was necessary to differentiate between such isolated 'islands' of memory and the beginning of continuous remembering (*see also* Gronwall and Wrightson, 1980). A further point is that it may be difficult to estimate relatively brief periods of PTA with any degree of precision, because of uncertainty about the exact chronology both of the accident itself and of subsequent events. Even when they had exhausted all potential sources of information, including the statements of witnesses as well as ambulance and hospital records, Gronwall and Wrightson (1980) found that the most detailed classification of PTA possible was 'less than 5 min', 'between 5 and 30 min' and 'more than 30 but less than 60 min', and they concluded that it was difficult to measure PTA duration accurately when it was less than an hour.

Gronwall and Wrightson had devoted considerable time and energy to carrying out a prospective study of PTA, involving repeated interviews every 15 minutes from the patients' admission until the return of continuous memory and full orientation. Providing such routine yet skilled observation of individual patients is clearly not practicable in most clinical settings. Because of this consideration Russell (1932; *see also* Russell, 1971, p. 12) advocated the use of retrospective assessment of PTA following the restoration of continuous normal memory. This was also taken to provide a means of distinguishing between the occurrence of isolated 'islands' of memory and the return of continuous memory and full consciousness which marks the true end of PTA (Russell and Nathan, 1946; Symonds and Russell, 1943). In Gronwall and Wrighton's study retrospective assessments were concordant with their own prospective assessment of PTA in 75 per cent of the total sample of 67 patients with minor closed head injury. The likelihood of any discrepancy was not affected by the timing of the retrospective interview anywhere between one week and three months after the original accidents. Moreover, when 36 of the patients received a second retrospective interview 2–3 months after the first, only four produced different estimates of PTA duration on the two occasions. These results tended to confirm Russell and Nathan's (1946) assertion that retrospective estimates of PTA remained relatively constant over time, and contradicts a suggestion by Sisler and Penner (1975) that the duration of PTA varies on repeated assessment.

In principle, patients' retrospective reports may tend inadvertently to incorporate information concerning the earlier stages of their recovery which has subsequently been provided by relatives or nursing staff (Levin *et al.*, 1982a, p. 75). Against this idea, however, Gronwall and Wrightson found that nearly all discrepancies in the retrospective assessment of PTA arose from patients giving progressively *longer* estimates of PTA duration. Such discrepancies clearly could not be the result of confabulation to 'fill the gap', as Gronwall and Wrightson themselves noted, nor could they result from the incorporation of second-hand accounts. (Nor, incidentally, do they constitute 'shrinkage' of the sort observed in the case of RA.) Gronwall and Wrightson did however suggest that these discrepancies might reflect the patients' increasing confusion between their own veridical memories and what they had subsequently been told by eyewitnesses, or changes in their criteria for deciding whether apparent memories were genuine experiences or merely second-hand information. Another problem is that, unless the patients' progress has been continuously monitored, it may be difficult to establish the veracity of their retrospective reports. Indeed, these may in principle be far from accurate (especially with regard to their chronology) given the unfamiliar and depersonalized context of a hospital ward. A final point is that in the absence of any standardized procedure for measuring disturbances of consciousness one might well be inclined to question how different examiners could be expected to produce consistent measures of PTA duration (Levin *et al.*, 1979b).

PTA Scales

In order to handle these problems, a number of researchers have tried to develop objective, quantifiable techniques for measuring the duration of PTA. These include a concurrent assessment of a patients' orientation (that is, basic awareness of time and place) of the sort contained in the Wechsler Memory Scale (WMS: Wechsler, 1945), which also includes subtests evaluating story recall, memory span, the recall of simple visual designs and paired-associate learning (*see* Chapter 4, pp. 101–2):

1 What year is this?
2 What month is this?
3 What day of the month is this?
4 What is the name of the place you are in?
5 In what city is this?

Groher (1977) administered the WMS to 14 patients with severe closed head injuries who had been unconscious for an average of 17 days. They were tested 'after regaining consciousness or as soon as they demonstrated an ability to tolerate a one-hour testing session . . . In the majority of cases, this was a one-week period' (p. 214). The Orientation subtest was scored out of a maximum of six, presumably having been supplemented by the question, 'What day of the week is this?' The head-injured patients were profoundly impaired on this subtest: their average score was less than one question answered correctly. They were also impaired on all the remaining subtests of the WMS, implying a generalized memory dysfunction. What is perhaps more surprising is that they continued to be impaired on the Orientation subtest through four successive retests on the WMS during the subsequent 120 days, so that they were on average still only able to answer three questions correctly nearly five months after their accidents. Groher also presented data for 14 comparable patients who showed persistent language and memory disorders more than a year after they had sustained a closed head injury; across five successive testing sessions, they consistently achieved an average of only about four items correct on the Orientation subtest. Since these patients were undoubtedly beyond the phase of PTA, these results suggest that the assessment even of a simple awareness of time and place among head-injured patients is by no means a straightforward matter (*see also* Kapur, 1988, p. 19–20).

On the basis of an earlier brief test of temporal orientation (Benton *et al.*, 1964), Levin *et al.* (1979b) developed the Galveston Orientation and Amnesia Test (GOAT); this contains 12 questions covering simple biographical information, the circumstances of the patient's injury, and the patient's knowledge of the current time, place and situation. The Test yields a global index of amnesia and disorientation out of a possible maximum score of 100, together with separate estimates of retrograde and anterograde amnesia (defined in terms of the latest memory before the head injury and the earliest memory after the injury). The GOAT is intended to be administered at least once a day, though in coma the GOAT score is zero (Levin *et al.*, 1984). The duration of PTA is defined as the period in which the total GOAT score is less than or equal to 75 (the borderline level of performance according to a standardization group of patients who had recovered following mild closed head injury). In a second series of 52 adult patients with closed head injuries, those cases in whom this period extended beyond two weeks tended to show evidence of diffuse or bilateral mass lesions on angiography or computerized tomography, and especially of compressed ventricles as the result of brain swelling. In this study, the duration of PTA according to the GOAT was found to be inversely related to eye opening, motor responses and verbal responses on the day of admission according to the Glasgow Coma Scale, which was taken to demonstrate the broad validity of the GOAT. However, in a subsequent study, Levin *et al.* (1984) found only a rather weak relationship between the duration of coma and the duration of PTA according to the GOAT among 50 consecutive admissions with severe closed head injuries; in particular, there were several cases who showed prolonged PTA in spite of relatively brief periods of coma. Levin *et al.* concluded that there might be other important determinants of the duration of PTA than the duration of coma.

A similar procedure to the GOAT was developed by Artiola i Fortuny *et al.* (1980), but this also contained a simple, objective memory test for the examiner's face and name and for three pictured objects. The patients were tested daily, and the end of PTA was defined as the first of three consecutive days on which each patient correctly identified the three original objects out of a set that also contained five distractor items. Estimates of PTA duration obtained from 80 patients in this study produced a very similar distribution to independent estimates that were obtained from the same patients by neurosurgical staff using traditional clinical methods. The correspondence between measures of PTA and orientation obtained using this technique was said to be 'close', and it was claimed to offer an efficient and rapid means of detecting slight deterioration in a patient's condition that might require urgent clinical or surgical treatment. Subsequently, Shores *et al.* (1986) extended this test to produce the Westmead PTA Scale. This contained two questions concerning biographical information, five questions to test the patient's orientation for time, date and place, two questions on the examiner's face and name, and three questions on the retention of pictured objects. The end of PTA was defined as the first of three consecutive days on which each patient answered all 12 questions correctly. This Scale is claimed to have shown a high degree of inter-rater reliability and have been satisfactorily used with only a minimum of training by medical staff, nurses and occupational therapists;

moreover, the duration of PTA according to the Scale was found to be a much better predictor of the neuropsychological outcome following severe closed head injury than duration of coma according to the Glasgow Coma Scale (Shores, 1989). In common with the procedures devised earlier by Levin *et al.* (1979b) and by Artiola i Fortuny *et al.* (1980), this Scale was developed primarily for clinical rather than experimental use, and it therefore combined the assessment of amnesia with that of orientation. This was in accordance with the view expressed by Russell (1932) that in order to be considered to have recovered full consciousness following a closed head injury the patient should be *both* fully orientated *and* reliably capable of laying down new memories (E. A. Shores, personal communication). Nevertheless, as Newcombe (1982) concluded, there remains the need for a more comprehensive research instrument that would measure separately the different aspects of continuous autobiographical memory as well as orientation for person, time and place.

In their prospective analysis of PTA, Gronwall and Wrightson (1980) administered an orientation questionnaire every 15 minutes after the patients had arrived at the accident and emergency department. They were scored out of a maximum of 18 points on their name, address and date of birth, the year, month and day of the week, and where they were and why they were there. Each of a control group of 12 patients without head injuries who were also tested in the accident and emergency department achieved at least 17 points on this questionnaire, and so a score of 16 or less was taken to signify disorientation. In the case of the patients with minor head injuries, there was a significant relationship between the recovery of full orientation and the return of continuous memory, such that the proportion of dis-orientated cases was greater among 13 patients who were tested before the return of continuous memory than among 44 patients tested after the return of continuous memory (as confirmed at subsequent interviews). Nevertheless, eight patients were still disorientated after the return of continuous recovery, while five patients showed persistently impaired recall of ongoing events despite normal orientation. Gronwall and Wrightson concluded that 'the proposition that the return of full orientation signals the end of PTA (Russell, 1971) is clearly untenable' (p. 57). It should however be clear from the account that was given earlier that for Russell this proposition was a matter of definition rather than one of empirical fact. The empirical claim which was made by Russell (1971) was simply the one quoted above, namely that 'the retro-spective assessment of the duration of the amnesic period is a remarkably good guide to the duration of loss of full consciousness' (p. 12). Cronwall and Wrightson made the claim that there was 'no consistent relationship' between the duration of anterograde amnesia and the duration of disorientation (p. 59), but they presented no evidence on this point and their own data would tend to refute such an extreme position (cf. also Sisler and Penner, 1975).

Theories of Post-Traumatic Amnesia

Early theoretical discussions of the nature of PTA emphasized the wide variety of psychological disturbances shown by head-injured patients during the acute post-traumatic phase. Schilder (1934) presented case material to argue that PTA was characterized by a generalized cognitive dysfunction, and he argued that this could be attributed to 'a confusion concerning the perception and synthesis of impersonal material' (p. 184). Symonds (1937) agreed that this played a large part, but considered that other features were equally important:

> There is profound disorientation in space and time, with a tendency to interpret the surroundings in terms of past experience. There is defect of perception and inability to synthesize perceptual data. Memory and judgment are grossly impaired. Thought is constantly impeded by persever- ation. Disturbance of the speech function is conspicuous. The mood is often elated and there is sometimes a push of talk resembling that seen in hypomanic states. (p. 1082)

He also mentioned 'the inability to distinguish clearly between figure and background in the thought process' (p. 1084). Subsequently, Ruesch and Moore (1943) tested 120 patients within 24 hours of their closed head injuries on a variety of simple cognitive tasks. Any pronounced impairment was mainly restricted to a serial subtraction test (*see also* Ruesch, 1944b). Schacter and Crovitz (1977) noted that this task depended upon intact immediate memory for its adequate performance, but Ruesch and Moore had found that the immediate memory spans of their patients were essentially normal. Nevertheless, the latter investigators had excluded any patients who appeared comatose, confused or delirious, and it was suggested by Mandleberg (1975) that they may have inadvertently confined their attention mainly to those who were fully conscious and out of PTA.

Like the theoretical discussions concerning the nature of RA, those concerning the nature of PTA have been based upon the traditional notions of consolidation and retrieval. For instance, Benson and Geschwind (1967) argued that PTA 'seems most likely to represent not a failure of retrieval but a failure to establish new memory traces' (p. 542). However, they did observe that the correlation between the duration of PTA and the residual duration of RA suggested that 'the retrieval process depends on the same system that is necessary for the laying down of new memories' (p. 542). Similarly, Yarnell and Lynch (1973) regarded their observations concerning PTA in the absence of impaired consciousness as providing further evidence for a specific effect of closed head injury upon the consolidation of new information in a long-term memory system. On the latter point, immediate memory span may well be preserved during PTA (e.g., Ruesch, 1944b; Ruesch and Moore, 1943; Schilder, 1934; but cf. Mandleberg, 1975), whereas measures of long-term memory typically show a pronounced decrement in performance; indeed, Shores *et al.* (1986) found no long-term retention at all on the part of head-injured patients tested on a verbal-learning task during PTA.

Gronwall and Wrightson (1980) attributed the fact that personally salient episodes occurring during PTA could sometimes be subsequently recalled to fluctuating levels of arousal during the post-traumatic period. However, as a theoretical concept, this has little explanatory power and even less heuristic value. An alternative interpretation of the phenomenon of 'islands' of memory is that the anterograde amnesia associated with closed head injuries may involve a retrieval problem. This is also the implication of evidence that, like RA, this amnesic state may perhaps be alleviated to some extent by the application of barbiturates (Russell and Nathan, 1946), hormonal preparations (Oliveros *et al.*, 1978) and hypnosis (Milos, 1975), although at least in the latter case there are considerable problems with much of the research to date, as was noted earlier (p. 76). In general, one possible reason for a retrieval deficit is that the relevant experiences are represented in memory but are not encoded or organized in a way that would permit efficient retrieval using the usual forms of memory search.

The specific notion that post-traumatic memory disorders result from a failure to establish an adequate organizational structure in memory was considered by Fodor (1972). When compared with a control group of accident victims, patients tested soon after closed head injury were found to be impaired in the recall of organizationally related test items when tested after a short delay (though not when tested immediately). Fodor concluded that closed head injury yielded a reduced capacity for using organizational structure in the material to be remembered. However, these results cannot be seriously accepted, because they are subject to a number of major methodological criticisms and because the published account of this experiment omitted key information about the experimental procedure (*see* Brooks, 1984; Schacter and Crovitz, 1977). Most important, Fodor included no independent measure of PTA other than her patients' performance on the criterion task, and so it is far from clear whether all of her patients were indeed tested within the period of PTA. In addition, their performance in the immediate recall test was subject to a ceiling effect, whereas their performance in the delayed recall test on the unrelated test items was subject to a floor effect. In contrast to Fodor's results, a subsequent study by Dunn and Brooks (1974) showed that head-injured patients tested during PTA used both phonemic and semantic structure in a normal fashion. This was taken to imply that PTA did not implicate a qualitatively different pattern of memory encoding, although more recently Brooks (1984) advocated caution in attempting to generalize from these findings because they were based upon the results of just five head-injured patients.

One final point is that it would be exceedingly naive to characterize PTA purely as a state of confusion or disorientation. Patients who have sustained a closed head injury leading to a relatively long period of unconsciousness may demonstrate a stage of recovery marked by thrashing, combativeness, yelling and excessive movement (*see* Hayden and Hart, 1986). By virtue of their confusion patients in this agitated state may have little insight into their condition. It may therefore give rise to considerable distress on the part of their relatives or carers and also constitute a major challenge to professional rehabilitation workers (Gans, 1983; Malkmus, 1983).

Disorientation and Cognitive Impairment

Mandleberg (1975) compared a group of severely head-injured patients tested during PTA with a matched group of severely head-injured cases out of PTA on the Wechsler Adult Intelligence Scale (WAIS: Wechsler, 1955). This contains six Verbal subtests (Information, Comprehension, Arithmetic, Similarities, Digit Span and Vocabulary) and five Performance subtests (Digit Symbol, Picture Completion, Block Design, Picture Arrangement and Object Assembly). The former patients produced a generalized impairment which was more pronounced on the Performance subtests than on the Verbal subtests. There were no significant differences between the two groups of patients when they were all retested out of PTA, which demonstrated that they were essentially equivalent in their general intellectual capacity. It was concluded that PTA was a qualitatively distinct phase of recovery from closed head injury characterized by a general disorder of cognitive ability.

However, this investigation suffers from the opposite problem of interpretation to that raised in connection with the study by Ruesch and Moore (1943). The patients tested within PTA undoubtedly had very severe injuries (their mean duration of PTA was 110 days), and it is conceivable that some had not recovered full awareness on assessment. In this regard, it is relevant that the impairment shown by these patients extended to the Vocabulary subtest of the WAIS, which tests a knowledge of word meanings. Tests of this sort are normally assumed to be somewhat less vulnerable to disruption by brain damage, and are often used as an index of a patient's premorbid level of attainment, provided that there is no evidence of any dysphasia (Milberg *et al.*, 1986). For instance, Babcock (1930) argued that differences in premorbid intellectual level 'are shown in interests, in the data to which one spontaneously attends, and especially in the vocabulary. Words when once learned are not quickly forgotten, and remain as indications of the ability a person once had . . . ' (p. 5). Nelson and McKenna (1975) found that patients with dementing diseases produced significantly poorer performance on the Vocabulary subtest of the WAIS than a group of normal control subjects, and they concluded that vocabulary-type tests were affected by generalized intellectual deterioration. Nevertheless, the average age-scaled score of their dementing subjects (10.2) was at the normal level, which suggests that the control patients in this study (who were patients with extracerebral disorders and nonacademic employees of a university college) may have been atypical in terms of their knowledge of word meanings.

The two groups of subjects in Nelson and McKenna's study showed no sign of any difference in their scores on the Schonell Graded Word Reading Test, and the researchers concluded that reading ability was potentially a better indicator of premorbid level of functioning than vocabulary level. Nelson and O'Connell (1978) therefore devised the New Adult Reading Test (NART) as a measure of premorbid attainment, and it is nowadays routinely used in the UK for just this purpose. In the study that was carried out by Shores *et al.* (1986), no difference was found between head-injured patients tested during PTA (roughly seven weeks after their injuries) and head-injured patients tested out of PTA (roughly 33 weeks after their injuries) in terms of their standardized scores on the NART: both groups achieved normal scores on this test. Nevertheless, results analogous to those of Mandleberg (1975) were obtained by Bond and Brooks (1976) using alternative tests of verbal and nonverbal intelligence. Seven patients with severe head injury were assessed during PTA on both the Mill Hill Vocabulary Scale (Raven, 1962) and the Progressive Matrices test (Raven, 1960). In comparison with published normative data, these patients were substantially impaired on both tests, although more so in the case of the latter. This tends to confirm Symonds' (1940) notion that PTA implicates a generalized impairment of intellectual function.

Benson *et al.* (1976) described three patients who had suffered closed head injuries and who demonstrated a persistent disorder of orientation for place, relocating their hospital at a different though personally significant geographical location, despite the fact that their memory for ongoing events had largely recovered. The converse pattern was described by Gronwall and Wrightson (1980), who found a number of patients who demonstrated persistently impaired retention of ongoing events despite normal orientation. The latter researchers had interviewed patients with mild closed head injuries on a number of occasions after their arrival in the accident and emergency department in order to determine separately the patients' level of orientation and the recall of ongoing events. Although Gronwall and Wrightson had obtained a significant relationship between the recovery of normal orientation and the return of continuous memory, their results led them to question whether post-traumatic disorientation and PTA were really functionally equivalent (*see also* Sisler and Penner, 1975).

Papanicolaou *et al.* (1984) demonstrated a physiological correlate of PTA in the form of the P-300 component of the human average evoked potential. This is a characteristic feature of the electrophysiological response to a distinct and infrequent stimulus interspersed within a regular series of otherwise constant, regularly occurring stimuli (such as physical tones). Its precise latency, though typically around 300 msec following stimulus presentation, is thought to be an index of cognitive efficiency: it is sensitive to manipulations of processing capacity but appears to be independent both of intrinsic stimulus information and also of reponse selection (Pritchard, 1981). Papanicolaou *et al.* found that the P-300 latency was significantly delayed in eight patients who were still in PTA according to their scores on the GOAT in comparison with ten patients who were normally orientated after recovery from PTA. Since the latter group did not differ significantly from a control group of seven hospital staff, it was concluded that the P-300 latency was not merely a function of the severity of a closed head injury, but was a specific physiological index of cognitive function in PTA.

Finally, to the extent that PTA constitutes a state of disorientation with regard to time, place and situation, it is interesting to consider whether the duration of PTA could be influenced by the therapeutic method known as 'reality orientation', which is more usually employed in the care of confused geriatric patients. As Moffat (1984) explained, this method 'aims to maintain or retrain a person's awareness of time, place and current events by incorporating this information in staff interactions with the patient. This structured conversation may be assisted by classroom sessions, the use of external aids, repetition and possibly by specific behavioural training' (p. 82). Corrigan *et al.* (1985) proposed that the cognitive deficits shown by head-injured patients during PTA could be ameliorated by their participation in reality orientation groups (*see also* Bond, 1979). Unfortunately, their research study did not include any control patients, and consequently the improvements which they described in certain individual cases might have arisen merely from the spontaneous remission and termination of PTA itself. Indeed, Shores *et al.* (1986) reported that this amnesic state severely constrained the amount of 'carry-over' that could be achieved from one therapeutic session to the next; in contrast to this state of affairs, they noted that marked changes in behaviour and response to therapy could be obtained once their patients had emerged from PTA. It also has to be added that the benefits of reality orientation therapy obtained in more carefully designed studies with other groups of patients have been extremely modest and of limited clinical value (*see* e.g., Hanley *et al.*, 1981). Instead, it has been suggested that the most fruitful approaches to direct remediation of cognitive and behavioural disturbances during post-traumatic amnesia are those which concentrate on structuring the patients' environment in order to minimize the impact of their confusion (Hayden and Hart, 1986).

Concluding Summary

Following the cessation of coma, patients with closed head injury show a characteristic impairment of memory function. This takes the form of: (a) a specific inability to remember events that were experienced during a short interval immediately before the injury itself (retrograde amnesia or RA); and (b) a specific inability to retain information about experienced ongoing events (post-traumatic amnesia or PTA). The duration of RA and the duration of PTA appear to vary with each other and with the severity of the injury, as measured by the duration of coma.

RA develops within a few minutes of a closed head injury even when the patient has not lost consciousness. The duration of RA is difficult to measure with any degree of accuracy, and it is subject to 'shrinkage' during the course of the patient's recovery. The transient component of RA is usually attributed to a failure of retrieval processes, and this is supported by evidence that it can be alleviated by drugs or hypnosis. The residual component that persists indefinitely after the injury is usually attributed to the disruption of memory consolidation. RA does not appear to affect the retention of information within short-term memory, and there is a suggestion that memory for general knowledge and for learned skills is also well preserved. These considerations imply that RA is a selective impairment of long-term episodic memory.

The state of PTA is marked by disorientation and anterograde amnesia; the duration of the latter according to retrospective questioning is taken to be an estimate of the duration of the former. Because of difficulties in accurately measuring the duration of PTA, a number of standard scales have been developed that assess recall of the circumstances of the injury, basic awareness of current time and place, and continuous autobiographical memory. PTA predominantly involves a specific failure to consolidate new information in long-term memory; however, it also implicates a generalized though less pronounced impairment of intellectual function and behavioural problems may be evident. Reality orientation and other forms of cognitive retraining seem to be less effective in the remediation of these problems than restructuring the patient's environment.

Chapter 4

Memory Function

Even after the return of normal awareness and orientation, and even after the period of profound memory loss described in the previous chapter, many patients with closed head injuries continue to complain of a wide variety of disabling symptoms. As Symonds (1962) noted, these *sequelae* tend to be predominantly psychological in nature. Most particularly, a significant proportion of head-injured patients continue to report an impaired ability to remember. Tooth (1947) gave a more detailed account of the nature of this impairment: 'This complaint is usually described by the patient as absentmindedness: inability to recall names, faces, telephone numbers, and, in the Services, orders. Many patients with this complaint mentioned that they had to rely on a notebook for facts which they would formerly have retained in memory' (p. 6).

Russell (1934) found that 25 per cent of all patients with closed head injuries reported 'loss of memory or mental ability' during a period of at least two months after leaving hospital, though this was much more common among older patients. One or two studies have suggested that the incidence of memory impairment might be only around 10 per cent of all patients admitted to hospital with head injury in the case of both adults (Lidvall *et al.*, 1974) and children (Klonoff and Paris, 1974). However, the true figure is likely to be much greater than this. Oddy *et al.* (1978b) administered a sympton checklist to patients with severe closed head injuries roughly six months after their accidents. 'Trouble remembering things' was both the symptom that was most frequently reported by the patients themselves (38 per cent of the sample) and also the symptom most frequently attributed to the patients by their relatives (44 per cent of the sample). Similarly, Rimel *et al.* (1981) found that roughly 59 per cent out of 424 patients with minor closed head injuries complained of impaired memory three months after their accidents, while interviews with their family members and close friends 'indicated an even greater problem with the patients' memory than the patients recognized or were willing to admit' (p. 224). A study of just 20 head-injured patients by McLean *et al.* (1983) also produced reports of 'memory difficulties' in 35 per cent of the sample when they were assessed three days after their accidents and in 40 per cent of the sample when they were reassessed a month later.

Some writers have been sceptical about the validity of such subjective reports of memory dysfunction (e.g., Schacter and Crovitz, 1977), but several investigators have chosen to take this seriously as a research issue. Almost all of their work has been concerned with the long-term consequences of closed head injury, however, and their findings will therefore be considered in detail together with other aspects of recovery and rehabilitation in Chapter 7 (*see* pp. 237–40). The present chapter will be concerned rather with whether measurable disturbances of memory function persisting beyond the period of post-traumatic amnesia (PTA) can be confirmed by objective psychometric testing. It will be useful to consider this matter separately with regard to minor closed head injuries and with regard to severe closed head injuries.

Memory Function Following Minor Head Injury

Empirical Findings

The first systematic follow-up study of memory function in patients with minor closed head injury was carried out by Conkey (1938). Her patients were 25 cases of simple concussion, including some with no apparent loss of consciousness. Most of them were kept in hospital for more than two weeks, but this seems to have been standard practice at the time. (Indeed, with reference to cases of simple concussion, a consultant at the Edinburgh Royal Infirmary mentioned in 1934 that 'following Dr [W. R.] Russell's advice it was now a routine practice to keep these cases for three weeks in hospital': *see* Russell, 1934, p. 141.) When tested on up to five occasions after their accidents and compared with a control group of normal subjects of similar age and educational, economic and social status, the head-injured patients showed a general cognitive impairment which tended to resolve over a period of 34 weeks following the injury. Most particularly, these patients demonstrated a persistent and pronounced decrement in performance on tests of learning and remembering, and this appeared to be associated with a specific deficit in the acquisition of new memories. Conkey argued that much of the generalized impairment of cognitive functioning which had been produced by her patients could be attributed to this deficit, which following Goldstein (1936) she ascribed to 'the impairment of the ability to perceive abstract relationships' (p. 53) in the material to be remembered.

As Brooks *et al.* (1984) pointed out, the control subjects in Conkey's study were tested only once, and so strictly speaking they did not match the head-injured patients in terms of their overall level of practice or familiarity with the test procedures. However, in order to evaluate the effects of hospitalization on performance, Conkey tested a second control group which consisted of surgical patients examined once in hospital and once out of hospital with an interval which was roughly equivalent to that between the first and second testings of the head-injured patients. There was virtually no difference between the levels of performance which these control patients achieved at the two sessions, which indicated 'that the effect of hospitalization on performance is little or nothing' (p. 23). Indeed, these patients tended if anything to produce better results at the first session; as Conkey pointed out, this suggests that any effects of the subjects' familiarity with the test situation were counterbalanced by the effects of novelty at the first session or of indifference at the second. In short, it is unlikely that the results produced by Conkey's head-injured patients were contaminated by practice effects.

Three more recent studies have considered the performance of patients with minor closed head injuries on tests of recognition memory. (Such tasks will be considered in more detail on pp. 109–12.) Levin *et al.* (1976b) compared nine head-injured patients who had been conscious on their admission and throughout their hospitalization with 23 control patients suffering from peripheral neurological disorders in terms of their short-term memory for random shapes with a forced-choice recognition procedure. Unfortunately, their results were subject to a ceiling effect: only one of the head-injured patients and only two of the control patients made any errors on this task. Subsequently, Hannay *et al.* (1979) assessed 19 patients with mild closed head injuries who had been conscious on admission and throughout their period of hospitalization on a continuous memory task for line drawings of familiar living things. They showed no sign of any impairment in terms of their corrected recognition scores in comparison with a control group of 19 patients with diverse somatic complaints. Payne-Johnson (1986) used the same task as Hannay *et al.* to compare 20 patients with closed head injuries of varying degrees of severity with 15 other accident victims. The 11 patients with relatively mild head injuries were tested within three days of their admission to hospital. Their performance on the continuous memory task was no better than that of the more serious cases, and the head-injured patients as a group were significantly impaired in comparison with the control patients.

A number of researchers have studied the performance of head-injured patients using the selective reminding procedure (Buschke, 1973; Buschke and Fuld, 1974). This is a modified multitrial free-recall task in which only the items that have not been recalled on a given trial are presented again for learning on the subsequent trial: that is, the subject is 'selectively reminded' of the items not recalled on the previous trial. The encoding of items into long-term storage is supposed to be shown by their correct recall on two consecutive trials (and therefore in the absence of their presentation on the second of the two trials); the consistent retrieval of items from long-term storage is supposedly shown by their correct recall on subsequent trials (that is, without any further 'reminding'). However, the selective reminding procedure yields a number of other indices of immediate and delayed recall and recognition. The strengths and weaknesses of this test in the context of neuropsychological assessment have been discussed by Loring and Papanicolaou (1987).

McLean *et al.* (1983) used the selective reminding procedure within an assessment battery to compare 20 patients tested three days and one month after closed head injuries with 52 normal control subjects of a similar age and background. The head-injured patients were found to be significantly impaired on the measures of immediate retention at the 3-day test but not at the 1-month test. Nevertheless, the duration of PTA had been less then 24 hours in the case of nine of these patients, and the latter were not significantly impaired on any of the measures at either test. The small size of this sample obviously makes it difficult to come to any serious conclusion on the basis of these data, but an unpublished study by Levin and Eisenberg had also found that the performance of 46 patients with mild closed head injury was within the normal range on the selective reminding procedure at a 16-day follow-up (*see* Levin *et al.*, 1982a, pp. 109–12). Similarly, Barth *et al.* (1983) found no overall impairment on the Wechsler Memory Scale (*see below*, pp. 101–2) in 70 patients with minor closed head injuries tested three months after their accidents.

Gentilini *et al.* (1985) administered a battery of cognitive tasks to 50 consecutive cases of mild head injury (defined as a loss of consciousness lasting less than 20 min) and 50 normal controls drawn from among their relatives and friends. The battery included immediate memory span, a word recognition test and a free-recall test using the selective reminding procedure. The head-injured patients, who were tested roughly a month after their accidents, were not significantly impaired either in terms of their overall performance on the battery as a whole or in terms of their performance on any of these three memory tests. Gentilini *et al.* concluded: 'if there is structural damage after mild head injury, it generally recovers from the neuropsychological standpoint within one month after the trauma' (p. 139). A multi-centre investigation by Levin *et al.* (1987c) considered 57 patients with minor closed head injury (defined as a loss of consciousness lasting 20 min or less) in terms of their performance on memory span, the free recall of a list of animal names using the selective reminding procedure, and the reproduction of visual geometrical designs. When compared with a control group of 56 healthy volunteers, the head-injured patients were found to be impaired on all three tasks (and especially on the verbal-memory task) when tested a week after their accidents, but not when retested a month afterwards.

Levin *et al.* (1987a) carried out a similar investigation of 20 patients with minor closed head injuries, who received computerized tomography and magnetic resonance imaging (MRI) as well as neuropsychological assessment. The baseline performance of these patients (conducted on average nine days after their injuries and within 24 hours of the MRI scan) was impaired with reference to a group of 13 normal controls on free recall using the selective reminding procedure and on a spatial analogue of that task. Those patients with MRI-defined lesions within the temporal lobes tended to show an even greater degree of impairment on both tasks at the baseline examination than those with lesions within the frontal lobes. Moreover, the magnitude of the impairment on these tasks was significantly related to the size of lesions within the right temporal lobe, though not to the size of lesions within the left temporal lobe. Those patients who were subsequently available for retest at one month and three months after their injuries showed a reduction in the size of their lesions on serial MRI and a concomitant improvement in their performance on the cognitive tasks, but they continued to be impaired on the verbal-memory task.

One problem is that several of these studies compared the performance of head-injured patients across repeated testing with the performance of a normal control group on a single administration of a free-recall test using the selective reminding procedure. However, this procedure shows a significant practice effect even when alternative materials are used at different sessions (*see* Hannay and Levin, 1985), and any improvement on the part of the head-injured patients can therefore be attributed merely to the effects of practice. A second problem is that the comparison groups in these studies consisted of normal, healthy individuals who had not been involved in major accidents. As will be explained later in this chapter (pp. 121–4), any decrement on the part of the head-injured patients can therefore be attributed as much to the anxiety-producing effects of involvement in a major accident and of rapid and unanticipated admission to hospital as to the specific effects of the injury itself upon cerebral function.

In a careful analysis of the neuropsychology of moderate head injury, McMillan and Glucksman (1987) made the following proposal:

> Ideally a control group should differ from a head-injured group only by not having sustained a brain injury. Hence a comparison group should control for the physical damage, shock, stress and disability arising from the injury. Controls should also belong to a population that has a similar likelihood of sustaining a head injury. (p. 393)

In order to control both the nonspecific aspects of accidents involving a head injury as well as 'at risk' factors or predisposing characteristics of the victims of such accidents, McMillan and Glucksman employed control subjects who had sustained an orthopaedic injury (usually involving an arm fracture or sprain). They assessed 24 patients with moderate head injury (defined by a duration of PTA of between one and 24 hours) and 20 patients with orthopaedic injury within seven days of their accidents, and found no difference between these two groups on tests of associative learning, narrative recall and visual reproduction. The patients in this study also described their everyday memory abilities using a Subjective Memory Questionnaire (Bennett-Levy and Powell, 1980), and the resulting ratings were found to be significantly lower in the case of the head-injured group. Nevertheless, when each patient was assessed by a relative or close friend, the ratings of everyday memory ability that were given to the head-injured patients were not significantly different from those that were given to the orthopaedic controls. These results suggest that the specific effects of minor closed head injury upon the brain mechanisms subserving human learning and memory tend to dissipate within the first week following the injury.

Theoretical Interpretations

Some researchers have attempted to interpret the putative impairment of patients with minor closed head injuries in learning and remembering in terms of contemporary theories of normal memory function. In principle, such a strategy can provide clinicians with a more sophisticated analysis of the difficulties and problems encountered by their patients, and at the same time it provides researchers with a novel body of empirical data with which to validate, refine and develop their theories (Richardson, 1982). As mentioned in the previous chapter, a theoretical distinction between 'short-term' and 'long-term' memory became prevalent during the 1960s, but it was also the source of much controversy. As a way of resolving such debates, Waugh and Norman (1965) proposed a new model based on a phenomenological distinction made originally by William James. According to this, the current contents of consciousness constituted a *primary memory*, a short-term store of limited capacity that permitted instantaneous encoding and retrieval; once material was no longer the focus of conscious attention, however, it might still be retained within a *secondary memory*, a long-term store of indefinitely large capacity that required effortful encoding and retrieval. The covert repetition (or 'rehearsal') of items being held temporarily within primary memory was considered to be the sole mechanism by which material could be entered into secondary memory; in the absence of rehearsal, material could not be stored in any permanent form and would thus be forgotten (*see* Figure 4.1). Finally, performance in tests of long-term retention was taken to depend only upon secondary memory but both forms of storage might contribute to performance in tests of short-term retention.

One source of evidence taken to support this account of human memory came from the analysis of free recall, in which subjects attempt to recall a list of items in any

Figure 4.1   The theory of primary and secondary memory

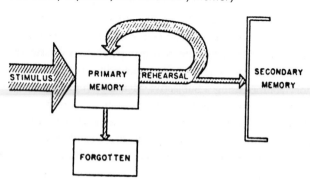

Source: Waugh, N. C. and Norman, D. A. (1965) 'Primary memory', *Psychological Review*, 72, pp. 98–104. Reprinted with permission.

order that they wish. In an immediate recall test, performance tends to be relatively good on the first few items presented (the so-called 'primacy effect'), relatively poor across the items in the middle of the list, and especially good on the last few items presented (the so-called 'recency effect'). However, if the recall test is delayed by some intervening activity, even if only for a few seconds, performance on the last few items tends to be no better than on those in the middle of the list (Glanzer and Cunitz, 1966). These findings were originally taken to suggest that the recency effect in immediate free recall reflected the contribution of a transient form of storage (that is, short-term storage or primary memory), whereas the residual performance throughout the list seen on both immediate and delayed free recall reflected the contribution of a relatively permanent form of storage (that is, long-term storage or secondary memory).

Parker and Serrats (1976) used this analysis to interpret the memory performance of 108 patients with closed head injuries, including 38 cases with PTA lasting 24 hours or less. These patients were tested on the free recall of lists of words at one month and three months after their injuries, and then every three months thereafter. At the first test, more than 50 per cent of the patients with minor head injuries produced normal performance, and most of the remainder showed impaired performance extending throughout the lists of words. A few patients showed a more pronounced impairment on the early and middle list items. In all three cases the intrusion errors that the patients made (that is, the words produced at the time of recall which had not in fact been presented in the list to be remembered) tended to be items which had been presented and recalled correctly in earlier lists. However, nearly all of the patients achieved a normal level of performance during the first year after the injury. Parker and Serrats concluded that minor closed head injuries tended to produce a selective impairment of the long-term storage system. Unfortunately, they gave no information at all about the control group used in their study. More fundamentally, however, the two-component analysis of free recall which they used has been largely discredited. Baddeley and Hitch (1974) showed that, if subjects carry out this task while retaining a sequence of digits in their heads, performance is (not surprisingly) impaired, but the recency effect is preserved. This shows conclusively that the recency effect in free recall does not reflect the contribution of any limited-capacity short-term store. A more likely possibility is that it merely reflects an optional but prevalent strategy among practised subjects of recalling the last few items in a list first, leaving the remaining items vulnerable to decay and to output interference (Richardson and Baddeley, 1975).

Richardson (1979a) used a similar procedure to investigate the role of mental imagery in the performance of 40 cases of minor closed head injury (with PTA at most seven hours) and a control group of 40 orthopaedic patients. All of these patients were tested within a few days of their injuries on the immediate free recall of five lists of relatively concrete words and five lists of relatively abstract words, and then received an unexpected final recall test on all of the words presented. The overall results are shown in Table 4.1. The head-injured patients were found to be impaired with respect to the control subjects in the recall of lists of concrete words, but not in their recall of lists of abstract words. The orthopaedic controls produced superior performance on the lists of concrete words compared with the lists of abstract words, and this was consistent with a large amount of previous experimental research with normal subjects. However, the head-injured patients failed to show a significant advantage in their recall of concrete material with respect to their recall of abstract material. Within this head-injured sample, the magnitude of the difference between the recall of concrete words and the recall of abstract words for each individual patient varied inversely with the duration of PTA, but neither the site of the impact nor the incidence of concussion appeared to affect the test results. Finally, because the same pattern of results was obtained both in the initial, immediate recall test and in the final, delayed recall test, it was concluded that closed head injury gave rise to a specific impairment of long-term memory rather than of short-term memory.

Table 4.1   Mean per cent correct in free recall for head-injured patients and for orthopaedic control subjects on concrete and abstract material in initial and final testing

	Initial Testing		Final Testing	
	Concrete	Abstract	Concrete	Abstract
Orthopaedic controls	46.9	35.3	17.4	10.8
Head-injured patients	41.6	36.7	12.2	10.5

Source: Richardson, J. T. E. (1979) 'Mental imagery, human memory, and the effects of closed head injury', *British Journal of Social and Clinical Psychology*, 18, pp. 319–27. Reproduced by permission.

Richardson noted that his findings refuted the view that closed head injury resulted in an impairment of abstract thinking, because this would have predicted quite the opposite pattern of results: in other words, a more pronounced deficit in the case of abstract material than in the case of concrete material. Instead, he interpreted the results in terms of the 'dual coding' theory devised by Paivio (1971), in which 'images and verbal processes are viewed as alternative coding systems, or modes of symbolic representation' (p. 8). The superior performance of the control subjects in their recall of concrete items was attributed to their use of mental imagery either as an additional memory code or as a more effective memory code in the case of concrete material. Conversely, the failure of the head-injured patients to demonstrate a significant difference in their performance between concrete and abstract items was taken as evidence that imagery was not being effectively employed by these subjects. Richardson concluded that closed head injury gave rise to a selective impairment in the use of imagery as a form of elaborative encoding in long-term memory.

Further evidence on this matter was obtained from an analysis of the prior-list intrusion errors that had been produced by the head-injured and control patients in this study (Richardson, 1984b). The results are shown in Table 4.2. The control subjects showed a strong tendency to produce intrusion errors from previous lists that were of similar concreteness to the current list: that is, most intrusion errors that they produced in attempting to recall concrete lists came from earlier concrete lists, and most intrusion errors that they produced in attempting to recall abstract lists came from earlier abstract lists. Nevertheless, the head-injured patients showed no sign of this sort of effect: the concreteness of their intrusion errors was quite unrelated to the concreteness of the list that they were trying to recall. This appeared to confirm the notion that closed head injuries impaired retention by disrupting the normal encoding of the image-evoking quality of the material to be remembered.

Evidence that the effect of minor closed head injuries on memory was specific to the imaginal encoding of *verbal* material was obtained in two experiments by Richardson and Barry (1985). They eliminated the necessity for transforming verbal information into an imaginal representation by presenting the original material in a pictorial form (as unfamiliar faces or as line drawings of common objects). In neither case did head-injured patients tested within a few days of their injuries show any impairment in their retention of such material. Richardson and Barry then asked whether head-injured patients might be induced to encode verbal information using mental imagery by means of suitable training instructions. They therefore repeated the earlier study of free recall carried out by Richardson (1979a) with additional patients who were instructed to make up mental images that related together the things described by the words in each list. Previous experimental investigations had shown that instructions of this sort give rise to substantially enhanced performance in normal

Table 4.2   Numbers of prior-list intrusion errors given by head-injured patients and orthopaedic control subjects in the immediate free recall of concrete and abstract lists of words

	Concrete lists	Abstract lists	Total
Control patients			
Concrete intrusions	58	28	86
Abstract intrusions	20	58	78
Total	78	86	164
Head-injured patients			
Concrete intrusions	37	31	68
Abstract intrusions	46	45	91
Total	83	76	159

Source: Richardson, J. T. E. (1984) 'The effects of closed head injury upon intrusions and confusions in free recall', *Cortex*, 20, pp. 413–20. Reproduced by permission.

Table 4.3   Mean per cent correct in free recall for head-injured patients and for orthopaedic control subjects on concrete and abstract material in initial and final testing, under standard learning instructions and imagery mnemonic instructions

	Initial Testing		Final Testing	
	Concrete	Abstract	Concrete	Abstract
Standard Instructions				
Orthopaedic controls	51.8	40.9	18.8	13.3
Head-injured patients	40.8	39.7	10.3	11.2
Imagery Instructions				
Orthopaedic controls	56.6	48.8	22.3	10.2
Head-injured patients	54.5	47.5	20.5	9.1

Source: Richardson, J. T. E. and Barry, C. (1985) 'The effects of minor closed head injury upon human memory: Further evidence on the role of mental imagery', *Cognitive Neuropsychology*, 2, pp. 149–68. Reproduced by permission.

subjects. When given these relatively simple instructions, Richardson and Barry found that both head-injured patients and orthopaedic controls produced better performances with concrete items than with abstract items, and indeed there was no sign of any difference between the two groups in their level of retention (*see* Table 4.3). In short, instructions to use imagery in learning lists of single words increased the head-injured patients' performance to the level demonstrated by the normal control subjects, and they reinstated the effect upon recall of the concreteness of the items to be remembered.

Richardson and Barry concluded that the effects of closed head injury on human memory should be regarded as a functional deficit attributable to the patients' failure to adopt the optional strategy of constructing interactive images. One might say that the problem which is exhibited by these patients lies not so much in their ability to remember *per se*, nor in their ability to use mental imagery or any other mnemonic strategy, but in their efficient and spontaneous use of such strategies. In other words, the effects of minor closed head injury appear to be principally upon *metamemory*: that is, the strategic knowledge of how, when and where to employ mental imagery and other mnemonic techniques in order to support effective learning and remembering in everyday life (Pressley *et al.*, 1987).

Memory Function Following Severe Head Injury

Given that even a minor closed head injury may give rise to deficits in learning and remembering that persist beyond the period of PTA, it is not surprising that more severe cases also exhibit this sort of impairment. There have been many clinical reports of such impairment since Russell's seminal paper in 1932, but in these accounts it is typically not clear how memory performance or deficits of memory performance were assessed. Nevertheless, in the last 20 years a considerable amount of formal research has been devoted to the study of learning and remembering in head-injured patients beyond the period of PTA, and most of this work has involved patients with severe closed head injuries. It is now beyond any doubt that such patients manifest a generalized impairment of episodic memory (that is, the retention of particular biographical events and episodes). Such an impairment has been observed in a variety of tasks, with both verbal and pictorial material, and with both lists of unrelated words as well as coherent narrative.

The Wechsler Memory Scale

This research was to some extent made possible by the development of standardized tests of memory function for use in a clinical setting. Until quite recently, the most widely used instrument in this connection was undoubtedly the Wechsler Memory Scale (WMS: Wechsler, 1945), which contains seven subtests:

1　Personal and Current Information (regarding the patient's age, date of birth and major Government figures);
2　Orientation (with respect to date and place);
3　Mental Control (assessed in terms of simple counting and recitation tasks);
4　Logical Memory (recalling the gist of two short pieces of narrative);
5　Memory Span (recalling sequences of digits in both a forward and a backward direction);
6　Visual Reproduction (drawing simple geometric figures from memory); and
7　Associate Learning (a multitrial paired-associate learning task).

An age correction factor is added to the patient's total score across the seven subtests to yield a 'Memory Quotient' (MQ). This index was intended to be broadly analogous to, and directly comparable with the patient's Intelligence Quotient (IQ) according to the Wechsler-Bellevue Intelligence Scale (Wechsler, 1944), the predecessor to the Wechsler Adult Intelligence Scale (WAIS: Wechsler, 1955). Since the MQ was in fact standardized against the Wechsler-Bellevue Performance scores of 100 normal adult subjects, it is not surprising that among normal subjects the MQ is very highly correlated with the IQ. There also seems to be a high degree of communality among the various subtests of the WMS. When neurological or psychiatric patients are tested, however, there may prove to be discrepancies between the IQ and MQ, and the structure of the WMS breaks down into two and possibly three major factors: the first is measured by the Mental Control and Memory Span subtests, the second is associated with the Logical Memory, Visual Reproduction and Associate Learning subtests, while a third may be associated with the Personal and Current Information and Orientation subtests (*see* Skilbeck and Woods, 1980). Both the absolute MQ and the relative discrepancy between the IQ and the MQ are affected by brain damage, but a selective impairment on the WMS is most clearly observed in patients with lesions of the left medial temporal lobe. All these issues are discussed in detail in a review paper by Prigatano (1978).

The factorial structure of the WMS that has emerged from the study of clinical patients makes excellent sense in terms of current assumptions in theorizing about human memory. Atkinson and Shiffrin (1968) accepted the general distinction between long-term storage and short-term storage, but they argued that the latter should be regarded not simply as a temporary store of information but as a *working memory* responsible for a variety of additional control processes such as rehearsal, encoding, decision making and retrieval. Baddeley and Hitch (1974) demonstrated that performance in a variety of cognitive tasks was disrupted by making subjects perform them whilst holding a sequence of digits or consonants in their heads, and they took these findings to support the notion of working memory as a flexible, limited-capacity processing system. This idea has proved very influential in subsequent work with both normal and brain-damaged subjects (Baddeley, 1986). The subtests of the WMS that were identified with the first of the factors mentioned above are clearly measures of the efficiency of working memory as that concept has been described in recent experimental research. In contrast, the subtests of the WMS that were identified with the second of those factors are obviously measures of the efficiency of long-term or permanent memory (cf. Russell, 1975).

IQ and MQ Following Severe Head Injury

The first systematic study of persistent memory disorders in patients with severe closed head injury was carried out by Dailey (1956), who used the Wechsler-Bellevue Intelligence Scale as well as the WMS in the psychological assessment of 31 patients with post-traumatic epilepsy roughly five years after their injuries. There was no control group in this study, nor were any summary statistics given, but the severity of the original injury, as measured by the durations of post-traumatic unconsciousness, was reported to show a substantial correlation with the discrepancy between IQ and MQ. Subsequently, Black (1973) compared 50 patients with closed head injuries and 50 patients with penetrating missile wounds of the brain on the WAIS and the WMS. The latter group achieved a mean IQ of 95.5 and a mean MQ of 90.5, which Black considered to be 'within normal limits'. The patients with closed head injuries achieved a mean IQ of only 84.5 and a mean MQ of only 79.1, representing a significant deficit in both cases. However, as Corrigan and Hinkeldey (1987) noted, the discrepancy between IQ and MQ was obviously very similar in the two groups.

An unpublished investigation by Prigatano found a mean (IQ–MQ) discrepancy of +10.07 in 15 patients with traumatic head injury, compared with a mean (IQ–MQ) discrepancy of −2.42 in 11 psychiatric controls (*see* Prigatano, 1978). Gronwall and Wrightson (1981) administered the WMS to 71 head-injured patients with durations of PTA from a few seconds to several days. Those patients in whom PTA had lasted more than 24 hours achieved lower MQs than the remainder of the sample.

Timming *et al.* (1982) classified 30 patients with severe head injuries into four distinct groups according to the results of computerized tomography. When they were assessed at discharge roughly 13 weeks after their injuries, all four groups were severely impaired on both the WAIS and the WMS. The deficit on the WMS seemed to be most pronounced in the case of patients with focal intracranial lesions (haematomas) and those with enlarged ventricles. However, detailed statistical comparisons could not be made among the groups because some patients were too impaired to be given one or both tests; in particular, fewer than half of the total number of patients were able to carry out the WMS at the time of their discharge. Corkin *et al.* (1985) described five cases of chronic global amnesia resulting from closed head injuries. Their average IQ on the WAIS was 98.0, and none achieved less than 90; however, their mean MQ was 75.8, representing a mean (IQ–MQ) discrepancy of +22.2, and all of them scored less than 90 on this test. Nevertheless, Solomon *et al.* (1986) reported a mean discrepancy of only +3.14 in 126 patients with closed head injury; they tentatively suggested that diffuse or generalized lesions might normally be associated only with relatively small discrepancy scores.

Corrigan and Hinkeldey (1987) compared 38 patients with closed head injuries and 21 patients who had suffered cerebrovascular accidents on the WAIS and WMS. These latter patients achieved a mean IQ of 93.81 and a mean MQ of 94.67, but those with closed head injuries achieved a mean IQ of 89.05 and a mean MQ of 79.92. The corresponding (IQ–MQ) discrepancy scores (i.e., −0.86 and +9.13) proved to be significantly different by a simple pairwise test (implying that head-injured patients were selectively impaired in terms of memory function), though not when age, education and time since onset were taken into account as possible confounded variables. In 1981, however, the Wechsler Adult Intelligence Scale–Revised (WAIS–R) had appeared (Wechsler, 1981). Corrigan and Hinkeldey presented data from a further 98 patients who had suffered traumatic head injuries and another 52 patients who had suffered cerebrovascular accidents on the WMS and the WAIS–R. The latter patients achieved a mean of IQ of 87.79 and a mean MQ of 102.73, while those with closed head injuries achieved a mean IQ of 82.24 and a mean MQ of 85.31. The corresponding (IQ–MQ) discrepancy scores were still significantly different, but this was now because the patients with cerebrovascular accidents produced a mean MQ that was substantially *larger* than their mean IQ.

The pattern of results that Corrigan and Hinkeldey found with stroke patients has been obtained with other populations as well. Prifitera and Barley (1985) measured the IQs and the MQs of 120 psychiatric inpatients, using the WAIS for half of the sample and the WAIS–R for the other half. The subjects who received the WAIS produced a mean IQ of 102.93 and a mean (IQ–MQ) discrepancy of +2.40, but those who received the WAIS–R produced a mean IQ of only 96.15 and a mean (IQ–MQ) discrepancy of −6.12. Since previous studies had shown differences of a similar magnitude between the WAIS and the WAIS–R (i.e., Prifitera and Ryan, 1983; Wechsler, 1981, p. 47), Prifitera and Barley argued that the mean IQ on the WAIS–R and the mean MQ on the WMS did not reflect equivalent levels of intellectual performance. Corrigan and Hinkeldey noted that their own results showed a difference of 6–7 points between the mean IQ values produced by the WAIS and the WAIS–R. They offered no explanation for this result, however, and suggested that it could not explain the (IQ–MQ) discrepancy of −14.94 which they had obtained in stroke patients using the WAIS–R.

Nevertheless, Larrabee (1987) pointed out that the WAIS itself yields mean IQs which are roughly 4–5 points lower than those generated by the Wechsler-Bellevue Intelligence Scale, on which of course the WMS was standardized (*see* Wechsler, 1945), Larrabee attributed this to the general pattern for successive standardizations of intelligence tests to yield lower scores when they are administered to the same groups of subjects. In discussing this general pattern, Flynn (1984) noted yet another problem with the Wechsler-Bellevue Intelligence Scale, namely that it had been standardized on an urban sample and therefore yielded mean IQs for the general population that were probably 3–4 points too low. The upshot of all this is that an (IQ–MQ) discrepancy of anywhere between −10 and −16 is entirely to be expected if the WAIS–R and the WMS are used with normal samples of subjects. Larrabee (1987) also provided further reasons for questioning the practical utility of making direct comparisons between the IQ and the MQ.

The validity of the MQ and of the WMS itself has come under scrutiny for a number of reasons. Indeed, Prigatano (1978) listed several serious weaknesses of the WMS as a psychometric instrument:

> They include (1) no scaled or standard scores available for individual subtests; (2) problems of scoring the Logical Memory subtest and the need to take into consideration the tendency of the patient to guess or not to guess on the test; (3) lack of norms for a large representative sample . . . (4) lack of good numerical determinations of the test-retest reliability of the MQ scores in normals; (5) lack of information as to the distribution of Full Scale IQ minus MQ scores, especially in individuals with Superior IQ scores; and (6) a need for restandardization of the MQ scores with the WAIS Full Scale IQ (or the now-being-standardized WAIS–R) as opposed to the Wechsler-Bellevue. (p. 828)

Prigatano concluded that 'the WMS needs to be improved substantially if it is to continue as a viable measure of memory function' (*loc. cit.*).

Further Studies Using the Wechsler Memory Scale

One strategy for dealing with these problems has been to amend the WMS where necessary and submit it to more careful psychometric evaluation. Russell (1975) devised a new version of the WMS using just the Logical Memory and Visual Reproduction subtests, but supplemented by an additional retention test after a 30-min delay. This then provided indices of short-term memory, long-term memory and percentage retention on both tasks, but these were not combined into a total memory score. Poorer performance was generated on all six measures by a heterogeneous sample of 75 brain-damaged patients than by a control sample of 30 normal subjects, and within the brain-damaged group all six measures were found to show a substantial correlation with the patients' Average Impairment Ratings on the Halstead-Reitan battery (*see* Chapter 5, pp. 143–4). Although this latter group contained 15 cases of closed head injury and eight cases of open head injury, Russell did not report their data separately. A new set of norms based upon a much larger sample of normal and brain-damaged subjects has recently been published (Russell, 1988).

In contrast to the strategy that was adopted by Russell, other researchers have tried to improve the usefulness of the original WMS in neuropsychological assessment by adding further items and forms of assessment (Milberg *et al.*, 1986). Nevertheless, there are a good many residual problems with all these variants of the WMS (*see* Loring and Papanicolaou, 1987). Some attempt to handle these problems was made in the Wechsler Memory Scale–Revised (WMS–R) which was recently published (Wechsler, 1987). This incorporates: an extended and modified battery of subtests; scoring procedures for indices of Verbal Memory, Visual Memory, Delayed Memory and Attention-Concentration, as well as a General Memory index; and validation material involving several clinical groups. Results from a sample of head-injured patients were included in the test manual, but no information was provided on the severity of their injuries or its relationship with objective memory performance. The WMS–R is now widely used in North America and the UK, but at the time of writing has not yet been employed in published research on the effects of closed head injury.

An alternative strategy has been to continue to employ the WMS or its constituent subtests as a research tool in spite of its evident clinical limitations. The use of an appropriate control group would then obviate the need to rely upon normative data that are generally agreed to be of doubtful validity. This approach was adopted by Brooks (1972), who used the Logical Memory, Visual Reproduction and Associate Learning subtests of the WMS, together with tasks requiring the reproduction of a complex geometrical drawing and the continuous recognition of geometrical shapes. He tested 26 patients with PTA lasting a minimum of two days and an average of 46 days roughly six months after their injuries, and compared them with a group of orthopaedic outpatients. The head-injured patients were impaired on all of the tests except Visual Reproduction, and they also showed more pronounced forgetting over a 30-min interval of the material used in the Logical Memory and Associate Learning tasks. Brooks (1976) reported a similar study in which the entire WMS was administered to 82 patients with severe closed head injury and 34 orthopaedic patients. The head-injured patients produced poorer performances on all the subtests except Visual Reproduction, although they produced only slightly fewer errors on the Mental Control task and were not significantly impaired when recalling the digits in the order of presentation (i.e., forward) in the Memory Span task. Their most pronounced deficits were on the immediate and delayed versions of the Logical Memory and Associate Learning tasks; they also showed more pronounced forgetting than the control patients on the latter subtest, though not on the former subtest. Similar profiles on the subtests of the WMS were described: by Levin and Peters (1976) in the case of a single patient suffering from prosopagnosia (that is, an inability to recognize the faces of familiar people) following severe head injury; by Corkin *et al.* (1985) in five cases of chronic global amnesia resulting from closed head injury; and by Levin and Goldstein (1986) in comparing 12 cases of severe closed head injury with ten normal controls.

Groher (1977) administered the WMS to 14 patients with severe closed head injuries who had been unconscious for an average of 17 days following their accidents. They were tested after they had regained consciousness and at four successive intervals of 30 days thereafter. On all seven of the subtests, they were profoundly impaired at the first testing session, but showed considerable subsequent improvement. Their performance was evaluated as being 'within normal limits' on the Mental Control, Logical Memory and Memory Span subtests by the third testing session (i.e., two months after their head injuries), and on the Personal Information subtest by the final session (i.e., four months after their head injuries). Their average MQ increased from 58.3 at the first session to 74.7 at the final session, but they showed persistent deficits on the Orientation, Visual Reproduction and Associate Learning subtests. Groher also administered the WMS over five testing sessions to a similar group of patients who had sustained their head injuries at least a year before. They showed no sign of changes in their performance on any of the constituent subtests, and Groher therefore concluded that the improvement shown by the previous group of patients was an accurate reflection of their recovery which was not contaminated by practice effects.

Kear-Colwell and Heller (1980) administered the WMS to 70 patients with closed head injuries and 116 subjects from the general population. They then carried out a factor analysis of the scores on the seven WMS subtests, which yielded three oblique factors. The head-injured patients were significantly impaired on all three factors, but particularly so on the factor which was defined by the Logical Memory and Associate Learning subtests. Indeed, when the contrast between the groups was incorporated in the factor analysis as a dichotomous variable, it showed a substantial loading on that factor and no relation at all with the other two factors. Gronwall and Wrightson

(1981) obtained a somewhat different solution from the results of 71 head-injured patients with PTA lasting between a few seconds and several days, but this may have been the result of using an orthogonal (Varimax) solution to estimate factors which are quite likely to be correlated with one another. A similar solution was obtained when the duration of PTA was included as a variable but the factor analysis was restricted to those cases in whom PTA had lasted for at least one hour; however, the duration of PTA produced only a modest loading on each of the three factors extracted. Finally, Cullum and Bigler (1985) compared 16 head-injured patients who had undergone craniotomy for the treatment of subdural haematoma with 16 head-injured patients who had not suffered a haematoma on the WMS. The former group achieved a significantly lower mean MQ (69.94 versus 81.56), which resulted mainly from lower scores on the Logical Memory and Visual Reproduction subtests, and especially from lower scores on the Associate Learning subtest.

Other Procedures for Assessing Memory Function

Apart from the subtests of the WMS, researchers have used a variety of other procedures for evaluating learning and memory in patients with severe closed head injuries. When assessing their subject with traumatic prosopagnosia, Levin and Peters (1976) tested his performance on repeated learning trials on sequences of digits that exceeded his immediate memory span (and therefore demanded the use of long-term storage). Unlike normal subjects, this patient never managed to exceed or equal his memory span in his performance on this task. Lezak (1979) found that most of a sample of 24 patients were impaired on the Rey Auditory-Verbal Learning Test when tested within the first six months after traumatic brain injury, although she provided no clinical information about the severity of their injuries. Brooks and Aughton (1979b) found that patients with severe head injuries were profoundly impaired on a paired-associate learning test devised by Inglis (1959) in which subjects had to learn just three pairs of unrelated words, and the magnitude of their impairment was directly related to the duration of PTA (*see also* Brooks and Aughton, 1979a; Brooks *et al.*, 1986b). Gronwall and Wrightson (1981) compared 20 patients with closed head injury and 30 normal controls on the Visual Sequential Memory subtest from the Illinois Test of Psycholinguistic Abilities, which is a more difficult test of the immediate reproduction of geometrical figures than the Visual Reproduction subtest of the WMS. The head-injured patients were severely impaired on this task, but their scores were very highly correlated with those on a serial addition task, and Gronwall and Wrightson considered that it added little new information. Sunderland *et al.* (1983) administered a battery of memory tests to 33 patients with severe head injuries (PTA lasting between two days and 90 days) between two and eight months after their accidents. In comparison with a control group of 37 orthopaedic patients, they showed an impairment across most of the tests of episodic memory and also on a test of speed of access to semantic memory, though not on a multiple-choice vocabulary test.

Sunderland *et al.* also devised a retrospective questionnaire and a daily checklist to be completed both by each patient and independently by a close relative concerning the patient's memory failures in everyday life. The relatives of the head-injured patients reported significantly more memory failures than the relatives of the control subjects. In both groups the most commonly reported memory failures were:

> Finding that a word is 'on the tip of your tongue'. You know what it is but can't quite find it.
> Forgetting something you were told a few minutes ago. Perhaps something your wife or a friend has just said.
> Forgetting something you were told yesterday or a few days ago.
> Forgetting where you have put something. Losing things around the house.

However, the head-injured patients themselves did not report significantly more memory failures than the orthopaedic control patients, and there was essentially no relationship between the performance of individual subjects in either group on the formal memory tests and the total number of memory failures reported either by the patients themselves or by their relatives. Sunderland *et al.* suggested that any residual memory problems might have been obscured by a tendency for both the head-injured patients and their relatives to compare the patients' condition at the time of assessment with the major cognitive dysfunction suffered during the comparatively recent period of PTA and the very early stages of recovery. Nevertheless, they also suggested that the absence of correlations between 'objective' performance and 'subjective' reports was also due to differential exposure to cognitive demands:

> Having only just returned home, the most severely injured recent patients were less often back at work and may have been sheltered by relatives from cognitively demanding situations. Few memory errors will be made in an environment that makes few demands on memory, despite the poor performance of these patients on objective tests. The less seriously injured recent patients were more often back at work or were at least likely to be taking on domestic duties and to be venturing out, thus exposing themselves to problems and thereby making errors. Such a difference in exposure would tend to cancel out any subjective-objective correlations that might otherwise have occurred. (p. 353)

Many investigators have used tests of free recall incorporating the selective reminding procedure (Buschke, 1973; Buschke and Fuld, 1974) which was described earlier in this chapter (pp. 93–4). Levin and Eisenberg (1979a, 1979b) assessed head-injured children and adolescents within a few weeks of their accidents, and found a significant degree of impairment on both storage and retrieval in comparison with normative data; this was especially pronounced in patients who were still comatose on admission to hospital. The unpublished study of Levin and Eisenberg (Levin *et al.*, 1982a, pp. 109–14) found deficits on this task among adolescents with severe head injuries at 40 days after injury (well after their state had improved to within normal limits according to the GOAT). Patients with diffuse lesions or with mass lesions involving the left hemisphere according to computerized tomography were substantially impaired; however, those with mass lesions involving the right hemisphere performed as well as patients with mild head injuries (i.e., within the normal range). In addition, among the patients with lesions of the left hemisphere, those with lesions infiltrating the temporal lobe performed less well than those whose lesions spared the temporal lobe, who in turn performed as well as the patients with lesions of the right hemisphere.

Gronwall and Wrightson (1981) assessed 20 head-injured patients in whom PTA had lasted between two and 56 hours roughly 26 days after their injuries. These patients were impaired on a test of free recall using the selective reminding procedure in comparison with a group of 30 normal controls, and within the group of head-injured patients there was a negative relationship between recall performance and the duration of PTA. Levin *et al.* (1982b) administered a similar test to 30 head-injured children and 30 head-injured adolescents; in each age group, half of the patients had sustained severe injuries (defined by a Glasgow Coma Scale score on admission of 8 or less), while half had sustained minor injuries (defined by a Glasgow Coma Scale score of more than 8). In both age groups the patients with severe injuries produced poorer performances than those with minor injuries, while there was no difference between the two age groups in terms of the proportion of cases who were impaired in comparison with age-matched normal controls.

McLean *et al.* (1983) examined 11 patients with a PTA lasting more than 24 hours. These patients were impaired relative to 52 normal control subjects when tested three days after their injuries on a variety of measures of retention, but not when retested one month later. Nevertheless, there is a distinct possibility that many of these patients were still in PTA at the first assessment, since they were also significantly impaired on the orientation section of the GOAT. An alternative explanation of their deficit at this time is that they were still suffering from the nonspecific effects of involvement in a major accident followed by rapid and unexpected admission to hospital (*see below*). Moreover, the small size of this sample makes it hard to rely upon the negative results obtained at the 1-month follow-up. In contrast, Shores *et al.* (1986) found a significant impairment on free recall using the selective reminding procedure in 20 patients with severe closed head injuries tested roughly 33 weeks after their accidents when compared with 20 other accident victims undergoing orthopaedic treatment.

Instead of tests of *recall*, in which the subjects are required to reproduce the items that were to be remembered, some researchers have used tests of *recognition*, in which the subjects have to identify those items among a larger set that includes some 'distractor' items which have not been previously encountered. Both sorts of test require explicit memory for the occurrence of an episode in the recent past, but there is now considerable evidence that recognition and recall depend upon distinct (though overlapping) sets of cognitive processes (e.g., Mandler, 1980). As mentioned above, Brooks (1972) used a continuous recognition test involving simple geometrical figures that had been devised by Kimura (1963). The head-injured patients were found to be impaired in terms of their corrected recognition scores, calculated as the difference between the total number of correct recognitions (i.e., identifying a previously presented item as 'old') and the total number of 'false positive' errors (i.e., identifying a distractor item as 'old'). Brooks (1974b) obtained similar results in a subsequent study in which he tested 34 patients with severe closed head injury roughly 12 months after their accidents on the same continuous recognition test. The head-injured patients in this study also tended to produce more 'false negative' errors (i.e., identifying a previously presented item as 'new') than the controls, but the two groups did not differ in terms of the number of false positive errors.

The study by Levin *et al.* (1976b) that was mentioned earlier included 15 patients with severe closed head injuries. Those who had been comatose for less than 24 hours were not impaired either relative to the patients with mild head injuries or relative to the control patients with peripheral neurological disorders. However, those patients who had had persistent coma, neurological deficits, aphasic disturbances, or signs of brain stem involvement were more likely to show an impairment on this task with respect to the control group of patients with peripheral neurological disorders. Levin and Peters (1976) asked their single case of traumatic prosopagnosia to learn a list of 48 unrelated nouns. His performance was essentially normal when he was asked to recognize 24 of the original nouns immediately after presentation of this list, but it was severely impaired relative to a group of six normal controls when he was tested on the other 24 nouns after a delay of 30 min. Alexandre *et al.* (1979) carried out a study whose methods and results were broadly similar to those of Brooks (1974b) with 50 cases of severe head injury and 25 normal controls; half of the patients with a closed head injury in this study had been surgically treated for intracranial haematoma, but there was no difference in performance between these patients and the nonoperated cases of closed head injury.

The investigation by Hannay *et al.* (1979) which was also mentioned earlier in this chapter included 28 patients with severe head injuries. They produced poorer performances in terms of their corrected recognition scores and more false positive errors than either the patients with mild injuries or the control patients with somatic complaints. However, they made relatively few false negative errors (in other words, they correctly identified nearly all of the previously presented items). When evaluated across all of the patients in this study, the duration of coma was found to be negatively correlated with the number of correct responses although it failed to show any significant relationship with either sort of error. The same task was used by Levin *et al.* (1981b) to compare 32 patients with severe head injuries and 78 control patients with somatic or psychiatric symptoms, but in this study all of the subjects underwent computerized tomography to evaluate the magnitude of ventricular enlargement. Dilation of the ventricles was not significantly related to the incidence of memory impairment on this task, but it was significantly related to the incidence of impairment on free recall using the selective reminding procedure. Levin *et al.* (1982b) administered a continuous recognition task to children and adolescents with severe and minor closed head injuries, and found that the patients with severe injuries exhibited impaired recognition performance in comparison with those with minor head injuries, but that there was no difference between the two age groups in terms of the proportion of cases who were impaired in comparison with age-matched normal controls.

In the study by Sunderland *et al.* (1983) that was mentioned above, the patients with head injuries showed significant deficits on both Kimura's (1963) continuous recognition task and a test of recognition memory for unfamiliar faces, although not on a forced-choice word-recognition test in which performance approached a ceiling for both the patients and their controls. Corkin *et al.* (1985) used both verbal and nonverbal versions of Kimura's continuous recognition task in assessing five patients with chronic global amnesia following severe head injuries. All five of these cases were regarded as impaired on both versions of the task in terms of their corrected recognition scores. Indeed, Corkin *et al.* noted that head-injured patients seemed to be particularly impaired on these tasks in comparison with amnesic patients with other aetiologies. Finally, as was mentioned earlier in this chapter, Payne-Johnson (1986) used the same task as Hannay *et al.* (1979) and found that patients with both mild and more severe head injuries were impaired, but that there was no difference between these subgroups.

Brooks (1974b) suggested that the poor performance of the head-injured group in his own study might have been caused either by reduced initial learning or by a strategy of increased caution, but he concluded that the data were not available to distinguish between the two alternatives. Subsequently, however, Brooks (1974a) analysed the performance of his original subjects in terms of the framework of signal detection theory. The head-injured patients produced a significantly lower mean value of the parameter d', an index of recognition sensitivity, and a significantly higher mean value of the parameter β, an index of response bias. Brooks concluded that severe head injuries produced poorer memory efficiency but also a more cautious response criterion. Richardson (1979b) criticized Brooks' arguments with specific reference to the validity of d' and β as indices of sensitivity and response bias; he suggested that, when the theory was applied in an appropriate manner, severe head injury was shown to produce an impairment of recognition sensitivity with no concurrent change in response bias. Similar arguments were put forward by Hannay *et al.* (1979), who concluded from their data that head-injured patients tended to set a *less* stringent criterion in a recognition memory task (that is, they were *more* likely to guess 'old'). In short, patients with severe head injuries are uniformly very impaired in recognition memory tasks; however, research to date is quite inconsistent as to whether they are more cautious, less cautious, or relatively unbiased when compared with normal controls.

Most of the formal procedures which have been described so far stem from laboratory research on human learning and memory and may not provide an accurate assessment of head-injured patients' abilities in daily life. The Rivermead Behavioural Memory Test was developed by Wilson (1987, chap. 5) to diagnose impairment in everyday memory functioning and to monitor change resulting from treatment for memory difficulties. It contains 11 subtests which were designed to provide analogues of a range of everyday memory tasks that appeared to be troublesome for brain-damaged patients, and were selected on the basis of the types of memory failure reported by the patients in the study by Sunderland *et al.* (1983) and on the basis of behavioural observations of patients in a rehabilitation settting:

1 Remembering a name
2 Remembering a hidden belonging
3 Remembering an appointment
4 Picture recognition
5 Prose recall
6 Remembering a short route
7 Remembering an errand
8 Orientation (based on the Orientation subtest and the Personal and Current Information subtest of the WMS)
9 Date
10 Face recognition
11 Learning a new skill

Each of these items was shown to discriminate effectively between a group of 25 patients assessed as having everyday memory problems and a separate group of 16 patients assessed as not having such problems by occupational therapists. (All 41 patients had brain damage, in 24 cases as the result of head injury.) The number of items performed correctly by each subject showed a highly significant difference between the two groups of patients, demonstrated excellent interrater reliability, test-retest reliability and parallel-form reliability, and was highly correlated both with therapists' observations of memory failures and with performance on standard tests of memory performance (including the Logical Memory test from the WMS), but not with measures of IQ according to the WAIS.

Many investigators have shown that the degree of memory impairment following severe head injury is directly related to the duration of PTA (Brooks, 1974a, 1976; Brooks and Aughton, 1979b, Brooks *et al.*, 1980; Dailey, 1956; Levin *et al.*, 1976b;

Parker and Serrats, 1976), although this relationship seems to be more pronounced in the case of older patients (Brooks, 1972, 1974b). The degree of impairment may also be associated with the level of consciousness on admission according to the Glasgow Coma Scale (Levin and Eisenberg, 1979a, 1979b), the duration of post-traumatic unconsciousness (Dailey, 1956; Groher, 1977; Hannay *et al.*, 1979; Kløve and Cleeland, 1972; Levin and Eisenberg, 1979a, 1979b; Levin *et al.*, 1982b; but cf. Brooks *et al.*, 1980), and with the incidence of neurological signs of brain-stem damage (Levin *et al.*, 1976b). On the basis of the discussion in Chapter 2, therefore, one might conclude that postconcussional disorders of learning and remembering are produced by rotational movement of the brain at the time of head impact. Conversely, measures of focal cerebral damage do not show a consistent relationship with the degree of residual impairment (*see* Brooks, 1975, 1976; Brooks *et al.*, 1980; Levin and Eisenberg, 1979a; Levin *et al.*, 1976b, 1982b). In particular, the extent of the memory disorder is not affected by the presence of skull fracture (Brooks *et al.*, 1980; Kløve and Cleeland, 1972; Levin *et al.*, 1976b; cf. Brooks, 1975). It is not clear whether dysphasia should be regarded as a focal neurological sign that affects the extent of memory impairment (Brooks, 1974b; Levin *et al.*, 1976a, 1976b; Thomsen, 1977; *see* Chapter 5, pp. 171–3), and the prognostic significance of intracranial haematomas has also still to be determined (*see* Alexandre *et al.*, 1979; Cullum and Bigler, 1985; Timming *et al.*, 1982). Indeed, in the study by Brooks *et al.* (1980), patients who had undergone surgical removal of a haematoma were found to perform significantly better on story recall than nonoperated patients, which was taken to reflect a bias in the selection of patients for neurosurgical treatment. This study found that the side of haematoma was irrelevant as a predictor of memory performance; there is however unpublished evidence suggesting that focal damage to the left temporal lobe may be important in this context (Levin *et al.*, 1982a, pp. 109–14).

Theoretical Interpretations

One theoretical interpretation of the effects of severe closed head injury upon memory function has been in terms of the two-store theory of memory that was originally proposed by Waugh and Norman (1965). In its most fully articulated version (e.g., Baddeley and Patterson, 1971), this model proposed that performance in immediate memory tasks was dependent both upon a relatively transient or short-term store of limited capacity that relied heavily on a phonemic (i.e., speech-based) representation of the information that was to be remembered, and upon a relatively permanent or long-term store of indefinitely large capacity that relied heavily on a semantic (i.e., meaning-based) representation of the information that was to be remembered. A study by Brooks (1975) used this theory to explore the nature of memory performance in 30 patients with closed head injuries and 15 other accident victims who were undergoing the treatment of limb injuries. Most of the head-injured patients were very severely injured, apart from five in whom the duration of PTA was 24 hours or less, and they were tested on average 15 months after their injuries. Brooks' conclusion was that the persistent memory impairment found after closed head injuries reflected a selective deficit in the ability to store new information in long-term memory, but it will be useful to consider in detail the evidence that led to this conclusion.

Brooks employed just two tasks in his investigation: the free recall of lists of unrelated common words, and immediate memory span for digits (both in the order of presentation and in the reverse order). The control patients were found to be superior to the head-injured patients in free recall, but there was no difference between the two groups in terms of the digit-span task, whether the items were recalled forwards or backwards. This implies that closed head injuries disrupt a component of the memory system which contributes to performance in free recall but is not involved in memory span. Levin and Peters (1976) similarly found that their single case of post-traumatic prosopagnosia had an intact memory span. However, in his subsequent study, Brooks (1976) found the head-injured patients to be impaired in the backwards digit-span task, although not in the forwards digit-span task. Thomsen (1977) reported a significant decrement in digit span following severe head injury, but as will be seen in a moment the appropriateness of her comparison group is open to doubt. Nevertheless, it has to be recognized that patients with severe closed head injuries will not necessarily show a clear dissociation between memory span and tests of long-term retention (Becker, 1975; Levin and Goldstein, 1986; Lezak, 1979). Indeed, when Brooks (1975) examined the influence of the time that had elapsed between head injury and psychological testing, the patients who had been tested within six months of their accidents produced significantly poorer performances in memory span than those who had been tested more than six months afterwards; no such difference was obtained in the measures of long-term retention. This would suggest that short-term memory is impaired by severe head injury but rapidly improves to a normal level, whereas long-term memory recovers much more slowly and exhibits a persistent residual impairment.

In Brooks' (1975) study, the patients' retention of half of the lists presented for free recall was tested immediately after their presentation, whereas that of the remainder was tested after a delay of 20 sec, during which the patients were required to engage in an irrelevant counting task. The patients were if anything more impaired in the delayed test than in the immediate test. Levin *et al.* (1976b) argued similarly that short-term recognition memory was rather less vulnerable to closed head injury than long-term recognition memory. Brooks (1972, 1976) noted similar patterns in immediate and delayed recall on subtests of the WMS. Within the tests of immediate free recall, Brooks (1975) noted that his head-injured and control patients tended to diverge mainly in their performance on the words presented in the early and middle serial positions of a list. This pattern was also noted in the study by Parker and Serrats

(1976), which included 70 patients with a PTA duration exceeding 24 hours. Like Brooks, they concluded that closed head injury gave rise to a selective deficit in the encoding of new information into long-term storage. However, it was noted earlier that the formerly prevalent view that the recency effect in free recall reflects the contribution of a short-term store has now been quite discredited. Fortunately, Brooks was able to provide independent data regarding the putative long-term and short-term components of recall by estimating their respective contributions from the order in which the items to be remembered were actually recalled. This confirmed that the head-injured patients were impaired on the long-term component but not on the short-term component of free recall.

Finally, Brooks also provided a detailed analysis of the errors made by his patients. The head-injured patients were found to have produced significantly fewer intrusion errors from previous lists, which was taken to mean that closed head injury affected the storage of information into long-term memory rather than the retrieval of information from long-term memory. However, Schacter and Crovitz (1977) argued that these results were equally consistent with the view that the items to be remembered were stored but for some reason could less readily be retrieved. (One idea might be that head-injured patients were more cautious.) Thomsen (1977) found that her patients with severe closed head injuries showed a greater tendency to produce intrusion errors from previous tests in their recall, while Richardson (1984b) found that minor closed head injuries produced no effect upon the total number of prior-list intrusion errors. Rather more convincing evidence was produced when Brooks asked four independent judges to classify the remaining errors in terms of whether they were similar to the items to be remembered with regard to their sound or their meaning. The two groups of patients did not differ in terms of the proportion of their errors that fell into the former category (i.e., acoustic confusion errors). However, the head-injured patients produced a very much smaller proportion of errors that fell into the latter category (i.e., semantic confusion errors). Richardson (1984b) failed to find this pattern in the case of patients with minor closed head injuries, and Brooks' analysis is complicated by the fact that the head-injured patients in his study tended to make more extra-experimental errors than the control patients. Indeed, Levin *et al.* (1979a) found that more than half of a sample of 27 patients with severe closed head injuries fell above the 96th percentile of a normal control group in terms of the number of intrusion errors made in learning a single list following the selective reminding procedure. Nevertheless, Brooks' results are consistent with the idea that severe closed head injuries tend to disrupt the storage of new information into a memory system that depends upon semantic coding.

The discussion thus far has implied that the rotational acceleration of the brain that is induced by a severe closed head injury gives rise to a selective impairment of the encoding of material into long-term storage. However, it is important to remember that qualitatively different forms of impairment can arise from the focal lesions that occur as the result of skull fractures or intracranial haematomas. A very interesting example of this was a patient reported by Warrington and Shallice (1970), who had suffered a left parieto-occipital fracture in a road accident and subsequently had to undergo surgery for the evacuation of a left parietal subdural haematoma. When assessed 11 years later, his performance in tests of long-term memory (including the Associate Learning subtest of the WAIS and a multitrial free-recall task) was essentially normal. However, his digit span was just two, and he proved to have a general impairment in the repetition of auditory verbal stimuli. Shallice and Warrington (1970) presented further evidence to substantiate the notion that this patient had a selective reduction in the capacity of short-term memory.

Because of epileptic seizures, the patient then underwent exploratory craniotomy enabling the extent of damage to be macroscopically visualized. Warrington *et al.* (1971) reported that 'the lesion was both to cortex and white matter, but mainly to the former, which in places was totally lacking, the white matter being exposed' (p. 378). Warrington *et al.* presented the findings of their postoperative assessment, in which the patient performed at or above the normal level on the Performance subtests of the WAIS and roughly within the normal range on the Logical Memory and Associate Learning subtests of the WMS. However, his performance was more variable on the Verbal subtests of the WAIS, where he was impaired on the Arithmetic subtest and especially on the Digit Span subtest.

At the time, following the specific proposals of Waugh and Norman (1965) and Atkinson and Shiffrin (1968), it was the conventional wisdom that information could only be encoded within long-term memory by being held and rehearsed within short-term memory. As Shallice and Warrington (1970) noted, the fact that their patient's long-term retention was essentially intact in the face of a gross impairment of short-term retention created grave difficulties for this view. As an alternative, they argued instead that short-term memory and long-term memory constituted functionally independent forms of storage (*see* Figure 4.2). Largely thanks to these research findings and also to evidence from other neurological patients with similar patterns of memory dysfunction, this is now very much the prevailing conception of the functional architecture of human memory.

Earlier in this chapter, it was suggested that a minor closed head injury produced an impairment of memory function by disrupting the use of mental imagery as a form of coding within long-term memory. A study by Thomsen (1977) compared 41 patients with severe closed head injuries and 21 control subjects on the multitrial free recall of a single list of ten concrete nouns and a single list of ten abstract nouns. The head-injured patients appear to have found the concrete list easier to learn than the abstract list, but no attempt seems to have been made to equate the words in the two lists on other relevant characteristics such as meaningfulness and frequency of occurrence. Be that as it may, the head-injured patients proved to be significantly impaired on the abstract list as well as on the concrete list. This result might tend to

Figure 4.2   Shallice and Warrington's (1970) theory of the relationship between the short-term store and the long-term store (R refers to the rehearsal loop)

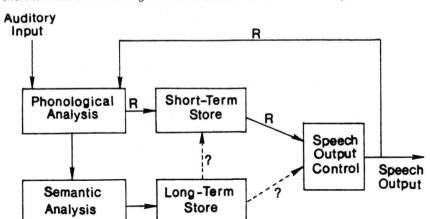

Source: Shallice, T. (1989) *From Neuropsychology to Mental Structure*, Cambridge, Cambridge University Press. Reprinted with permission.

suggest that the persistent and pronounced impairment of memory function that follows the occurrence of a severe closed head injury is not to be ascribed merely to an impairment in the use of mental imagery, because this idea had been predicated upon the finding of a *selective* decrement in the retention of concrete material. Nevertheless, Thomsen's control subjects were students from a college of further education, and it is quite possible that they were not really an appropriate comparison group. College students are very atypical of the general population in a range of characteristics, most obviously their age, intelligence, educational level and social class (Richardson, 1987). The control subjects used in Thomsen's study were in fact of a similar age range and occupational status to her head-injured patients, and they 'had not had any known damage to the brain' (p. 73). There was, however, no suggestion that any of this particular comparison group had ever been involved in serious accidents. This is an important point, and one that is worth considering in some detail.

Choice of Control Subjects

In the assessment of individual patients in clinical practice, it may occasionally be important to establish whether they are functioning at a lower level than their educational or occupational history would suggest, regardless of whether this is caused by the organic effects of head injury or to the broader social and psychological factors that are of necessity attendant upon an individual's involvement in a major accident. In these circumstances it will often be appropriate to use standard normative data in arriving at a formal evaluation. It may even be possible to arrive at an estimate of a patient's premorbid performance on the basis of specific biographical characteristics, such as age, education and occupation (*see* Barona *et al.*, 1984).

In some instances, of course, test results may be available from before the person's injury. These might be obtained as a formal aspect of the research methodology, as in the case of a recent investigation of head injuries among American college football players in which they had been systematically assessed during the preseason (Barth *et al.*, 1989). Alternatively, premorbid test results might be available by virtue of the choice of the population to be studied. This would be the case in studies of closed head injuries among the members of the armed services, who would have undergone routine psychological assessment in the course of their induction (e.g., Becker, 1975; Dresser *et al.*, 1973; Russell, 1981). It would also be likely in the case of research involving head-injured schoolchildren, who might well have received tests of mental or scholastic ability (e.g., Levin and Eisenberg, 1979a). Even so, premorbid data of this sort need to be considered with care and even scepticism (*see* Teuber, 1969). Once the psychologist wishes to go beyond the circumstances of the individual patient, however, and to make general statements concerning the effects of head injuries on mental function, whether for the purposes of assessment, rehabilitation or research, then the need arises to establish a suitable comparison group with which to compare the head-injured sample.

In experimental research, a control group is a group of subjects who are treated in an identical manner to those in the experimental group with the exception that they are not exposed to the manipulation which is under investigation. In other words, the two groups differ only with respect to the critical independent variable whose effect is being studied. This can normally be achieved by assigning individual subjects at random to one of the two groups, so that the experimental manipulation is systematically either imposed upon or withheld from subjects who are otherwise drawn from the same underlying population. In research in clinical neuropsychology, however, it is neither ethically permissible nor practically possible to allocate participants at random to control and experimental groups by systematically exposing them to or protecting them from disease or trauma. Membership of the two groups is therefore a 'classification' variable that is determined in advance of the research study in question rather than a 'treatment' variable resulting from the manipulations of the investigator, and it follows that research of this sort is intrinsically correlational rather than experimental in nature (*see* Ferguson and Takane, 1989, pp. 246–7). Under these circumstances the selection of a suitable control group will be of considerable importance, since the researcher will otherwise be seeking to attribute differences in performance between a clinical sample and a control group to some neurological indicator in the full knowledge that the two groups may well differ on many other relevant characteristics (Richardson, 1982).

In the case of research into the effects of closed head injury, it is normally considered necessary to select control subjects who are similar to the head-injured sample in every relevant respect, save that of having received a blow to the head (McKinlay and Brooks, 1984; McMillan and Glucksman, 1987; Rutter *et al.*, 1980). In particular, it is common for control subjects to be chosen from accident victims who have been admitted to hospital for orthopaedic treatment of major fractures, since these patients also have suffered traumatic injury resulting in rapid and unexpected hospitalization (Brooks, 1976; cf. Brooks *et al.*, 1984). This also allows for the fact that accident victims are not a representative or random subgroup of the general population, but appear to differ from the remainder of the population in certain important respects (Aitken *et al.*, 1982; Mandleberg and Brooks, 1975). In particular, as McKinlay and Brooks (1984) pointed out, the choice of orthopaedic cases as control patients means that they are 'drawn from a similar ''at risk'' population with the over-representation of the young, of males, and of the lower socioeconomic classes' (p. 96), unlike other potential comparison groups such as cardiac patients or those with severe burns (*see also* Chapter 1, pp. 24–7).

Of course, the use of orthopaedic patients as a control population also assumes that head-injured patients are broadly similar to other accident victims. One might seek to justify this on the grounds that whether or not an accident leads to a head injury (as opposed to an injury to some other part of the body) is often a matter of chance. Of particular relevance to the assessment of post-traumatic cognitive function is the relatively poor premorbid academic attainment of patients with closed head injuries (Haas *et al.*, 1987; Rutter *et al.*, 1980), and this seems equally to be a characteristic of other accident victims (Hall *et al.*, 1987; Wilmot *et al.*, 1985). Nevertheless, Brown *et al.* (1981) found that children with mild head injuries (unlike those with severe head injuries) showed a rate of premorbid behavioural disturbance that was markedly higher than that of children who had suffered orthopaedic injuries not involving the head.

In research on the effects of severe head injury, McKinlay and Brooks (1984) argued that the control subjects should have sustained a traumatic injury that was life-threatening in at least a proportion of cases and involved a significant degree of disability, leading to an associated reevaluation of life plans and the possibility of adverse psychological reactions. They suggested that orthopaedic patients 'are less severely injured and can be expected to make a more or less full recovery over a few months; adverse psychological reaction to disability would therefore be expected to be less marked and less prolonged' (p. 97). Instead, they argued that cases of traumatic paraplegia would come closer to meeting the requirements for appropriate control subjects (cf. Rosenbaum and Najenson, 1976). However, McKinlay and Brooks acknowledged that the disabilities of paraplegics were permanent and severe, which might make any psychological reactions particularly acute, and yet at the same time visible and public, which might mean that they were easier to accommodate and less subject to stigma than mental disabilities.

Brain Function in Orthopaedic Patients

The choice of orthopaedic patients as control subjects appears to be more appropriate in the case of research into the effects of minor closed head injury. Nevertheless, there are at least four different reasons why this might be expected to give only a rather conservative assessment of the effects of traumatic brain damage upon psychological function.

First, an accident victim might have received a head injury that was not sufficiently conspicuous to be noted on medical examination. For example, it would seem that as many as 50 per cent of patients admitted to hospital with spinal cord injuries also have closed head injuries (Silver *et al.*, 1980). Whether these are detected will depend upon the vigilance of the receiving medical staff (Kopaniky and Wagner, 1987) and the level of expertise in the unit to which they are admitted (Silver *et al.*, 1980). For instance, Davidoff *et al.* (1985) found that only 25 per cent of patients with traumatic spinal-cord injuries were assessed for PTA. They concluded that a closed head injury was a frequent concomitant of traumatic spinal-cord injury but that 'many of these closed head injuries remain undetected and their sequelae unevaluated' (p. 42). Kopaniky and Wagner (1987) also suggested that evidence of a possible head injury may be inadvertently dropped from the patient's medical record as the spinal cord injury becomes the major focus for medical attention. Equally, however, as Cope (1987) pointed out, it may well be very difficult to assess mental function in patients with spinal cord injuries since they 'are not only paralyzed but their initial course is also characterized by passivity and dependency' (p. 100).

Second, an accident victim whose orthopaedic injuries were sufficiently serious as to warrant emergency hospitalization might have received a bodily impact which transmitted an inertial loading to the brain even without a direct impact to the head (*see* Chapter 2). This may of course be evidenced by a loss of consciousness at the time of the accident and by a subsequent PTA. Hall *et al.* (1987) evaluated a consecutive series of 130 patients with spinal cord injury and found that 56 per cent were quadriplegic as the result of a high-energy deceleration accident, 36 per cent had lost consciousness at the time of their injuries, and 15 per cent had neurological indicators of significant brain stem or cortical damage. Wilmot *et al.* (1985) assessed 67 patients with traumatic spinal-cord injuries on a neuropsychological test battery, and found that 43 of them were impaired, seven of them profoundly so. Despite the fact that their physicians were aware of this study, only ten patients had been diagnosed as having a head injury or a cognitive problem (*see also* Hall *et al.*, 1987). Similar results were obtained in a prospective study of 30 patients with spinal cord injuries by Davidoff *et al.* (1987). In this case, 57 per cent of the patients had scores that were suggestive of cognitive impairment on the Halstead Category Test when they were assessed between 8 and 12 weeks after their injuries. When some of the patients studied by Hall *et al.*

(1987) received a follow-up assessment an average of 16 months after their injuries, precisely one half of them were found still to be impaired.

Third, even without causing mechanical damage to the brain, orthopaedic injuries can give rise to brain injury. The latter is often an 'occult' injury in the sense that its onset may be delayed and so the symptoms and signs of cerebral involvement may not be present at the time of admission. There are at least two major mechanisms by which this can happen. On the one hand, a blunt injury to the neck can lead to the intimal dissection of a major cerebral artery resulting in the occlusion of blood flow or focal cerebral infarction (*see* Kopaniky and Wagner, 1987). Lampert and Hardman (1984) noted this as an indirect source of brain damage in boxing. On the other hand, an injury to the spinal cord often gives rise to respiratory insufficiency with the consequent risk of nontraumatic hypoxic damage to the brain (Cope, 1987). By means of a similar mechanism hypoxia can also result from traumatic chest injury, as well as other disorders such as pulmonary oedema (Teasdale and Mendelow, 1984).

Finally, even relatively minor orthopaedic cases might be undergoing uncomfortable or distressing treatment, and this might affect their performance in psychometric testing. In this context, it is interesting that Rutter *et al.* (1980) found that some form of surgical intervention had been necessary in 21 per cent of children with moderate head injuries, in 25 per cent of children with severe head injuries, but in 57 per cent of children with orthopaedic injuries.

From a practical point of view, then, the possibility of concurrent cerebral injury has to be taken seriously in the management of traumatic orthopaedic cases. Moreover, any residual cognitive impairment will have important implications for the treatment and rehabilitation of such patients. In particular, such deficits may well impede the learning of new skills and information (Davidoff *et al.*, 1987), and, as Cope (1987) pointed out, they may well explain some of the psychological problems of patients recovering from spinal cord injuries that have been thought in the past to be purely characterological or psychodynamic in nature. For present purposes, however, the main point to bear in mind is that the use of hospitalized orthopaedic control subjects might tend in principle to underestimate the effects of closed head injuries upon cognitive function.

Physical Trauma and Psychological Function

Some researchers have used samples of normal, healthy volunteers as control subjects in evaluating the effects of closed head injury. Brooks *et al.* (1984) noted that this provided an estimate of the asymptotic level of performance which might in principle be approached during the course of recovery in head-injured patients, and that the normal, healthy working population might well provide an important frame of reference, especially for medico-legal purposes. Other investigators have used nonemergency hospital admissions as control subjects. As mentioned earlier in this chapter (pp. 92–3), Conkey (1938) tested a group of surgical patients both in hospital and out of hospital, and found no sign of any difference between the two testing sessions. Moreover, these control patients showed a similar pattern of performance to the normal subjects which she used as the comparison group in evaluating the effects of closed head injury, and this tends to confirm that hospitalization itself has little or no effect upon performance in psychological tests. Nevertheless, as Conkey herself acknowledged, 'none of these patients was suffering from physical trauma of any type' (p. 18), and so the results of her study do not distinguish between the effects of trauma in general and the specific consequences of traumatic brain injury.

As McKinlay and Brooks (1984) observed, the empirical phenomena that are observed and reported in patients with closed head injury 'will be a mixture of specific effects of brain injury and general effects due to reactions to injury, hospitalization, threat to life and so on' (p. 98). Unfortunately, little is known about the generalized effects of serious trauma and consequent emergency admission to hospital on psychological functioning. Richardson and Snape (1984) pointed out (as indeed is immediately apparent to anyone involved in the treatment and care of accident victims) that these events constitute a major source of stress which is predominantly expressed as a profound anxiety about oneself, one's family, one's job, and so on. The nature, complications and clinical management of this acute response to trauma have been discussed by Peterson (1986). Gronwall and Sampson (1974, Expt. I) evaluated ten hospitalized accident victims within 48 hours of admission, but more than 24 hours after anaesthesia and a minimum of 12 hours after medication. They performed as well as ten normal controls on a serial addition task, which Gronwall and Sampson took to mean that 'neither shock nor worry resulting from the accident, nor a period of hospitalization' produced a significant deficit on that task (p. 34). Nevertheless, quite apart from the small size of these groups and the relatively trivial nature of the task with which they were presented, Gronwall and Sampson were led to question the motivation of their normal control subjects, who were naval ratings detailed to participate in the study, and also whether the two groups were adequately matched in terms of their occupational status and ability.

In current experimental research, it is generally agreed that effects of situational stress upon cognitive performance are likely to be mediated by the amount of experienced anxiety or 'state anxiety' that is engendered by the situation in question (e.g., Eysenck, 1982, p. 96). The latter was defined by Spielberger (1972) as a condition 'characterized by subjective, consciously perceived feelings of tension and apprehension, and activation of the autonomic nervous system' (p. 39; *see also* Spielberger, 1966). It was claimed by Liebert and Morris (1967; *see also* Morris and Liebert, 1970) that state anxiety had both cognitive components ('worry') and autonomic components ('emotionality'), and that of these it was the former that was responsible for cognitive dysfunction. The evidence for this distinction is not entirely unequivocal (*see* e.g., Richardson *et al.*, 1977), but nowadays it is widely accepted that anxiety (and other affective states) may interfere with human cognition (*see* e.g., Eysenck, 1982, chap. 6; Messick, 1965). Eysenck (1982) made a specific theoretical assertion concerning the likely effects of state anxiety upon cognitive functioning:

> Worry and other task-irrelevant cognitive activities associated with anxiety always impair the quality of performance because the task-irrelevant information involved in worry and cognitive self-concern competes with task-relevant information for space in the processing system. (p. 99)

In particular, he proposed that the principal manifestation of the concurrent processing of task-irrelevant information should be a reduction in the available capacity of working memory. This idea is supported by the fact that state anxiety has a profound effect upon performance in tests of memory span (*see* Eysenck, 1979; Hodges and Spielberger, 1969).

Richardson and Snape (1984) suggested that the worries which are shown by accident victims were precisely the sort of task-irrelevant information that might be expected to preempt the limited processing space available within working memory. They compared two samples, each of 30 orthopaedic patients: one group was tested as in-patients within a few days of their accidents, while the other group was tested as out-patients several weeks later. The former group was found to be severely impaired in comparison with the latter group on the task that had been used by Richardson (1979a) to measure the free recall of lists of concrete and abstract words (*see* the first two rows of Table 4.4). This was true, however, only on the initial, immediate test, not on the final, cumulative test. This pattern of impairment was clearly to be attributed to a specific problem in the use of a short-term store or working memory, rather than to any disruption of long-term or permanent memory. In short, this was precisely the outcome that was to be expected on the basis of current understanding of

Table 4.4   Mean per cent correct in free recall for out-patient controls, in-patient controls, and patients with minor and severe closed head injuries on concrete and abstract material in initial and final testing

	Initial Testing		Final Testing	
	Concrete	Abstract	Concrete	Abstract
Out-patient controls	56.3	46.9	19.1	12.9
In-patient controls	47.0	36.1	17.0	10.6
Minor head injuries	44.9	37.8	9.9	9.5
Severe head injuries	37.3	35.0	6.0	6.5

Source: Richardson, J. T. E. and Snape, W. (1984) 'The effects of closed head injury upon human memory: An experimental analysis', *Cognitive Neuropsychology*, 1, pp. 217–31. Adapted by permission.

the effects of stress and anxiety upon learning and memory, but one which also has important implications for the choice of an appropriate control group in research into closed head injury.

As explained earlier in this chapter, working memory is construed as a flexible, limited-capacity processing system that is involved in a wide variety of cognitive functions. Nevertheless, the experimental findings that led Baddeley and Hitch (1974) to develop this notion indicated that it was not a unitary device, but should be conceptualized as a complex system consisting of a central executive processor together with a number of 'slave' subsystems. Considerable support has been obtained for this sort of account in subsequent research (Baddeley, 1986). Two hypothetical subsystems of working memory have received particular attention. One is a 'visuo-spatial sketchpad' that is assumed to be mainly responsible for the construction and manipulation of spatial and pictorial representations and hence to be an important component in the utilization of mental imagery (Baddeley, 1988). The other subsystem is a short-term phonological store or response buffer that is assumed to be involved in the immediate recall of verbal items. Imposing a concurrent memory load upon subjects engaged in a short-term verbal memory task preempts some of the limited capacity of this store and therefore reduces its contribution to the overall level of performance (Richardson, 1984a). However, the worries and cognitive self-concern that are associated with involvement in a major accident requiring emergency hospitalization would presumably be effectively registered within long-term or permanent memory, and would not need to be maintained or rehearsed within the phonological buffer store. In short, *pace* the assertions of Gronwall and Sampson (1974, p. 34), the cognitive disruption that is engendered by anxiety amongst accident victims should result from competition with task-relevant information for space within the central executive processor itself, and should therefore be manifested across a wide range of intellectual activities.

Imagery and Memory Following Severe Head Injury

Nevertheless, the results that were obtained by Richardson and Snape (1984) suggest that the effects of the stress caused by involvement in a major accident tend to dissipate within a few weeks. It is certainly true that any long-term residual impact of emergency hospitalization is likely to be minimal in the case of patients who have sustained severe closed head injuries. Effects of this sort are unlikely to have influenced the performance of the head-injured patients that were described by Thomsen (1977), since they were assessed at least one year after their accidents. It remains true, however, that these patients were not comparable in certain important respects with the sample of college students which Thomsen selected as control subjects. To respond to Thomsen's findings, therefore, Richardson and Snape used their recently hospitalized orthopaedic patients as controls in a replication of Richardson's (1979a) original study with a sample which included eight cases of severe closed head injury (defined as a PTA lasting longer than 24 hours) and 22 cases of minor closed head injury. Their results are contained in the last two rows of Table 4.4. The severely injured patients showed an even more pronounced impairment on the concrete items, but they were not impaired on the abstract items. While the patients with minor closed head injury still showed a modest difference in their recall of concrete and abstract material, those with severe closed head injury showed no difference at all. Thus, the conclusions of Richardson (1979a) seem to apply even to patients who have suffered severe closed head injuries. Provided that these patients are tested beyond the period of PTA, and provided that they are not suffering from any peripheral defects, their ability to recall lists of abstract words appears to be essentially normal. Richardson and Snape concluded: 'there is at present no reason to think that Richardson's imagery account is not entirely adequate as an explanation of the persistent disturbance of memory function which results from closed head injury' (p. 228). In this context it is intriguing that Thomsen (1977) herself suggested that some of her head-injured patients had not realized the difference between the concrete and abstract words, and had therefore been unable to visualize the former in attempting to learn them.

It is interesting to note that the pattern of results obtained by Richardson (1979a) and replicated by Richardson and Snape (1984) is not peculiar to patients with closed head injuries. Many groups of patients with either localized or generalized cerebral dysfunction show a normal superiority in their recall of concrete words relative to their recall of abstract words (Richardson, in press). However, Weingartner *et al.* (1979a, 1979b; *see also* Caine *et al.*, 1977) found that patients with Huntington's disease showed no sign of any difference in their recall of the two types of word. Some of these patients were asked to provide imageability ratings of individual words, and their judgements broadly reproduced the mean ratings generated by large normative samples. Weingartner *et al.* concluded that Huntington's patients were sensitive to the varying imageability of words but failed to use this attribute when encoding material for later recall. Weingartner *et al.* (1979a) also found no difference in the recall of concrete and abstract words on the part of normal volunteers given intramuscular injections of scopolamine, which is an acetylcholine receptor blocker that is well known to disrupt memory function. Because of the similarity between these data and those which had been obtained with Huntington's patients, Weingartner *et al.* raised the question whether the memory impairment in Huntington's disease was caused by some disorder of acetylcholine-mediated neurotransmission. Nevertheless, Sitaram *et al.* (1978) also found no difference between the recall of concrete and abstract words in normal volunteers who had been given a single oral dose of choline (which gave rise to an *increase* in the overall level of recall performance). It is important, too, to note that all of these studies employed the selective reminding procedure, and that none of these findings is replicable when more conventional testing procedures are employed (Richardson, in press).

It is equally pertinent to enquire whether the memory deficits shown by head-injured patients are really confined to the use of mental imagery in memory tasks. Earlier in this chapter it was noted that instructions to use mental imagery can alleviate the memory impairment seen in patients with minor closed head injury (*see* Richardson and Barry, 1985), and that the underlying problem is thus one of metamemory rather than of memory itself. In this case, there is no reason to assume that the effects of head injury are solely confined to the strategy of employing interactive imagery. Indeed, Marschark *et al.* (1987) have argued that concrete and abstract words differ not just in terms of their imageability but also in terms of the relative ease with which they can be subjected to relational processing. Though originally intended to explain apparently problematic findings concerning the retention of narrative, the latter proposal yields a very coherent analysis of the effects of concreteness and imageability both in paired-associate learning (Marschark and Hunt, 1989) and in free recall (Marschark and Surian, 1989). This prompts a quite different sort of account of the effects of a closed head injury upon learning and memory (M. Marschark, personal communication): namely that head-injured patients fail to engage in relational processing during the presentation of word lists unless they receive instructions that specifically encourage them to do so (for instance, by constructing interactive images).

A study carried out by Levin and Goldstein (1986) is of direct relevance to this theoretical proposal. These researchers compared 12 patients with severe closed head injury and ten normal controls on the multitrial free recall of word lists designed to measure the use of semantic organization in learning and remembering. The head-injured patients were found to be impaired not just in the amount that was recalled, but also in measures of categorical clustering and subjective organization. Indeed, an index of the consistency of order of recall between successive trials was below the level of chance in the head-injured patients (*see also* van Zomeren, 1981, p. 111). These results obviously cannot be handled by an account based upon the subjects' use of mental imagery, but they are entirely consistent with an analysis in terms of relational organization. An intriguing task for future research is to determine whether the deficits identified by Levin and Goldstein can be attenuated or perhaps even abolished by instructing head-injured patients to engage in appropriate organizational activities.

Concluding Summary

An impairment of learning and remembering is the most frequent subjective complaint and the most prominent residual deficit among patients who have sustained a closed head injury. Provided that it is sufficiently serious to warrant hospitalization, even a minor closed head injury can produce a measurable decrement on tests of memory function that persists beyond the period of post-traumatic amnesia. Nevertheless, in the latter case the magnitude of any such impairment is relatively slight, and it appears to resolve within the first few weeks following the closed head injury. It is certainly very doubtful whether a minor closed head injury gives rise to any major handicap in a patient's everyday remembering. This transient disruption of learning and remembering can be attributed to a selective impairment in the use of mental imagery as a form of elaborative encoding in long-term episodic memory which can be abolished by the administration of imagery mnemonic instructions.

Severe closed head injury gives rise to a more pronounced and more persistent memory dysfunction that is manifested across a wide variety of tasks. It can be readily demonstrated on the Wechsler Memory Scale and its constituent subtests, especially when the patients are retested on the Logical Memory and Associate Learning tasks after a 30-min delay. The magnitude of this impairment varies directly with the severity of the injury, but is not consistently related to measures of focal cerebral damage, and is also largely independent of the incidence of memory failures in daily life. Memory dysfunction following severe head injury can also be ascribed to a selective impairment in the use of mental imagery as an elaborative memory code, though there is evidence that it involves a more widespread disruption of relational processing in long-term storage.

Attempts to evaluate different theoretical accounts of the effects of closed head injury upon memory function have been bedevilled by problems over the choice of an appropriate control group. Involvement in a major accident followed by rapid and unexpected admission to hospital engenders anxiety, and the resulting cognitive self-concern leads to a reduction in the available capacity of a short-term store or working memory. This can be manifested across a wide range of cognitive tasks, but is conceptually distinct from the specific effects of brain injury. These considerations tend to motivate the choice of orthopaedic patients as a suitable control population, although for a number of different reasons this might provide only a conservative assessment of the effects of closed head injury upon psychological function.

Chapter 5

Cognition and Language

Apart from the faculty of memory, the cognitive abilities of human beings include those of perception, attention, communication, comprehension, thinking and reasoning. In considering the nature of post-traumatic amnesia (PTA) in Chapter 3, I suggested that the immediate phase of recovery from a closed head injury involved a generalized impairment of cognition, the most obvious aspect of which happened to be an anterograde memory disorder. Given that even mild cases of closed head injury can demonstrate a measurable reduction in the ability to learn and remember that endures (at least for a limited time) beyond the period of PTA, it is important to determine the incidence and severity of persistent disorders in other aspects of cognition. In fact, as this chapter will explain, head-injured patients do tend to show impaired performance across a wide range of intellectual functions. Disorders of this sort may well prove to be a source of considerable personal distress both to the head-injured patients themselves and to their close relatives and friends. However, in addition such disorders will also be a primary determinant of the level of activity and employment that is open to head-injured patients. In other words, the incidence and severity of persistent cognitive dysfunction is likely to constrain the ability of individuals recovering from closed head injury to return to their previous lifestyles and occupations.

In this chapter, I shall discuss the general nature of the cognitive impairment that is shown by head-injured patients and its relationship to various possible prognostic indicators. I shall then go on to consider the relative vulnerability of verbal and nonverbal cognitive functioning, as measured by formal psychometric instruments. Finally, I shall review what is known about the disorders of language and communication that tend to result from closed head injury.

Cognitive Function

Early Studies

The first systematic study of intellectual abilities following closed head injury was that reported by Conkey (1938), who administered an extensive battery of psychological tests to 25 patients with simple concussion. The results of the tests that were specifically concerned with memory function were described in the previous chapter (pp. 92–3). Conkey classified the remaining tests into three levels of difficulty or 'levels of mental functioning'. Both the magnitude of the patients' impairment at the initial examination 2–3 weeks after their injuries and the rate of recovery to a normal level of performance were a direct function of task difficulty. However, Conkey suggested that the three groups of tests differed from each other in terms of the *nature* of the impairment in question. Simple tests of orientation, personal information and recitation produced impaired performance largely because the head-injured patients took an appreciably longer time to carry out the tasks than normal controls. Rather more complicated tests tended to produce poorer performance because they often depended upon the use of 'old knowledge and associations' (or what would nowadays be characterized as the retrieval of information stored within 'semantic memory': Tulving, 1972). The most complex tests emphasized high-level reasoning and problem solving, and Conkey suggested that her head-injured patients had failed on these latter tasks because they were deficient in 'the use of symbolism, the perception of logical relations and the ability to abstract' (p. 39).

In each category of test, however, the performance of the head-injured patients approached that of normal controls over a period of 34 weeks, although there was some suggestion of a slight residual impairment in the case of the tests of intermediate difficulty. Unfortunately, the interpretation of Conkey's findings is complicated by the very high attrition rate across the test sessions among her head-injured patients. She ascribed this to the fact that a large number of her subjects 'belong to the "unfortunates" of society and are unreliable and shiftless', and she characterized it as a 'weeding out process . . . in which the more reliable and more desirable individuals were obtained for study' (p. 20). It could however equally be argued that it is the patients who have made a good recovery and returned to their previous employment who are unwilling to take time away from their work or other responsibilities to participate in repeated testing sessions purely for the sake of clinical research. In a study of 1248 patients reported by Rimel and Jane (1983), for example, 74 per cent of the survivors were regarded as having made a good recovery by the time of their discharge from the primary care hospital; however, of the 79 per cent of the survivors who returned for a 3-month follow-up session, only 66 per cent were regarded as having made a good recovery. Moreover, in a recent study of patients with minor head injury where only 37 per cent of the original sample returned for a follow-up evaluation, it was noted that 'reluctance to miss a day of work and the necessity of travelling a long distance (despite reimbursement for travel expenses) were the chief reasons cited by patients who declined a follow-up examination' (Levin *et al.*, 1987c, p. 236). Nowadays, patient drop-out for whatever reason is recognized as a serious methodological problem in longitudinal research (*see* Brooks *et al.*, 1984).

Ruesch and Moore (1943) tested 120 patients within 24 hours of their closed head injuries on a variety of simple cognitive tasks. As mentioned in the previous chapter, any pronounced deficit was chiefly restricted to a task that required the subjects to count backwards repeatedly by seven from 100. The likelihood of complete failure in this task was increased in those patients with bloody spinal fluid (which is suggestive of the occurrence of a subarachnoid haemorrhage) or a history of alcoholism. A subset of 85 of the original patients was retested on this task on each of the three subsequent days, and they showed an improvement in their overall accuracy, although not in the time taken to carry out the task. Ruesch (1944b) subsequently incorporated the earlier tasks into a more extensive psychometric battery, which he then administered to 90 other patients with closed head injuries. Of these, 40 were tested within the first 48 hours after their accidents, whereas the remaining 50 cases 'could not be tested until a later date, mostly because of lack of cooperation and prolonged disturbance of consciousness within the first two days after admission' (p. 485). There were however no significant differences in performance between the two groups. A subset of 53 of the original patients underwent repeated testing over the weeks following their injuries, and they showed some slight improvements, most commonly on the serial subtraction test and a psychomotor search test. Ruesch concluded that as the result of closed head injury 'mental speed is retarded, the ability to keep up a sustained effort is reduced, and judgment in general is defective' (p. 494).

Ruesch *et al.* (1945) presented similar findings in 49 patients tested within four weeks of sustaining a head injury and 79 patients tested more than four weeks afterwards (in many cases more than one year afterwards). It is nevertheless important to note that no control subjects were used in the latter studies, and that impaired performance on a particular test was simply inferred from the observation of a subsequent improvement on that test. Similar arguments were used by Chadwick *et al.* (1981a; *see also* Rutter, 1981):

> It is a general rule with acute damage to the brain that the intellectual deficit is greater immediately after the damage and that progressive improvement occurs during the following months. The presence of this pattern of recovery, therefore, provides a strong indication that the initial deficit was a consequence of the acute damage. Conversely, the absence of any recovery phase provides strong circumstantial evidence that the initial deficit was *not* due to acute brain damage. (pp. 52–3)

Gronwall and Sampson (1974, p. 22) pointed out that the procedure used by Ruesch confounded improvements due to the recovery of cognitive function with improvements due to practice; indeed, the tests on which Ruesch found an improvement on repeated testing were just the sort of task on which one might expect practice effects. However, this criticism does not apply to the study by Chadwick *et al.*, in which comparisons were made with a control group of orthopaedic patients who followed the same testing schedule, thus enabling any effects of recovery to be differentiated from those of practice.

Ruesch (1944b) went on to experiment with a number of other tasks designed to evaluate mental speed (naming colours and reading the names of colours), spatial thinking ability, flicker fusion and tachistoscopic recognition. He found no statistically significant differences on these tasks between 33 patients with simple concussion and 15 patients with more severe injuries involving subdural haematomas or skull fractures, though he noted that some of the tasks required a good deal of alertness and that the latter patients had consequently been tested much later after their accidents. As Denny-Brown (1945b) observed, these findings indicated 'that the type of disorder early in the course of a mild head injury was not distinguishable from the type of disorder in a comparable stage of recovery from a severe injury with prolonged unconsciousness' (p. 469).

In a subsequent study, Ruesch (1944a) evaluated simple visual reaction time and the tachistoscopic recognition of three-digit numbers among 25 patients with recent head injuries, 32 chronic cases with persistent post-traumatic symptoms and 25 hospital employees as control subjects. The recently head-injured patients were found to be significantly impaired on both tasks, while the chronic cases were impaired in the case of simple visual reaction time but not in the case of tachistoscopic recognition. The transient 'delayed apperception' shown by the recently injured patients in tachistoscopic recognition was inversely related to their performance on the Wechsler-Bellevue Intelligence Scale, and Ruesch suggested that it was 'an expression of intellectual impairment' (p. 248). One problem with this study, as van Zomeren (1981, p. 16) pointed out, is that the head-injured subjects were considerably older than the control subjects. Nevertheless, Ruesch concluded that visual examination methods had 'a definite place in clinical procedures, since they may reveal defects and show improvement where other methods fail' (p. 250). A more recent study by Hannay *et al.* (1982) found that tachistoscopic recognition was related to the severity of closed head injury, as indexed by the duration of coma, though significantly so only when the stimuli were presented within one or other visual hemifield rather than centrally.

An Information-Processing Framework

In the absence of an articulated theoretical framework for discussing the processes involved in human cognitive performance, these early studies rested upon a purely *a priori* classification of the psychological tests that were to be used and a largely intuitive description of the resulting findings. One notable exception to this was a paper by Goldstein (1943). On the basis of his experience with patients who had suffered brain damage as the result of gunshot wounds sustained during wartime (*see* Goldstein, 1942, chap. 5), Goldstein described a battery of psychological tasks based upon laboratory research that would be useful in evaluating cognitive disturbances following concussion as the result of closed head injury. The battery comprised: a self-paced continuous addition task in which subjects had to add together pairs of digits printed on a sheet of paper; tests of simple and choice reaction time; a block-design test of abstract thinking; and the recognition of tachistoscopically presented words and objects. The continuous addition task was intended to provide a measure of the subject's 'general performance capacity' (p. 331). In the case of the reaction-time tasks, Goldstein provided the following rationale: 'if the subject shows normal behavior in the single [i.e., simple] reaction test but definite deviation in the choice reaction test, both as to protracted reaction time and fluctuation with more or less errors, it is an indication of impairment of the higher mental capacities' (p. 232).

Norrman and Svahn (1961) administered a battery of psychometric tests to 24 patients more than two years after they had sustained severe closed head injuries. They proved to be significantly impaired on a three-choice reaction-time task, in comparison with both normal subjects and a control group of psychiatric patients, but they showed no sign of an impairment on a test of simple reaction time. Moreover, among the head-injured patients the mean choice reaction time was correlated with clinical ratings of the severity of residual neurological signs, but the mean simple reaction time was not. However, these patients were also impaired on tests of finger identification and finger dexterity, which suggests that their deficit in the test of choice reaction time might have been the result of response competition rather than of reduced 'general performance capacity'.

Choice reaction-time tasks came to be used frequently by experimental psychologists during the 1950s and 1960s. This was prompted by the notion of the individual subject responding to external stimuli as being somewhat akin to a communication channel that had a limited capacity for processing and transmitting information during a particular period of time (e.g., Broadbent, 1958). The classical demonstration of human beings' limited information-processing capacity was Hick's law: the finding that the response latencies in a choice-reaction-time experiment varied with the number of alternative possible stimuli, and more specifically that they increased as a direct logarithmic function of the number of alternatives (Hick, 1952). Miller (1970) evaluated performance on this task in the case of five patients with severe closed head injuries in whom PTA had lasted for more than a week; they were tested between three and 12 months after their injuries, at which time they had no residual motor deficits. These patients produced slower response latencies than a group of five normal control subjects, and the magnitude of their impairment increased directly with the number of possible alternative stimuli. Miller argued that the effect of a closed head injury was to slow down the individual's decision-making and information-processing abilities, and that it could not be ascribed to any disruption of sensory or motor processes. Clearly this is entirely in accord with Ruesch's (1944) informal suggestion that 'mental speed is retarded' in head-injured patients (p. 494).

Klensch (1973) measured simple reaction time to auditory stimuli and to visual stimuli and two-choice reaction time to combinations of stimuli in both modalities. Similar increases in all three measures were found in the case of 76 patients with minor closed head injuries when compared with a heterogeneous group of 125 normal control subjects that consisted of students of medicine and psychology together with healthy patients who were undergoing routine electroencephalographic monitoring. The increases in question were relatively slight in overall magnitude, though contrary to the impression given by Klensch they were highly significant in every case. However, as van Zomeren (1981, pp. 19–20) pointed out, the simple and choice reaction-time tasks that were employed in this study were not strictly comparable with one another in terms of the cognitive processes being tapped. In particular, the choice reaction-time task required that the subjects made a response to the particular combination of a tone and a white light but no response either to a red light (with or without a tone) or to a tone or a white light in isolation. (The two simple reaction-time tasks by definition required a response to be made on every trial.) It is obvious that such a procedure yields a measure of reaction time only on a proportion of the total number of trials, and it may also increase the variability of that measure substantially in comparison with the conventional paradigm where the subjects are required to make one of two positive responses on each trial.

An elaborated version of the information-processing analysis of human behaviour was produced by Broadbent (1971). First, just as in his earlier formulation (Broadbent, 1958), attention in the form of a selective filter intervened between the sensory representation of incoming information and the limited-capacity central processing system. Second, however, the information that was subsequently received by the latter system might have been degraded by neural 'noise' during the course of its transmission, and was therefore more appropriately described as 'evidence'. Third, particular responses were associated with different evidential inputs to the limited-capacity processing system by a process of 'categorizing'. Finally, by a process of 'pigeon-holing' the system could assign either more or fewer evidential inputs to each possible response. By this means, response selection could be modulated by motivational influences and by prior information held within short-term memory. The relationships among these three strategies of processing are shown in Figure 5.1. According to Broadbent (1971), 'Filtering varies the strength of transition *a* (solid arrow), relative to transitions *b*, *c* and *d* (dotted arrows). Pigeon-holing varies the strength of *p* (solid arrow), relative to *q* (dotted arrow)' (p. xiv). Gronwall and Sampson (1974) carried out a series of experiments to apply this model to cognitive performance in head-injured patients.

Figure 5.1 *The relationship between category states, evidence, and the outside world according to the model of Broadbent (1971)*

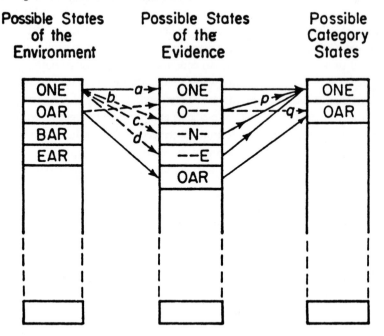

Source: Broadbent, D. E. (1971) *Decision and Stress*, London, Academic Press. Reprinted with permission.

Gronwall and Sampson's Experiments

Their first experiment made use of a paced auditory serial addition task (PASAT: Sampson, 1956), in which the subjects were presented with a random series of digits and were required to report the sum of each number and the number that had immediately preceded it. As Gronwall and Sampson (1974) noted, 'PASAT thus yields an estimate of the subject's ability to register sensory input, respond verbally, and retain and use a complex set of instructions. He must also hold each item after processing, retrieve the held item for addition to the next digit, and perform at an externally determined pace' (p. 26). The task was administered to ten cases of 'mild concussion' in whom PTA had lasted less than an hour and to ten cases of 'severe concussion' in whom PTA had lasted between one hour and seven days; they were all tested within 48 hours of admission, as soon as they were capable of responding to simple questions, and testing was repeated every 24 hours until their discharge from hospital, with a final retest about five weeks later. Their performance was compared with that of ten accident victims and ten normal controls. All of the subjects were able to perform an unpaced version of the task without error, which suggested that the demands being made upon memory and general intellectual skills were well within the capabilities of head-injured subjects.

However, the patients with severe concussion proved to be severely impaired on the PASAT itself relative to the other three groups. This deficit was more pronounced at the first test, when half of these patients were still apparently in PTA (Gronwall and Sampson, 1984, pp. 33–4), but was still apparent at the final retest five weeks later. The patients with mild concussion were significantly impaired relative to the accident victims at the first test but not at the final retest. The latter result might of course have reflected the process of recovery from a minor head injury, but Sampson (1961) had found a marked practice effect on the PASAT with normal volunteers, which he had attributed to 'central integrating mechanisms' being better able to handle briefly presented task-relevant information (p. 194). More recently, Barth *et al.* (1989) also found a large practice effect on the PASAT in the case of 48 uninjured control subjects. In fact, as Miller (1979) observed, it is simply not clear whether the two groups in Gronwall and Sampson's study had been matched effectively in the amount of practice which they had received on the task.

Comparable data from a much larger sample of 80 patients with minor head injuries were subsequently presented by Gronwall and Wrightson (1974). Seventy-five of these patients achieved PASAT scores within the normal range at a retest 30–35 days after their accidents, and the remaining five patients received an unspecified number of weekly retests until their scores too were within the normal range. This progressive improvement in performance was interpreted as a manifestation of the spontaneous process of recovery, but the possibility of practice effects was clearly as great as in the previous study. Gronwall and Sampson (1974) concluded from their results that concussion affected the rate of human information transmission. Since the interstimulus interval had been systematically varied within each administration of the task, it was possible to estimate the time needed by each group to produce a correct response at the first test: this was 3.2 sec for the accident victims, 3.5 sec for the normal controls, 3.9 sec for the patients with mild concussion and 14.3 sec for the patients with severe concussion.

Gronwall and Wrightson (1975) used the PASAT to investigate the effects of multiple concussion upon human information processing. They tested 20 head-injured patients with a history of a previous head injury requiring admission to hospital, although neither injury had resulted in skull fracture and there was no clinical evidence of cerebral contusions or intracranial haematoma. Ten of these patients had suffered relatively mild injuries, with PTA lasting less than an hour, whereas the remaining patients had suffered more severe injuries, with PTA lasting 1–24 hours. They were individually matched with 20 patients who had been admitted to hospital for the first time with head injuries of a similar severity. Not surprisingly, when initially tested within 48 hours of their accidents these head-injured patients were substantially impaired on the PASAT in comparison with a group of 60 normal control subjects. This was true even of those who had sustained just a single mild head injury, though they did perform better than those patients who had recently sustained more severe head injuries. In addition, the patients who had a history of a previous head injury were significantly impaired relative to those who had no such history, both in terms of their initial level of performance on the PASAT and in terms of the number of days that elapsed before their performance approached normal levels. These results confirmed the earlier observation that even a minor closed head injury impairs human information-processing capacity, but they also demonstrated that this impairment is both greater and longer-lasting in the case of patients who have suffered a previous concussional head injury.

The second of the experiments that were described by Gronwall and Sampson (1974) sought to measure choice-reaction time in one situation where the visual stimuli and manual responses were physically adjacent and therefore highly compatible and in a second situation where the stimuli and responses were linked by a verbal label and were thus less compatible with each other. In the compatible condition, any variation in the response latencies with the number of alternatives could be attributed to variations in movement time, in line with previous experimental research. Moreover, in this condition 12 patients with minor closed head injury (PTA lasting less than 10 min) showed no increase in either reaction time or movement time compared with 12 normal control subjects. However, in the incompatible condition, the response latencies systematically increased with the number of alternatives, indicating that significant demands were being made on central processing capacity. In this case, the head-injured patients produced significantly slower responses when tested within 24 hours of admission to hospital, but not when retested five weeks later. The results of this experiment were taken to confirm the results of the first study when using discrete rather than paced stimulus presentation, and also to show that neither response production time nor movement time was significantly slowed by concussion. Gronwall and Sampson concluded that closed head injury gave rise to a temporary deficit either in the effective channel capacity or in the use of the pigeon-holing mechanism.

In their third experiment, 12 patients with mild concussion together with 12 normal control subjects were asked to repeat aloud short recorded messages that were masked by white noise. When the messages were merely sequences of unrelated words, the performance of both groups of subjects was adversely affected by the level of white noise, but the head-injured patients showed no sign of any impairment in this task. This was taken to mean that concussion had no effect on either the perception of spoken material or the storage of that material within short-tem memory. However, when the messages were second- or fourth-order statistical approximations to English, the patients with mild concussion were found to be significantly impaired when tested within 24 hours of their admission to hospital, but not when retested roughly five weeks after their discharge. A detailed analysis of the subjects' errors suggested that the two groups had made similar use of partial evidence (as shown by the occurrence of auditory confusion errors) and of pigeon-holing (as shown by the effect of correct responses and inter-word associations upon the probability of correctly repeating subsequent items in a message). However, unlike the control subjects, the head-injured patients had been unable to take advantage of linguistic redundancy in order to enhance their probability of reporting the initial items in the messages which they heard. Gronwall and Sampson argued that the reduced information-processing capacity of patients with mild concussion meant that they were unable to analyse new incoming evidence and simultaneously to modify their responses to previous stimuli.

In accordance with this analysis, two further experiments showed that the effects of mild concussion could be mimicked by making normal subjects engage in a concurrent secondary task that made demands upon their central processing capacity. In the first of these studies, the subjects carried out the message repetition task while sorting cards bearing letters of the alphabet into four trays. In the second study they carried out the PASAT while performing a two-choice reaction-time task. In both experiments the pattern of results produced by subjects carrying out the primary task with and without a concurrent secondary task was qualitatively very similar to the results produced by subjects with mild concussion tested on admission to hospital and at follow-up five weeks later. A final experiment tested the possibility that head-injured patients had a reduced channel capacity because they were processing irrelevant stimuli as the result of impaired 'filtering'. Five patients with mild concussion and five normal controls carried out a dichotic listening task in which different recorded passages of text were presented to each ear via headphones. The subjects' task was to 'shadow' or repeat aloud the message read to the left ear; however, at a certain point the two passages were switched between the two tracks, so that the previously correct message became the incorrect message (and vice versa). In previous research using this procedure subjects had typically reported a few words from the original (but now incorrect) message before reverting to the correct ear (e.g., Treisman, 1960). In comparison with the normal controls, the head-injured patients produced poorer performances when tested within 24 hours of admission to hospital but not when retested 31 days later. Unfortunately, none of the subjects produced any intrusion errors from the irrelevant message following the switch of the passages between the two ears. However, the control subjects were more likely to make errors of omission following the switch, whereas the patients with mild concussion made no more omissions than elsewhere in the experiment. The patients' informal comments tended to confirm the notion that they had found it relatively easy to ignore the irrelevant message. Gronwall and Sampson concluded that the impairment shown by the head-injured patients in this dichotic listening task was the result of reduced channel capacity rather than enhanced distractability.

Further Research on Choice Reaction Time

Van Zomeren and Deelman (1976) carried out further investigations of simple and choice reaction time in head-injured patients. In their first experiment, 20 patients with severe closed head injuries were assessed on average about three months after their accidents. They were found to be impaired in comparison with 20 normal control subjects, but the magnitude of this impairment varied with task complexity. Also, the reaction times produced by these head-injured patients in the most complex (four-choice) conditions were significantly correlated with the duration of coma. In a second experiment, simple and four-choice reaction times were compared in three groups, each of 11 head-injured patients tested between three and six months after their accidents, who were differentiated by the duration of their unconsciousness: less than one hour, between one hour and one week, and longer than one week. The results confirmed that the effect of task complexity increased with the severity of the closed head injury. In the third and final experiment, the latter relationship was replicated, albeit in an attenuated form, when patients with severe closed head injuries were tested roughly two years after their accidents. Van Zomeren and Deelman concluded that patients with severe closed head injuries were impaired in the higher aspects of information processing, and they presented tentative findings that this might be linked to a deficiency in the availability of one or more neurotransmitters. Van Zomeren and Deelman (1978) presented similar results in the context of a 2-year follow-up study of head-injured patients and concluded that head injury influenced the rate of information transmission in the central nervous system.

Subsequently, van Zomeren (1981, pp. 38–49) presented further data to show that the increased effect of task complexity in head-injured patients was associated with slower decision making, rather than with any deficit in motor performance. Nevertheless, in another experiment he showed that subjects with severe closed head injuries were impaired in their movement time in a reaction-time task, and that they were more impaired than normal control subjects by irrelevant stimuli within the same broad framework of attention (pp. 119–123). These irrelevant stimuli were presented in close proximity to the critical stimuli and were physically identical to them. Other results led van Zomeren to conclude that their distracting influence within the information-processing system should be localized at the level of response selection, and that the effects of closed head injury on human cognition should again be attributed to a reduced processing rate. Van Zomeren et al. (1984) discussed the effects of closed head injury in terms of a theoretical distinction put forward by Shiffrin and Schneider (1977) between *automatic* and *controlled* information processing. They concluded that head-injured patients might be said to suffer from 'attentional' deficits in the specific sense that they showed a slower rate of controlled processing, but that they showed no evidence of any deficits of focused or selective attention, nor (with the exception of those cases with very severe head injuries) any deficits in tonic alertness in tasks that demanded sustained attention (cf. Brouwer and van Wolffelaar, 1985). They also speculated that a reduced capacity for information processing might explain certain aspects of the deficits in learning and remembering shown by head-injured patients, but they acknowledged that residual memory deficits were occasionally seen in patients whose information-processing capacity (as determined from reaction-time tasks) was essentially normal.

Miller and Cruzat (1981) noted the small size of the sample in Gronwall and Sampson's (1974) final experiment and the relatively mild nature of the patients' injuries. They carried out a more rigorous study of the effects of irrelevant information upon cognitive performance in 15 cases of severe closed head injury (with PTA lasting between 5 and 84 days), 15 cases of minor head injury (with PTA lasting between a few seconds and 24 hours), and 15 normal controls consisting of hospital staff or patients without neurological disorders. All of the head-injured patients were said to be 'well out of PTA at the time of testing', but otherwise no information was given with regard to the time after their injuries when the head-injured patients were tested. The subjects were required to sort packs of cards into two piles according to whether there was a letter A or a letter B on their faces. The cards in different packs contained zero, one, four, or eight irrelevant letters distributed at random across their faces. The times taken to sort a pack of cards increased with the amount of irrelevant information for all three groups of subjects. The patients with minor closed head injuries were not at all impaired on this task, while those with severe closed head injuries showed a substantial deficit. There was however no sign of an interaction between the effects of head injury and of irrelevant information. This implied that the relatively poor performance of the patients with severe head injuries was caused not by poor selective attention but rather by a central processing deficit.

Recent Studies of Information Processing after Head Injury

For practical reasons, Gronwall and Sampson (1974) did not include a control group of orthopaedic accident cases in most of their experiments. They justified this step on the grounds that their initial experiment had found that 'concussion and not shock as a result of an accident produced a deficit on PASAT' (p. 40). As mentioned in the previous chapter, Gronwall and Sampson expressed doubts about the motivation of the 'normal controls' used in that experiment (who were naval ratings detailed to participate by their superior officer), and they also suggested that these subjects might have been atypical in their occupational status since they were generally unskilled (p. 36). This means that it is still very much an open question whether involvement in a major accident combined with rapid and unexpected hospitalization itself gives rise to cognitive deficits.

Nevertheless, it is very interesting to note that the nature of the dysfunction that was posited by Gronwall and Sampson to be the underlying cause of cognitive impairment following closed head injury is equivalent to the disturbance of short-term memory that was postulated by Richardson and Snape (1985) to be the consequence of involvement in a major accident (*see* Chapter 4, pp. 123–4). From both perspectives performance was assumed to be impaired by virtue of a reduction in the available capacity of working memory: for Gronwall and Sampson the hypothesized deficit was associated with the central executive functions of working memory; for Richardson and Snape it was expressed in terms of the storage capabilities of working memory. The experiments by Gronwall and Sampson (1974) and by Miller and Cruzat (1981) demonstrated that the reduction in the available capacity of the working memory system which results from closed head injury was not caused by any impairment of selective attention (in other words, by a failure to filter out irrelevant external stimuli). However, they do not rule out the possibility that it is caused by attention being devoted to task-irrelevant information which is retrieved from long-term memory. According to Richardson and Snape, the latter was precisely the nature of the cognitive impairment that would be induced by traumatic anxiety.

Gronwall and Wrightson (1981) carried out a factor analysis using a Varimax solution of the results obtained from 71 patients with closed head injury on the PASAT and the constituent subtests of the Wechsler Memory Scale (WMS: Wechsler, 1945). Three factors were extracted, on one of which there were significant loadings associated with the PASAT and also a combined score on Personal Information and Orientation, but not with any of the other subtests of the WMS. The other factors were identified with learning and memory and with general knowledge and verbal competence. Gronwall and Wrightson then administered the PASAT in a battery of other tests to 20 head-injured patients whose PTA had lasted between two and 56 hours roughly 26 days after their injuries. Their scores on the PASAT were found to be very highly correlated with those on the Visual Sequential Memory subtest from the Illinois Test of Psycholinguistic Abilities, but they were not significantly related to three different measures of performance derived from a recall test using the selective reminding procedure. These researchers concluded that the deficit in information-processing ability which was measured by the PASAT 'is related to performance in memory tasks only when the tasks require complex processing, or where time constraints are imposed' (p. 894).

Sunderland *et al.* (1983) administered a four-choice visual reaction-time test to 33 patients with severe head injuries (in whom PTA lasted for between two and 90 days) between two and eight months after their accidents. To measure the motor component of this task, they also asked the subjects to press the response keys in rapid succession for one minute without reference to the stimulus lights. In comparison with the control group of 37 orthopaedic patients, the head-injured patients were found to produce significantly longer latencies on both tasks. A number of studies of head-injured children have also demonstrated reductions in finger-tapping rate and other indices of motor speed (Chadwick *et al.*, 1981a, 1981b; Klonoff and Low, 1974; Klonoff *et al.*, 1977; Levin and Eisenberg, 1979a, 1979b; Winogron *et al.*, 1984). Nevertheless, in the data presented by Sunderland *et al.* the increase in choice reaction time among head-injured patients was on average 113 msec, while that in their finger-tapping time was only of the order of 31 msec. This suggests that most of their impairment in choice reaction time was to be attributed to central (that is, cortical) factors rather than to peripheral (that is, motor) ones.

A study by MacFlynn *et al.* (1984) used a four-choice test of visual reaction time to monitor the recovery of cognitive function in 45 patients with minor closed head injury. When tested within 24 hours of their admission to hospital and again six weeks later, the mean reaction time of these cases was impaired in comparison with that of other patients drawn from the same general practices, although there was a clear improvement in the performance of the head-injured patients between these two sessions. When 28 patients were retested six months after their injury, they showed no sign of any impairment. However, no significant difference was found at any of the three sessions between those head-injured patients in whom PTA had lasted for less than 15 minutes and those in whom PTA had lasted for longer than 15 minutes. Moreover, MacFlynn *et al.* acknowledged that the apparent improvement of the head-injured patients in their study might simply have reflected the effects of practice on the reaction-time task, since these patients were tested two or three times whereas their control patients were tested only once.

Gentilini *et al.* (1985) compared 50 patients with mild head injury (defined as a loss of consciousness lasting less than 20 min) tested one month after their accidents with 50 normal controls recruited from amongst their friends and relatives. The head-injured group was found to be significantly impaired on a visual search task in which they were required to cancel instances of one, two or three digits from a 13 x 10 array. These patients were not however impaired on any of five other tests of memory and cognition, and Gentilini *et al.* suggested that this result might have been a Type I error (that is, a result that was significant by chance, leading to the incorrect rejection of a true null hypothesis). One of the other tests in this battery was a simple card-sorting task that made similar demands upon cognitive processing resources to the PASAT. In this task, the subjects were asked to sort an ordinary pack of playing cards into the four suits as quickly as possible, but while sorting each card to name the value and suit of its immediate predecessor. A single score was assigned that took into account both the speed and the accuracy of their sorting. Despite the apparent complexity of this task, there was no significant difference between the scores obtained by the two groups of subjects. Subsequently, Gentilini *et al.* (1989) compared another group of 48 patients with mild head injury and 48 normal controls on their original visual search task. When tested one month after their accidents, the groups differed significantly in terms of their response time but not in terms of their accuracy. In another study, Gentilini *et al.* showed that patients with mild head injury were significantly impaired in their choice reaction time for stimuli presented either to the left or to the right of a central fixation point. Although these researchers interpreted these findings in terms of 'a specific impairment of attention' (p. 174), they are much more consistent with the idea that head-injured patients suffer from a reduced central information-processing rate.

The multi-centre study by Levin *et al.* (1987c) considered 57 patients with minor closed head injuries and 56 normal controls in terms of their performance on the PASAT. The head-injured patients were found to be impaired when tested a week after their accidents, but not when retested one month or three months later. Once again, however, the increased performance of the head-injured patients on retesting might merely have reflected the effects of practice on the PASAT, since the control subjects were tested on only a single occasion. Moreover, since the latter were normal individuals who had not been involved in accidents, even the initial, transient impairment that was shown by the patients with closed head injuries can be attributed to the generalized anxiety-producing effects of their involvement in a major accident which had necessitated rapid and unexpected hospitalization. The same observation can be made with regard to an earlier investigation by Waddell and Gronwall (1984) that involved nine cases of minor closed head injury. When these patients were assessed using the PASAT on average 12 days after their injuries, they were clearly impaired in comparison with a control group of normal subjects, despite the fact that they had been regarded as 'neurologically intact' by the accident and emergency department and had not been admitted to hospital.

As mentioned in the previous chapter, the question of the appropriate comparison group was directly addressed by McMillan and Glucksberg (1987). Their study involved 24 patients with moderate head injuries (in whom PTA had lasted between one and 24 hours) and 20 patients with orthopaedic injuries who were all tested within seven days of their accidents. The choice of the latter comparison group was intended to ensure that it controlled for 'the physical damage, shock, stress and disability arising from the injury' (p. 393) as well as for certain 'at risk' factors for injury such as age, sex, social class and employment status. The head-injured patients were found to be impaired on the PASAT when the digits were presented at a relatively fast rate (one every 2 sec), but not when they were presented at a relatively slow rate (one every 4 sec). This was taken to support the view that head-injured patients exhibited a reduced rate of information processing. However, most of the head-injured patients in this study had been involved in road accidents or assaults, whereas most of the control patients had merely suffered falls (and all of them had sustained simple arm fractures or sprains). McMillan and Glucksberg acknowleged that the impairment shown by their head-injured patients on the PASAT might have resulted from higher levels of anxiety associated with their involvement in more serious accidents. It is consistent with this notion that 55 per cent of the head-injured patients but only 32 per cent of the orthopaedic patients were prescribed analgesic drugs during their hospitalization.

The Halstead-Reitan Battery

The higher executive functions which have been discussed so far in this chapter, and especially those concerned with decision making and with the organization of behaviour, are usually linked by neuropsychologists to the physiological structures of the frontal lobes, and a wide variety of psychological tests have been developed for the purpose of measuring brain impairment in these regions, usually with mixed success (*see* e.g., Lezak, 1982; Stuss and Benson, 1984; Walsh, 1978, chap. 4). For instance, the battery of tests originally developed by Halstead (1947) and revised by Reitan (1966) contains a number of subtests that are supposedly sensitive to frontal damage, including a complex sorting task, the Halstead Category Test (*see* Reitan, 1986, for a discussion of the battery's theoretical and methodological foundations). The proportion of tests in the battery on which a patient produces performance below a certain standard can also be used as a global index of impairment (Reitan and Davison, 1974). Kløve and Cleeland (1972) administered the Halstead battery to 100 head-injured patients, and found that the overall Impairment Index was significantly correlated with the duration of unconsciousness, though only when assessed during the first three months after the injury. It was also significantly greater in patients who had undergone surgical treatment of intracranial haematomas. Performance on the Category Test was also significantly related to the duration of unconsciousness, but only when administered more than six months after the injury. Klonoff and Paris (1974) found that the overall performance of head-injured children on an adapted version of the Halstead-Reitan battery was more strongly related to the duration of PTA than to the duration of unconsciousness.

Dikmen and Reitan (1976) administered the Halstead-Reitan battery to 34 patients with 'significant head injuries' soon after their accidents and again 12 and 18 months later (*see also* Dikmen *et al.*, 1983). Most of the psychometric measures derived from the battery showed an initial impairment followed by highly significant improvements across the three testing sessions, especially during the first 12 months. To control for practice effects, a subgroup of 23 head-injured patients was compared with normal control subjects matched for their educational levels who received a similar schedule of testing. The degree of improvement shown by the head-injured patients was generally greater than the effects of practice shown by the control subjects, significantly so in the case of seven of the 14 measures studied. Finally, the patients' neuropsychological status at the 18-month follow-up was correlated with characteristics of the head injury and the patients' early neurological condition, but especially with the results of early neuropsychological assessments.

Dye *et al.* (1979) compared 48 head-injured patients in whom the duration of coma had been on average two days with 16 other accident victims who had not sustained head injuries. The two groups were significantly different on most of the subtests and on the overall Impairment Index of the Halstead-Reitan battery, and the degree of impairment on the part of the head-injured patients was a direct function of their initial neurological status. Long and Webb (1983) also described findings of impaired performance on the Halstead-Reitan battery among patients with closed head injuries, and concluded that the battery 'appears to be highly sensitive to the type of impairment experienced by head trauma patients and to subtle effects present during the chronic phase of recovery that are not directly observable' (p. 56).

Rimel *et al.* (1981) presented preliminary findings from an assessment of 69 patients roughly three months after they had sustained minor closed head injuries associated with a period of coma not exceeding 20 minutes, a Glasgow Coma Scale score on admission of 13 or more, and a period of hospitalization of 48 hours or less. They concluded that 'mild neuropsychological impairment was evident on the vast majority of the Halstead-Reitan Neuropsychological Test Procedures, including the tests of higher level cognitive functioning, new problem-solving skills, and attention and concentration' (p. 226). Barth *et al.* (1983) provided more information from this project. Forty-four of the patients tested demonstrated mild to severe impairment on the Halstead-Reitan battery. This tended to be more pronounced among older patients and those with fewer years of formal education, and it was associated with impaired performance on other psychometric tests concerned with problem solving and memory. Nevertheless, it was not associated with deficits in tests of sensory processing or motor performance, and it was not correlated with either the duration of unconsciousness or that of PTA (though, as Barth *et al.* pointed out, the latter variables had a somewhat restricted range in their sample of patients and were difficult to ascertain precisely).

Further Research on Higher Executive Functions

Other tasks designed to evaluate the functioning of the frontal lobes include Nelson's (1976) modified card-sorting test, Benton's (1968) test of verbal fluency, in which subjects are required to produce as many words as possible beginning with a specified letter within 1 min, and an analogous test of design fluency (Jones-Gotman and Milner, 1977), in which subjects are required to invent novel designs. Levin *et al.* (1987a) included these three tasks in a comparison of 20 patients with minor closed head injuries and 13 normal control subjects. The performance of the head-injured patients at their initial assessment (on average nine days after their injuries) proved to be significantly impaired on all three tasks. The amount of damage to the frontal lobes, as estimated by means of magnetic resonance imaging, showed a significant correlation with performance on the design fluency test, but not with performance on the other two tasks. Nevertheless, performance on all three of the tests showed a significant relationship with the amount of damage to the *temporal* lobes. Those patients who were available for retest one month after their injuries were still impaired on the verbal fluency test, but the relatively few cases who were subsequently available for a further retest three months after their injuries did not show a significant impairment on any of the three tasks. However, given the very small sample size and the possibility of practice effects across the three testing sessions, it is difficult to interpret these latter findings. An impairment on the modified card-sorting test in patients tested some years after severe closed head injuries was found by Levin and Goldstein (1986), whereas Chadwick *et al.* (1981a, 1981b) found no sign of any impairment in verbal fluency among severely injured children tested a year after their accidents.

One further task that has been used to investigate processing speed and response selection is the colour-word test devised by Stroop (1935). This requires subjects to read aloud the names of colours and to name the colour of ink in which stimuli are printed. Their response latencies are found to be slower (more so in the second case) when the stimuli are the names of colours printed in a different colour of ink, and this effect is usually attributed to competition or interference between the alternative responses that are evoked by the stimuli. Van Zomeren (1981, pp. 83, 86) cited two unpublished studies, one with adults, the other with children, demonstrating that head-injured patients were impaired to roughly the same extent across the various conditions of the Stroop test. In other words, closed head injuries give rise to a reduced rate of information processing but do not have any specific effect upon attentional selectivity. At a follow-up session a year after their accidents, Chadwick *et al.* (1981a, 1981b) found that neither severely injured children nor mildly injured children were significantly impaired on this task. McLean *et al.* (1983) administered the two incongruent-colour conditions to 20 patients with closed head injuries and 52 normal control subjects. The nine patients with minor head injuries (indicated by a period of PTA lasting less than 24 hours) failed to show any significant impairment in either task. The 11 patients with severe head injuries were impaired when tested three days after their accidents, more so in terms of naming the ink colours than in terms of reading the colour names, but did not show a significant impairment in either task when retested one month afterwards.

Unfortunately, there are two major difficulties in trying to interpret the results of the study by McLean *et al.* First, as mentioned in the previous chapter, the patients with severe head injuries were also significantly impaired on the orientation section of the Galveston Orientation and Amnesia Test at their first assessment, and it is quite possible that they were still in PTA at this time. Second, these patients were significantly different from the control subjects in terms of the difference between the overall times to carry out the two Stroop conditions, which McLean *et al.* characterized as a measure of 'distractibility'. However, since these researchers failed to include the control conditions of the Stroop test (that is, reading colour names printed in a neutral ink and naming the ink colours in which neutral stimuli were printed), their results can be attributed to a deficit in naming colours rather than in selective attention. Indeed, it will be pointed out later in this chapter that head-injured patients do tend to suffer from naming disorders. Conversely, there is no independent evidence that closed head injuries give rise to any specific or disproportionate impairment of attentional selectivity (cf. Gentilini *et al.*, 1989; Gronwall and Sampson, 1974, Expt. VI; Miller and Cruzat, 1981; van Zomeren, 1981, p.86).

In short, in patients with minor closed head injury, it is possible to demonstrate a persistent disturbance of cognitive function that affects their performance in a wide variety of intellectual tasks and which can be attributed to a reduction in their central processing capacity. The tasks in question include several psychometric tests intended to be sensitive to lesions of the frontal lobes, which is of course entirely consistent with what is known about the probable sites of traumatic cortical damage (*see* Chapter2, pp. 45–7, 59–60). Among patients with severe closed head injury there tends to be an even more pronounced and widespread impairment of their cognitive abilities (e.g., Vigouroux *et al.*, 1971). This impairment may extend even to fairly simple mental abilities, such as counting backwards and giving items of general information (Brooks, 1976; Conkey, 1938), and in very severe cases can constitute a persistent condition of post-traumatic dementia (Denny-Brown, 1945b; Symonds, 1937). The latter was well documented as a progressive and relatively stereotyped disorder among ex-professional boxers before the introduction of stricter medical controls in boxing (Roberts, 1969).

When considered across all head-injured patients, the magnitude and extent of their intellectual impairment is related to several prognostic indicators. First, at an empirical level the degree of cognitive deficit tends to be correlated with the duration of coma (Brink *et al.*, 1970; Levin and Eisenberg, 1979a, 1979b; Levin *et al.*, 1977b; Ruesch, 1944; van Zomeren and Deelman, 1976, 1978; Winogron *et al.*, 1984). However, Kløve and Cleeland (1972) found that this relationship only held within the first three months after the head injury, and that it was no longer significant when the effects of other clinical variables were taken into account. Second, a few studies have found that the degree of cognitive impairment after closed head injury may be related to the depth of coma on admission to hospital according to the Glasgow Coma Scale (Levin and Eisenberg, 1979a, 1979b; Winogron *et al.*, 1984). Third, the degree of cognitive deficit is related to the duration of PTA (Chadwick *et al.*, 1981a; Gronwall and Sampson, 1974, Expt. I; Gronwall and Wrightson, 1981; Ruesch, 1944; van Zomeren and Deelman, 1978). Fourth, the degree of cognitive deficit is related to the incidence of positive neurological signs, diffuse electroencephalographic abnormalities or abnormalities revealed by computerized tomography, and intracranial haematomas, but not to the incidence of skull fractures or measures of acute intracranial pressure (Dye *et al.*, 1979; Kløve and Cleeland, 1972; Levin *et al.*, 1977b; Ruesch, 1944b; Ruesch and Moore, 1943; van Zomeren and Deelman, 1978; Winogron *et al.*, 1984).

Verbal and Nonverbal Intelligence

The Wechsler Adult Intelligence Scale

In the context of neuropsychological assessment, the obvious way in which to evaluate acquired disorders of cognitive function is by means of formal psychometric testing on standardized intelligence scales. The most widely used test is undoubtedly the Wechsler Adult Intelligence Scale (WAIS: Wechsler, 1955). As mentioned in Chapter 3, this consists of 11 subtests:

Verbal subtests:	*Performance subtests*:
Information	Digit Symbol
Comprehension	Picture Completion
Arithmetic	Block Design
Similarities	Picture Arrangement
Digit Span	Object Assembly
Vocabulary	

The raw scores on the individual subtests are transformed into a common scale between 0 and 19, and the total of the scaled scores is converted to an Intelligence Quotient (IQ) by comparison with the total scores achieved by a standardization sample of the appropriate age-range. Separate Verbal and Performance IQs may be obtained by summing the scaled scores on the relevant subtests, or else a Full scale IQ may be derived from the scaled scores on all eleven subtests. In 1981, the Wechsler Adult Intelligence Scale–Revised (WAIS-R) was published; some of the original test items were replaced, the order of the constituent subtests was changed, and a new set of population norms was produced (Wechsler, 1981).

Newcombe and Artiola i Fortuny (1979) have argued that conventional psychometric testing has considerable shortcomings in the context of the evaluation of psychological deficits in patients with brain lesions:

> In particular, intelligence tests (with or without a risky juggling of subtest scores) are flagrantly inadequate as measures of intellectual handicap following brain injury . . . Intelligence tests tend to measure well-practised skills in a highly structured setting. They were not designed to measure the effects of brain injury and their limited capacity to do so depends, to some extent, on the age at which the injury was sustained . . . [The] coarse grain of these tests, eminently suitable for screening, is not sensitive to the subtler problems of attentional control and fatigue associated with brain injury. (p. 183)

Other writers have noted that the WAIS continues to be used widely in neuropsychological research even though it was designed for a different purpose

(Lezak, 1987; Parsons and Prigatano, 1978). Nevertheless, many researchers have turned to tests such as the WAIS in order to determine the effects of closed head injury on human cognition.

In the earliest study of this sort, Ruesch (1944b) administered four tests from the Wechsler-Bellevue Intelligence Scale (the predecessor to the WAIS: Wechsler, 1944) to 70 patients between one and three months after closed head injuries. The mean IQ prorated from the scaled scores on these four tests was 94.5, which was essentially what was expected on the basis of the patients' educational background. Cole (1945) reported preliminary findings from 119 patients in the same series when they were similarly tested on portions of the Wechsler-Bellevue Intelligence Scale roughly six months after their discharge from hospital. Only four cases achieved poorer performances than had been expected on the basis of their educational background, and in each case the patient's psychiatric history cast some doubt on the validity of the latter estimate. Cole concluded: 'We are therefore not certain of a single clear example of continued intellectual impairment in this selected group of patients' (p. 477). However, Cole also presented informal data showing that head-injured patients suffered from a transient impairment in the speed with which they could perform coordinated actions, such as tying knots, buttoning and unbuttoning a coat, or dealing playing cards. In this context, it is interesting that Chadwick *et al.* (1981a, 1981b) found an impairment in manual dexterity among head-injured children which persisted for at least a year after their accidents. Ruesch *et al.* (1945) employed a slightly different set of four subtests from the Wechsler-Bellevue to assess 128 patients with head injuries. The mean prorated IQ was 96 in the case of 49 patients tested within four weeks of their accidents and 107 in the case of 79 patients tested more than four weeks (in most cases more than a year) afterwards. The difference between these means was statistically significant, but it is obvious that both are within the normal range.

Subsequently, Dailey (1955) administered the Wechsler-Bellevue Intelligence Scale to 31 patients with post-traumatic epilepsy about five years after their head injuries. No results were presented concerning their Full Scale IQs, but their Verbal IQs were found to be negatively related to the duration of post-traumatic unconsciousness, even when variations in their premorbid intellectual status were taken into account by controlling for the number of years of education. Black (1973) administered the WAIS to 50 patients with closed head injuries and obtained an average Full Scale IQ of 84.5; as mentioned in Chapter 4, this was significantly poorer than the mean IQ achieved by 50 cases with penetrating brain injuries and significantly impaired in comparison with a population mean of 100. Bond (1975, 1976) reported findings on the WAIS from 40 patients with severe head injury at intervals between three and more than 24 months after their accidents. Those who were tested within the first six months showed a pronounced decrement in Full Scale IQ that varied with the duration of PTA. Subsequently, those patients in whom PTA had lasted for less than 12 weeks achieved mean IQs that were within the normal range; however, those in whom PTA had lasted for more than 12 weeks continued to demonstrate impaired performance with little sign of any restitution of function. Across the entire sample of patients, there were significant negative correlations between Full Scale IQ and clinical ratings of the degree of neurophysical, mental and social disability.

Dye *et al.* (1979) found a mean Full Scale IQ of 88.0 on the WAIS among 48 head-injured patients, but a mean IQ of 101.3 among 16 control patients drawn from other accident victims who had not sustained head injuries. Levin *et al.* (1981a) assessed 21 patients with severe head injury who had been aphasic during their initial hospitalization. Those who showed a persistent generalized disruption of language function at least six months later were substantially impaired in terms of both their Verbal IQ and their Performance IQ, while those whose language function had returned to normal showed no sign of any deficit on the WAIS. Rimel *et al.* (1981) administered the WAIS to 69 patients with minor closed head injuries roughly three months after their accidents; no quantitative data were presented, but they apparently found 'no significant differences from established norms' (p. 226). In contrast, Timming *et al.* (1982) assessed 30 patients with severe head injuries before their discharge roughly 13 weeks following their accidents and found an average Full Scale IQ among the 19 patients who completed the WAIS of only 76.3. When considering five cases of chronic global amnesia resulting from closed head injuries, Corkin *et al.* (1985) found an average Full Scale IQ on the WAIS or the WAIS-R of 98.0, which was taken to be within the normal range. Finally, Solomon *et al.* (1986) reported a mean Full Scale IQ of 93.85 in 126 patients with closed head injury: this reflects a significant impairment for the sample as a whole, even though such a score would be within normal limits for an individual patient.

Some researchers have focused upon particular subtests of the WAIS. This has been motivated partly by the practical need to reduce the amount of time that would otherwise have to be devoted to administering the test in its entirety. With this aim in mind, various proposals have been made for abbreviating both the WAIS (e.g., Levy, 1968; Maxwell, 1957) and the WAIS-R (e.g., Cyr and Brooker, 1984; Roth *et al.*, 1984; Silverstein, 1982). As mentioned earlier, Ruesch (1944b) gave four subtests from the Wechsler-Bellevue Intelligence Scale (Similarities, Comprehension, Block Design and Digit Symbol) to 70 patients between one and three months after closed head injuries. Their average scaled scores were in each case between one half and one standard deviation below that expected in a normal population. There was no significant difference on any of the subtests between 17 patients who suffered complications such as intracranial haematoma, fractured skull, or bloody spinal fluid, and 53 patients with simple loss of consciousness.

In a very similar manner, Reynell (1944) selected six subtests from those described by Wechsler (1941): three of these tests (Vocabulary, General Information and General Comprehension) were chosen because they were expected to be relatively insensitive to brain damage, whereas the other three (Arithmetic Reasoning, Digit Retention and

Similarities) were chosen because they were expected to be particularly sensitive to brain damage. These tests were administered to 520 military personnel with head injuries (of whom 95 per cent were cases of closed head injury), and Full Scale IQs were prorated from their performance on each set of tests. In 117 patients, most of whom were cases of moderate or severe head injury (in the sense that they had suffered a period of PTA lasting at least 'a few hours'), the two estimates of IQ differed by ten points or more. The most conspicuous deterioration was in the ability to repeat sequences of digits backwards (cf. Lezak, 1979).

Similar results were found by Tooth (1947) in the case of 100 naval personnel with head injuries using five of the Wechsler subtests together with Kohs' blocks test and two sorting tests. Tooth's sample included an unspecified number of patients with gunshot wounds, but deficits on the Arithmetic Reasoning, Digit Retention and Similarities tests were most pronounced in the case of patients in whom the duration of PTA had been longer that 24 hours (who were more likely to have received closed head injuries). Nevertheless, Tooth found broadly the same pattern of deficit in 50 neurotic patients from a naval psychiatric clinic, which led him to the conclusion that 'this apparently specific type of differential failure is not peculiar to the head injuries and cannot, therefore, be exclusively determined by organic intellectual impairment' (p. 3). On the other hand, the magnitude of the impairment shown by the head-injured patients on the Similarities test was significantly greater among those who complained of memory disturbance and irritability following their accidents, which Tooth interpreted as evidence in favour of a physical basis. However, regarding the idea of looking for specific patterns of impairment across different tests he suggested that 'while group differences are clear enough, the deviation of individuals may be so slight or so variable that the method is of limited value in the assessment of the individual case' (p. 10).

Somewhat different findings were obtained in a much more recent study by Levin and Goldstein (1986), who compared 12 cases of severe closed head injury with ten normal controls. These head-injured patients were found to be significantly impaired in terms of their age-corrected scores on the Comprehension, Information and Digit Span subtests of the WAIS-R, though not on the Similarities subtest. Not surprisingly, they were also significantly impaired in terms of their Verbal IQs, prorated from their performance on these four subtests. Indeed, their average Verbal IQ of 86.7 was found to be 16.7 points below their average premorbid Verbal IQ, estimated from their age, race, sex, education and occupation, and across individual cases the degree of estimated intellectual deterioration tended to increase with the duration of impaired consciousness following their accidents ($r = +0.50$). Levin *et al.* (1987c) similarly compared 57 cases of minor closed head injury (defined as a loss of consciousness lasting 20 min or less) with 56 normal controls on the Digit Span and Digit Symbol subtests of the WAIS. The head-injured patients were found to be significantly impaired on both tasks when tested within a week of their accidents, but not when retested one month or three months later. However, as mentioned earlier in this chapter, the initial impairment shown by the head-injured patients in this study can be ascribed to the generalized anxiety-producing effects of their involvement in a major accident, and their subsequent improvement might merely reflect the results of practice. McMillan and Glucksman (1987) found no sign of any difference in performance on an abbreviated version of the WAIS-R administered within seven days of the accident between 24 patients who had sustained a moderate head injury and 20 patients who had sustained an orthopaedic injury.

Verbal IQ and Performance IQ

Wechsler's original distinction between Verbal IQ and Performance IQ was based largely upon an *a priori* classification of the corresponding subtests, and was not necessarily intended to correspond to qualitatively distinct forms of cognitive function. It has nevertheless received some empirical confirmation from studies that have reported factor analyses of the WAIS (Maxwell, 1960) and the WAIS-R (Canavan *et al.*, 1986). Vigouroux *et al.* (1971) presented data from 11 patients with severe closed head injury who had been tested on a psychometric battery including the Wechsler-Bellevue Intelligence Scale between 15 and 30 days after recovery of consciousness followed by retesting six months and 18 months later. Both their Verbal IQs and their Performance IQs showed some initial impairment with most recovery occurring within the first six months. There was however little apparent difference between the two IQ measures, and Vigouroux *et al.* concluded that 'the disturbances led to a generalized modification of mental functions' (p. 337). Nevertheless, subsequent research has tended to suggest that Performance IQs are more vulnerable to disruption as the result of a closed head injury than Verbal IQs.

A particularly well-designed study was reported by Becker (1975) in which ten patients with closed head injury were compared with a control group consisting of hospital staff and orthopaedic patients. Since the head-injured patients were enlisted in the US Navy, their premorbid IQs could be estimated from the General Classification Test scores that they had obtained on induction into service. It was therefore possible to show that the control group was well matched on this variable as well as other pertinent characteristics. The WAIS was administered to each head-injured patient within two weeks of their accidents and again about 10 or 11 weeks later. The control subjects were also tested on two occasions with the same intervening interval. The results are shown in Table 5.1.

The first point to note about these results is that the head-injured patients were impaired relative to the control subjects in terms of their Full Scale IQs and in terms of most of the constituent subtests, but that this impairment was rather more pronounced in the case of the Performance subtests than in the case of the Verbal

Table 5.1   Mean IQ and subtest scores for head-injured patients and controls on two successive administrations of the Wechsler Adult Intelligence Scale

	Head-injured		Control	
	Original	Retest	Original	Retest
Information	9.1	9.5	10.8	11.2
Comprehension	8.6	10.5	11.5	12.6
Arithmetic	8.2	9.5	9.7	10.6
Similarities	8.7	10.1	11.9	12.5
Digit Span	8.2	9.9	11.0	11.1
Vocabulary	9.6	10.3	11.1	11.3
Verbal IQ	93.7	100.7	106.0	109.2
Digit Symbol	6.4	8.0	11.4	12.7
Picture Completion	8.5	10.9	11.3	11.9
Block Design	6.6	9.9	11.6	11.8
Picture Arrangement	7.3	8.9	9.7	11.1
Object Assembly	6.1	8.9	11.8	13.3
Performance IQ	80.3	95.7	107.1	113.5
Full Scale IQ	87.1	98.4	106.9	111.9

Source: Becker, B. (1975) 'Intellectual changes after closed head injury', *Journal of Clinical Psychology*, 31, pp. 307–9. Copyright Clinical Psychology Publishing Company, Brandon, VT, USA, reprinted by permission.

subtests. This pattern of results has been obtained in other studies, which have also found that Performance IQs show a clearer correlation with independent neurological measures of the severity of a closed head injury than Verbal IQs (Bond, 1975, 1976; Corkin *et al.*, 1985; Dye *at el.*, 1979; Kløve and Cleeland, 1972; Levin *et al.*, 1982b; Mandleberg, 1975, 1976; Mandleberg and Brooks, 1975; Prigatano *et al.*, 1984; Timming *et al.*, 1982; cf. McMillan and Glucksman, 1987; Solomon *et al.*, 1986). Timming *et al.* found that Performance IQs were especially impaired in those patients whom computerized tomography had shown to have enlarged ventricles; indeed several of their patients who fell in this category were simply incapable of attempting the relevant subtests of the WAIS. Moreover, these findings are not merely an artefact of the specific materials or procedures involved in the WAIS, because similar results have been obtained in studies of intellectual deficits in head-injured children (Chadwick *et al.*, 1981a, 1981b, 1981c; Winogron *et al.*, 1984; cf. Woo-Sam *et al.*, 1970) that have used the Wechsler Intelligence Scale for Children (WISC: Wechsler, 1949).

In addition, several studies have used the Mill Hill Vocabulary Scale (Raven, 1962) together with Raven's (1960) Progressive Matrices test, which is a nonverbal test of problem solving and reasoning requiring the ability to conceptualize spatial and numerical relationships of an abstract nature. Although raw scores on these tests can be expressed as deviation IQ scores by comparing them with published norms (Peck, 1970), these tend to overestimate intelligence levels in the case of the Progressive Matrices test, perhaps because the general public is more familiar with visual problem-solving tasks nowadays than when the normative data were collected (*see* Newcombe, 1969, p. 48). As a result, estimates of mean IQ may differ by up to 10 points between the two tests even among orthopaedic control patients (Brooks and Aughton, 1979a, 1979b). Nevertheless, head-injured patients characteristically show a pronounced impairment on the Progressive Matrices test that increases with the severity of their injury according to the duration of PTA, whereas they show much less impairment on the Mill Hill Vocabulary Scale in comparison with orthopaedic control patients (Brooks and Aughton, 1979a, 1979b; Sunderland *et al.*, 1983) or with published normative data (Brooks *et al.*, 1980; cf. Bond and Brooks, 1976). However, Gentilini *et al.* (1985) found no impairment in the performance of 50 patients tested one month after sustaining minor head injuries on the Progressive Matrices test in comparison with a control group drawn from their friends and relatives.

The second point is that both groups of subjects showed a significant improvement on all three IQ measures but that the improvement demonstrated by the head-injured patients was not significantly greater than that shown by the control subjects. As Becker himself commented, 'This suggests, of course, that much of the "improvement" shown on retesting with the WAIS over relatively short time intervals must be attributed to practice and the experience of having taken the test' (p. 307). In fact, it has been known for a long time that IQ tests are susceptible to practice effects. This was formally demonstrated by Gerboth (1950), who tested 100 students on the two parallel forms of the Wechsler-Bellevue Intelligence Scale with an interval of four months between the two testing sessions. Subsequently Quereschi (1968) obtained similar findings in administering the WISC and the WAIS to 124 15-year-olds with a three-month interval between the testing sessions. Consistent with this formal evidence, the amount of improvement shown by the head-injured patients in Becker's own study was somewhat greater in the case of their Performance IQs than in the case of their Verbal IQs, but this also tended to be true of the control subjects. Indeed, the improvement which was shown by the head-injured patients was significantly greater than that shown by the control subjects on only two of the 11 subtests (Digit Span and Block Design). This outcome could be ascribed not so much to any particularly conspicuous improvement in the case of Becker's head-injured sample, as to the fact that his control sample showed virtually no improvement on these subtests at all. At least in the case of Block Design this result may be spurious, insofar as both Gerboth and Quereschi had found notable practice effects on this subtest. In the case of three of the remaining subtests (Comprehension, Picture Completion and Object Assembly), the apparently good improvement shown by the head-injured patients in Becker's study proved not to be significant when compared with the amount of improvement that was shown by the control subjects.

Becker suggested that his data should make clinicians very cautious about concluding that head-injured patients had recovered normal function simply because their IQs were back to premorbid levels. Equivalently, as Miller (1979) counselled, 'an IQ level consistent with what is known of the victim's abilities prior to the injury should not be used by itself as evidence of lack of any serious impairment' (p. 89). It certainly follows that longitudinal studies involving the repeated testing of head-injured patients (e.g., Black *et al.*, 1971; Bond, 1975, 1976; Bond and Brooks, 1976; Vigouroux *et al.*, 1971; Woo-Sam *et al.*, 1970) in themselves provide little or no information about the nature or the extent of recovery. However, Becker's data do not rule out the possibility of evaluating an individual patient's test performance over several occasions. Indeed, only by repeated testing during the post-traumatic period is it possible to assess the spontaneous recovery of cognitive function, the scope for treatment or rehabilitation and the efficacy of any therapeutic intervention with regard to the long-term outcome (Baddeley *et al.*, 1980; *see* Chapter 7, pp. 252–69).

Controlling for Practice Effects

The moral once again is that an appropriate comparison group must be identified which matches the head-injured patient or patients on *all* relevant respects. This includes their prior experience or familiarity not merely with the particular testing materials but with the broad assessment procedures, or what Baddeley *et al.* (1980) referred to as the patients' 'test sophistication'. As they explained with regard to the evaluation of learning and remembering, 'a subject given the same learning task but using different words will nevertheless improve his performance, developing better learning strategies or perhaps simply becoming more at ease in the test situation' (p. 140). The latter characteristics can obviously be controlled by administering a similar programme of repeated psychometric testing to the comparison group of choice (e.g., Dikmen and Reitan, 1976; Groher, 1977; Rutter *et al.*, 1980). Nevertheless, this is obviously a costly endeavour in terms of both time and resources (cf. also Brooks *et al.*, 1984) and may be vulnerable to motivational problems, leading to poorer performance and an increased likelihood of patients dropping out of the research programme (Baddeley *et al.*, 1980).

This approach was adopted by Klonoff *et al.* (1977), who compared each of 231 children admitted to hospital with head injuries with a normal control subject matched for age and sex; those under five years of age were assessed on the Stanford-Binet test, while those over five years of age were assessed on the WISC. The head-injured children were assessed during their initial hospitalization and at five annual examinations thereafter; the mean Full Scale IQs of 114 head-injured children who were assessed at both the initial session and the final session increased from 102.5 at the former to 112.3 at the latter. The control children were assessed in a similar way shortly after their referral and at five annual examinations thereafter; the mean Full Scale IQs of the control children that had been matched with the 114 head-injured children increased from 114.8 at the initial test to 120.4 at the final test. In other words, although both groups showed increases in their IQs over the six annual sessions, and although the difference between the two groups was significant at each examination, the magnitude of this difference progressively decreased.

The same approach was adopted by Chadwick *et al.* (1981a) in a further study of intellectual functioning in head-injured children. A group of 25 children with severe head injuries (defined by a PTA lasting longer than a week) and a group of 29 children with 'mild' head injuries (defined by a PTA lasting between an hour and a week) were compared with 28 children with orthopaedic accident injuries. All three groups received a short version of the WISC consisting of three Verbal subtests (Similarities, Vocabulary and Digit Span) and three Performance subtests (Block Design, Object Assembly and Coding). The Verbal subtests were carried out at an initial assessment and at a 1-year follow-up; the Performance subtests were additionally carried out at a $2\frac{1}{4}$ -year follow-up; and the severe head injury group and the control group were also examined on the Digit Span and Coding subtests at a further assessment four months after their accidents. The control group showed increases in both their prorated Verbal IQ (3 points in one year) and their prorated Performance IQ (9.4 points in $2\frac{1}{4}$ years). The children with mild head injuries showed a slight deficit in both their Verbal IQ and their Performance IQ in comparison with the control group thoughout the study. The children with severe head injuries showed a similarly modest deficit in their Verbal IQ, but a pronounced deficit in their Performance IQ which resolved to the level shown by the children with mild head injuries within a year (*see also* Chadwick *et al.*, 1981b). Chadwick *et al.* concluded that the deficit in the severe head-injury group was due to brain damage, whereas the deficit in the mild head-injury group was due to 'some other set of influences' (pp. 52–53). As Rutter (1981) subsequently elaborated this remark: 'Although the IQ scores of the children with mild head injuries remained below those of the control children, the lack of recovery implied that the cognitive deficit antedated the injury (and presumably was a function of their more disadvantaged social background)' (p. 1534).

In research studies, as opposed to therapeutic trials, it is possible to adopt a different strategy for evaluating practice effects. This was exemplified in a study by Mandleberg and Brooks (1975), who compared 40 patients with severe closed head injuries (in whom the duration of PTA was greater than four days) and 40 patients from a Department of Psychological Medicine. The head-injured patients were tested at roughly six weeks, five months, ten months and three years after their accidents, but for four different subgroups of ten patients the testing programme began at different points in this sequence. It was therefore possible to compare the four different groups at the three-year assessment, at which point the relevant patients had undergone testing on three, two, one, or no previous occasions. Since there were no significant differences between these four groups in their Verbal IQ, Performance IQ, or Full Scale IQ on the WAIS, Mandleberg and Brooks concluded that their sample of head-injured patients had not benefitted from the effect of practice. Comparisons among the head-injured patients at the four testing sessions and the control group showed that the head-injured cases were more impaired in their Performance IQs than in their Verbal IQs, that the former showed a slower recovery than the latter, but that all three IQ measures were within normal limits by the three-year follow-up assessment.

A similar approach was subsequently adopted by Mandleberg (1976). In the first part of this study, data were obtained from 51 patients who had been tested on the WAIS on four occasions, the last of which was up to six years after the original severe closed head injury. However, a further 98 patients had failed to complete the intended testing schedule, and these were divided into four groups according to which of the four occasions had been the first at which they had presented themselves for assessment. In the second part of the study, therefore, data were presented from these four groups solely with regard to the testing occasion in question. This involved a between-subjects comparison of patients who had not previously been tested, and Mandleberg claimed that it represented a replication of the first part of the study which eliminated potential practice effects. A statistical analysis was carried out on the data obtained at the final testing occasion, comparing the patients in the first part of the study (who had received the WAIS on three previous occasions) and those in the second part of the study (who had had no previous experience of the WAIS). Although there was a tendency for the former subjects to achieve higher scores, especially with regard to their Performance IQ, this proved not to be statistically significant, and Mandleberg suggested that concern regarding possible practice effects in serial testing on the WAIS might be misplaced.

It should be noted, however, that in these studies the effects of practice were evaluated by means of comparisons between different groups of subjects, whereas the effects of recovery were evaluated by means of comparisons within each subject's assessment profile. It is of course well known that between-subjects comparisons are less sensitive than within-subjects comparisons. Another problem is that Mandleberg's study was based on adventitious patterns of attendance, but it cannot be assumed that these were independent of the course of recovery. In particular, the patients who made a rapid recovery and returned to some form of employment might have been less willing or able to return for follow-up examination (cf. Levin *et al.*, 1987c); in this case, the patients in the second half of the study would be less likely to demonstrate any residual cognitive impairment, which would tend to counteract any effects of practice shown by those in the first half of the study. In general, it is highly improbable that those patients who respond consistently to follow-up requests and those who do so only sporadically are equally representative of the population of head-injured patients, as Mandleberg himself acknowledged. In the previous report by Mandleberg and Brooks (1975), it is simply unclear whether the different testing schedules were the result of a deliberate research strategy or irregular attendance on the part of the patients themselves. In the light of Becker's (1975) findings it is probably fair to suggest, as did Miller (1979), that Mandleberg and Brooks were probably a little too sanguine about the notion that practice effects could be ignored in the neuropsychological assessment of head-injured patients. Indeed, using a similar design, Brooks *et al.* (1984) reported significant practice effects in different groups of head-injured patients on the Progressive Matrices test and an associate learning test. Moreover, a colleague of Mandleberg and Brooks subsequently acknowledged that the final IQ scores achieved by their subjects were 'unusually high' and almost certainly attributable to the effects of practice (Bond, 1986, p. 357).

Vulnerability of Verbal IQ and Performance IQ

The greater vulnerability of Performance IQs than Verbal IQs appears not to be peculiar to patients with closed head injury but to be a general consequence of most organic brain disorders (Smith, 1975). For instance, a selective reduction in Performance IQ has been obtained in patients with spontaneously arrested congenital hydrocephalus (Richardson, 1978), and of course a similar pattern was noted in Chapter 3 in the particular case of head-injured patients tested during the period of PTA (Mandleberg, 1975). Alexandre *et al.* (1983) went so far as to use a discrepancy between Verbal IQ and Performance IQ of 20 points or more as one criterion for judging whether a head-injured patient was to be regarded as cognitively impaired. Researchers have offered a number of speculations as to the distinctive features of the Verbal and Performance subtests that would tend to give rise to such discrepancies.

Becker (1975) cited as 'the favored explanation' that Performance subtests 'depend heavily upon attention, concentration, immediate memory and present efficiency, rather than general knowledge, verbal fluency, education, experience, and long-term memory' (p. 309). This implies that short-term memory or working memory should be more vulnerable to organic damage than long-term or permanent memory, but the reverse is normally the case. To take an extreme example, patients who are clinically amnesic may often achieve normal scores on conventional tests of immediate memory span (Drachman and Arbit, 1966; Wechsler, 1917). Moreover, it was pointed out in Chapter 4 that the impact of closed head injury is most notable precisely in the area of long-term memory (pp. 114–5).

A different suggestion is that the Verbal and Performance subtests of the WAIS differ in terms of their structural complexity. As Mandleberg and Brooks (1975) commented, 'Verbal items can often be answered by a simple, readily elicited response, and to this extent the Verbal subtests may be regarded as structurally simpler than the Performance subtests, success on which appears to demand the integration of a number of complex functions including perception, learning, manual dexterity, speed, and attention' (p. 1125; *see also* Brooks *et al.*, 1984; Mandleberg, 1975). Brooks and Aughton (1979b) argued in a similar fashion that the Progressive Matrices test constituted a more complex task than the Mill Hill Vocabulary Scale. Nevertheless, in the absence of any independent criterion of structural complexity or any detailed functional analysis of the tasks in question, proposals of this sort have little explanatory power.

A third idea is that Verbal subtests tend to depend upon the retrieval of information from semantic memory whereas Performance subtests rely more upon the encoding of new information either in working memory or else in long-term episodic memory (cf. Brooks and Aughton, 1979b; Mandleberg, 1975). Babcock (1930) originally suggested on the basis of research with 'mentally deteriorated' individuals that 'for a long time after mental mal-functioning begins, old learning lasts practically unimpaired, except possibly for slowness of response, while ability to fixate new impressions shows weakness in varying degrees according to the degree of deterioration' (p. 5). In contrast to the sort of explanation that was offered by Becker (1975), this specifically predicts that Performance IQs are more likely than Verbal IQs to be disrupted by organic disorders that interfere with learning and remembering (cf. Conkey, 1938). Moreover the distinction being made here can be regarded as a special case of that drawn by Cattell (1973) between 'fluid' and 'crystallized' intelligence: the former reflects the ability to adapt to new situations, whereas the latter reflects the application of learned habits or principles. As a general rule, it seems to be the case that cognitive tests which measure fluid functions are more sensitive to brain damage than those which measure crystallized functions (e.g., Milberg *et al.*, 1986).

Finally, Newcombe and Artiola i Fortuny (1979) noted that most Performance subtests were timed, and they suggested that this factor in itself might account for differences in the rate of recovery of Verbal and Performance IQ. Van Zomeren (1981, p. 110) mentioned an unpublished study by Deelman which had shown that head-injured patients performed less well on timed intelligence tests than on tests conducted without a time limit, and he suggested that this was a confounded factor in the distinction between Verbal and Perfomance subtests of the WAIS. Similarly, Chadwick *et al.* (1981a) observed that 'timed measures of visuo-spatial and visuo-motor skills tended to show more impairment than verbal skills' (p. 49; *see also* Chadwick *et al.*, 1981b).

In fact, Babcock (1930) had originally proposed the hypothesis that mental deterioration as the result of organic damage could be measured by comparing performance on tests that emphasized the speed of response and demanded the formation of new memories with tests that were untimed and required only the retrieval of previous information. In more recent work, van Zomeren (1981, p. 110) claimed that head-injured patients suffered from a reduction in their available information-processing capacity, and that this would explain both their performance deficits on tasks in which processing time was crucial and their impairment on tasks which required the formation of new memory traces. Unfortunately, processing limitations would not explain the qualitative nature of the latter impairment: the idea of a reduction in cognitive capacity would be entirely consistent with the conclusion of Chapter 4 that head-injured patients show impaired relational organization in learning and memory, but it would not in itself motivate such a conclusion, and a connection between the two hypothetical mechanisms has yet to be demonstrated by empirical research.

The Left Hemisphere and the Right Hemisphere

The distinction between the Verbal and Performance subtests of the WAIS is of some theoretical interest, because it is commonly thought to map onto the functional asymmetry of the cerebral cortex. In particular, achievement in the Verbal subtests is assumed to depend upon the neural structures located within the cerebral hemisphere that is 'dominant' or specialized for language function (normally the left hemisphere), while achievement in the Performance subtests is assumed to depend upon neural structures within the nondominant cerebral hemisphere (normally the right hemisphere). Differential performance on the two groups of subtests on the part of patients with neurological deficits should therefore be very informative as to the anatomical lateralization of the underlying lesions. As Walsh (1978) expressed this idea:

> Patients with left hemisphere lesions will show relative impairment on the Verbal portions of the scales while conversely patients with lesions in the right hemisphere will show relative impairment on the Performance subtests. Furthermore, patients with diffuse damage will show no such differential effect. (p. 291)

A concrete example of this form of argument is contained within Levin and Peters' (1976) account of a patient with post-traumatic prosopagnosia: 'The finding that visuoconstructive skill was relatively deficient in comparison with verbal scores (Verbal Scale = 101, Performance Scale = 79) raised the question of right hemisphere dysfunction' (pp. 68–69).

However, until the advent of sophisticated medical imaging technology the empirical evidence for this interpretation of the Verbal-Performance distinction was quite unconvincing (*see* e.g., Walsh, 1978, pp. 291–2), and it was really little more than a convenient myth within psychometric testing. Some early investigations relating scores on intelligence tests to the results of computerized tomography (CT) were far from reassuring. Wood (1979) presented findings from 58 patients with unequivocal CT scans showing the presence of a cerebral tumour, taking a discrepancy of ± 18 points between their Verbal and Performance IQs as psychometric evidence for the presence and laterality of a lesion. Out of 22 patients with a tumour restricted to the left hemisphere, just four produced a relative deficit on the Verbal subtests of the WAIS, while another four showed a relative deficit on the Performance subtests. Out of 27 patients with a tumour restricted to the right hemisphere, none showed a relative deficit on the Verbal subtests, but only four produced a relative deficit on the Performance subtests. In short, only 16 per cent of unilateral lesions were correctly lateralized by means of a comparison between the patient's Verbal and Performance IQs, 8 per cent were incorrectly lateralized, and 76 per cent were not diagnosed at all. Wood concluded that 'the W.A.I.S. does not allow us to predict with any degree of confidence the presence, laterality or locus of a lesion' (p. 344; *see also* Warrington *et al.*, 1986).

In the case of patients with closed head injury, however, the picture is somewhat clearer. A study by Uzzell *et al.* (1979) compared CT findings and WAIS results in 26 patients with injuries of varying degrees of severity. The mean Verbal and Performance IQs for the eight patients with CT evidence of a left-hemisphere lesion were 72.1 and 80.8, respectively, while the mean Verbal and Performance IQs for the 13 patients with CT evidence of a right-hemisphere lesion were 96.4 and 78.9, respectively. The two groups differed significantly in terms of their verbal IQs but not in terms of their Performance IQs. A detailed analysis of the patients' age-corrected scaled scores on the individual subtests confirmed that the Verbal subtests differentiated the patients with left- and right-sided lesions, whereas the Performance subtests did not. An alternative procedure devised by McFie (1975) was used to compare the age-corrected scores on individual subtests with those obtained on the Vocabulary and Picture Completion subtests, regarded as reference tests to estimate the patients' premorbid abilities. In this analysis, the patients with left-sided lesions were more impaired on all of the Verbal subtests, significantly so in the case of the Similarities subtest, while those with right-sided lesions were more impaired on all of the Performance subtests, significantly so in the case of the Picture Arrangement and Digit Symbol subtests. Applying these two approaches to the test scores of individual patients showed that in the 21 cases of unilateral pathology the side of the lesion could be correctly diagnosed in 18 cases (86 per cent) and in 19 cases (90 per cent), respectively. These results were taken to confirm the broad validity of the Verbal and Performance subtests as measures of hemispheric function in head-injured patients with CT-documented lesions.

Nevertheless, it is interesting that similar results were not found in a study of head-injured children reported by Chadwick *et al.* (1981c). Each of these patients had sustained a unilateral compound depressed skull fracture, resulting in a torn dura and surgically verified damage to the underlying cerebral hemisphere (to the left hemisphere in 44 cases and to the right hemisphere in 53 cases). They were assessed on a test battery that contained four Verbal subtests and four Performance subtests from the WISC, and the results were prorated to generate estimates of Verbal IQ and Perfromance IQ. Performance on both measures was found to depend upon the presence of generalized damage, which was judged to have occurred (a) if the injury had led to unconsciousness for three days or more, (b) if there was evidence of cerebral oedema that required treatment, or (c) if there were definite motor signs that were either bilateral or ipsilateral to the side of injury. However, there was no significant difference between the cases with left-hemisphere damage and those with right-hemisphere damage with regard to Verbal IQ, Performance IQ, or any of the constituent subtests. This remained true even when the analysis was restricted to those children in whom there were neurological signs of motor abnormalities contralateral to the side of the injury, though the Full Scale IQs of these cases showed an appreciable impairment, which confirmed that their brain injuries were clinically significant. Few of the remaining measures in the test battery produced a significant difference between the children with lesions of the left and right hemispheres. Similar results were obtained by Levin *et al.* (1982b) in comparing severely injured children and adolescents in whom mass lesions had been visualized by CT within the left and right hemispheres. As Chadwick *et al.* noted, these findings are consistent with the proposition that the cognitive effects of lateralized brain injury show less differentiated patterns of performance in children because the cerebral hemispheres 'are less fixedly specialized in their functions during early and middle childhood than is the case in adult life' (p. 135).

Disorders of Language

Given that severe closed head injury can produce a widespread disruption of verbal as well as nonverbal cognitive functioning, it is of interest to enquire into the incidence, nature and severity of specific disorders of linguistic communication among head-injured patients.

The role of verbal responsiveness in the definition of coma and of consciousness was discussed in Chapter 1 (*see* pp. 14–6). Patients who remain comatose or in what Jennett and Plum (1972) called a 'persistent vegetative state' do not produce any communicative response whatsoever. A similar condition of prolonged speechlessness is that of *akinetic mutism*, although Jennett and Plum emphasized that in this condition postural adjustment and stereotyped withdrawal behaviour are usually possible. At a later stage of recovery, patients may still be totally mute, and yet prove to be capable of obeying simple commands. For example, Thomsen (1976) described a severely injured patient who never uttered a single word during the extended period of his hospitalization, nor indeed any other sound except for a loud 'A'. Nevertheless, this patient could spell out individual words by pointing to the correct letters, and he could also type single-word answers to simple questions.

Disorientation and anterograde amnesia during PTA are assessed from the patients' own verbal accounts of their awareness of recent experiences (*see* Chapter 3).

Occasionally, there may be a persistent condition of *reduplicative paramnesia*, which is typified by the patient's mistaken identification of his or her current geographical location as one that was personally significant in the past or more generally the misidentification of a person, place, or event for one that has been previously experienced (Benson *et al.*, 1976). Combined with a profound disorder of memory, confusion and confabulation during the period of PTA, this can be mistakenly construed as being symptomatic of a linguistic disorder. Conversely, however, a severe aphasic condition during these early stages of recovery can be confused with a persistent impairment of consciousness or a frank behavioural disorder (Stone *et al.*, 1978), and it may be difficult to assess less pronounced disorders of language function at this time. Among 50 head-injured patients examined by Levin *et al.* (1976a), the incidence of dysphasia was over 60 per cent among those who were still disorientated with respect to time, compared with 30 per cent among those who had achieved normal orientation. Groher (1977) tested 14 head-injured patients who had been in coma for on average 17 days. He used the Porch Index of Communicative Ability, which is a clinical test of gestural, verbal and graphic language skills. When tested roughly a week after regaining consciousness (presumably while still in PTA), these patients were grossly impaired in all three areas of communicative ability, although in comparison with other individuals with acquired language disorders their gestural skills were the most impaired and their verbal skills were the least impaired.

Aphasic Disturbances

In order to discuss the nature of persistent language disorders among patients with closed head injury, it is necessary to consider briefly the descriptive categories that are applied to cases of acquired aphasia. The dichotomy which was traditionally drawn in clinical practice was that between 'receptive' aphasia (defined as an impairment of comprehension) and 'expressive' aphasia (defined as an impairment of speech production). Geschwind (1971) argued that such a classification was misleading, and instead claimed that

> the most important distinction in disorders of language output is that between fluent and nonfluent aphasias. Patients with the latter produce little speech, which is uttered slowly, with great effort and with poor articulation. Characteristically the speech of such patients lacks the small grammatical words and endings, so that it may take on the quality of a telegram . . .
>
> By contrast, the patients with fluent aphasia effortlessly produce well articulated, long phrases or sentences with a normal grammatical skeleton, having normal rhythm and melody. Such patients often speak at a higher

rate than normal. The speech is abnormal, however, since despite the many words produced, it is often remarkably devoid of content.

> The abnormality of the speech output in the fluent aphasias is manifested primarily by failure to use the correct word, which is substituted for by circumlocutory phrases ('what you use to open a door'), by nonspecific words (like 'thing') or by incorrect words, so-called paraphasias, which are of two kinds. Verbal paraphasias consist of the substitution of one correct English word or phrase for another, sometimes related in meaning (e.g., 'knife' for 'fork'), sometimes totally unrelated (e.g., 'Argentinian rifle' for 'thumb'). Literal (or phonemic) paraphasias consist of the replacement of one or more sounds in otherwise correct words (e.g., 'spoot' for 'spoon'). (p. 655)

Geschwind's distinction between fluent and nonfluent forms of aphasia was rapidly accepted in research on acquired disorders of speech and language.

A detailed prospective study of aphasic disorders beyond the phase of PTA was reported by Heilman *et al.* (1971). All patients who were admitted to a major city hospital during a 10-month period with a diagnosis of closed head trauma received an aphasia screening examination once they were alert and cooperative. Those who showed any deficit were subjected to further investigation and assigned to a number of diagnostic categories:

> *Anomic aphasia* was defined as a fluent aphasia in which the patient demonstrates verbal paraphasias and circumlocutions, has normal comprehension and repetition, and has abnormal naming for all kinds of material especially to confrontation. *Wernicke's aphasia* was defined as a fluent aphasia with paraphasia, poor comprehension for spoken and written language, and poor repetition. *Broca's aphasia* was defined as non-fluent aphasia with good comprehension, which may improve slightly in repetition, series speech, and singing. *Global aphasia* was defined as a non-fluent aphasia with poor comprehension, poor repetition, and poor naming. *Conduction aphasia* was defined as a fluent aphasia with literal paraphasia, good comprehension, but very poor repetition and impaired naming. We defined *the syndrome of the isolated speech area* as a fluent aphasia with poor comprehension, but with excellent repetition and echolalia. (p. 266, italics added)

Out of the consecutive series of 750 head-injured patients, just 15 cases of aphasia were identified. One of these was excluded from further study because he met the diagnostic criteria only when lethargic, not when alert. A second patient was excluded because surgical treatment had been carried out before the aphasiological examination. Of the other 13 patients, nine had an anomic aphasia, while four had a Wernicke's aphasia, and no other type of aphasia was seen.

As implied in the definition quoted above from Heilman *et al.* (1971), anomic aphasia (also described as *amnesic, amnestic,* or *nominal aphasia*) is a relatively specific disorder of language function that is marked by an inability to identify objects or people by their names. This can typically be demonstrated in formal tests of object naming ('naming to confrontation'), but may also be reflected in the patient's spontaneous conversational speech. In both cases different sorts of anomic errors may be produced (the examples are taken from Levin, 1981):

1 semantic approximations (for instance, saying 'snout' for the tusks of an elephant);
2 circumlocutions (for instance, saying 'to make music' for the pedals of a piano);
3 concrete representations (for instance, saying 'orange' for a circle).

In contrast to this pronounced difficulty in word finding, the patient's ability both to comprehend and to repeat aloud spoken utterances may be essentially normal, as is illustrated by the individual cases described by Heilman *et al.* In addition, either through the nature of the errors or through the accompanying gestures and actions it may well be apparent that the patient understands perfectly well the use or function of the objects in question. On the other hand, Benson and Geschwind (1967) stressed that anomic aphasia after closed head injury was a generalized naming deficit that was not restricted to particular classes of objects or stimuli. They also argued that it was a direct consequence of focal brain damage and not simply one manifestation of memory disturbances, on the grounds that most patients with severe post-traumatic memory dysfunction do not suffer from anomic disorders. As an extreme example, Corkin *et al.* (1985) found no pronounced deficits of speech comprehension or production among patients with chronic global amnesia resulting from closed head injury.

Wernicke's aphasia (also described as *receptive* or *sensory aphasia*) is marked by an inability to comprehend both spoken language and written language (dyslexia). Among patients with severe closed head injuries it may be characterized by an impaired ability to repeat spoken utterances and by relatively fluent (indeed, unusually voluble) spontaneous speech in which incorrect words or phrases or even frank neologisms have been substituted (paraphasia). Newcombe (1982) has however noted the difficulty of giving an accurate assessment of a head-injured patient's problems in the area of speech comprehension. Subsequent research has confirmed that anomic aphasia and Wernicke's aphasia are the most common forms of language disorder in head-injured patients, whereas other forms of disorder are very uncommon. In particular, although it has been suggested that Broca's aphasia may result from closed head injury (Bakay and Glasauer, 1980, p. 108), this condition has been observed rarely if at all in the detailed clinical examination of consecutive series of patients (Levin *et al.*, 1976a; Thomsen, 1975, 1976). In contrast, as Levin (1981) pointed out, Broca's aphasia is a fairly common outcome of penetrating missile wounds of the brain (e.g., Alajouanine *et al.*, 1957). Turning to another form of acquired aphasia, one case of post-traumatic conduction aphasia (which as mentioned above is marked by a disproportionate impairment in repetition tasks) was reported by Warrington and Shallice (1970; Warrington *et al.*, 1971; *see* Chapter 4, pp. 115–6). Nevertheless, performance in tests of sentence repetition is normally preserved in cases of head injury (Levin *et al.*, 1976a, 1981a; Levin and Eisenberg, 1979a).

The results obtained by Heilman *et al.* indicate that clinical aphasia following closed head injury is relatively rare, occurring in about 2 per cent of all hospital admissions. (Conversely, head-injured patients may not figure at all in samples of neurological patients who are chosen retrospectively as instances of aphasia: Halpern *et al.*, 1973.) A previous study by Arseni *et al.* (1970) had similarly found just 34 cases of aphasia in a consecutive series of 1544 head-injured patients. These tended to be the consequences of assaults or accidental injury with a variety of objects rather than of traffic accidents or other causes (cf. Thomsen, 1974). The focal nature of the resulting brain damage was also shown by the high proportion (71 per cent) of these cases who had required surgical intervention for intracranial haematoma. Arseni *et al.* suggested in particular that post-traumatic aphasia was generally associated with lesions of the parietal lobe of the dominant cerebral hemisphere.

Heilman *et al.* (1971) reported that seven of their 13 aphasic patients had received a blow to the right orbito-frontal region of the cranium, whereas four had received blows to the left temporo-pariental region and two had no external evidence of trauma, though there seemed to be no relation between the site of impact and the nature of the aphasic disorder that had ensued. Although there was little direct evidence available as to the underlying structural pathology, Heilman *et al.* speculated from post-mortem evidence in other patients that 'contusion of the dorsolateral surface of the temporal lobe and temporoparietal junction is the most likely aetiology for these aphasias' (p. 269; *see also* Alajouanine *et al.*, 1957; and cf. Geschwind, 1971). The evidence that was reviewed in Chapter 2 (p. 46) indicates that contusions in these areas are extremely rare, which would account for the remarkably low incidence of aphasic disorders following closed head injury. The incidence of such disorders is not related to conventional clinical measures of the severity of head injury (de Morsier, 1973; Levin and Eisenberg, 1979a, 1979b; Sarno, 1980; cf. Heilman *et al.*, 1971). More specifically, as Levin (1981) noted, 'prolonged coma is neither a necessary nor sufficient condition for residual aphasia' (p. 455; *see also* Levin *et al.*, 1976a, p. 1069).

Subclinical Disturbances of Language

Nevertheless, subclinical manifestations of disordered comprehension and production of speech (or 'nonaphasic disorders of language': Prigatano *et al.*, 1986, p. 19) are common, especially in patients with severe closed head injuries. For instance,

Thomsen (1975) studied 26 patients who had been in coma for at least 24 hours, and found language disorders in 12 of these cases when assessed on average four months after their accidents. Naming errors and paraphasia were the most common deficits, while comprehension and writing problems were also observed, but symptoms characteristic of expressive disorders were rarely seen. Subsequently, Thomsen (1976) described a further 16 patients with severe closed head injuries in whom focal lesions due to intracranial haematoma or severe anoxia had been surgically verified. When examined on average 15 weeks after their accidents, 11 of these patients showed a wide variety of linguistic deficits, leading Thomsen to emphasize the 'multisymptomatic' nature of post-traumatic language disorders. In particular, nearly all of these patients demonstrated 'impaired analysis of speech, impaired analysis of reading, amnestic aphasia, verbal paraphasia, agraphia, and perseveration' (p. 363).

Levin *et al* (1976a) evaluated 50 head-injured patients on six constituent subtests of the Multilingual Aphasia Examination (MAE: Benton, 1967, 1969). They were tested 'after periodic monitoring of orientation to surroundings and time . . . had disclosed an absence or at least marked reduction of confusion' (p. 1063), although 38 per cent were still impaired on a test of temporal orientation (Benton *et al.*, 1964) when the MAE was administered. In comparison with 30 control patients with diverse somatic disease, they were impaired on tests of visual object naming and verbal fluency and also on the Token Test (De Renzi and Vignolo, 1962), though they were not significantly impaired on tests of sentence repetition, auditory comprehension, or reading comprehension. Duration of coma and signs of brain-stem involvement were negatively correlated with their performance on all six subtests, significantly so in the case of object naming, verbal fluency, auditory comprehension and reading comprehension, but their test performance was not related to the presence or absence of skull fracture, intracranial haematoma, or neurological findings of damage predominantly involving one or other cerebral hemisphere.

In the study by Groher (1977) mentioned earlier the 14 head-injured patients were reassessed on the Porch Index of Communicative Ability (PICA) at four successive intervals of 30 days after its initial administration. Their scores showed considerable improvement, but still reflected a significant impairment in both receptive and expressive language capabilitites even at nearly five months after their accidents. Nevertheless, although all the patients had initially shown marked anomia, their naming to confrontation proved to be normal at the final session. A comparison group of patients with long-standing disorders of language and memory showed no sign of any improvement across five testing sessions, and Groher therefore concluded that the improvement shown by his main group of patients was not simply the consequence of practice on the task. Groher asserted that the final status of his patients was unrelated to the duration of unconsciousness, but from the data shown in his Table 4 highly significant correlations emerge between the number of days in coma and the patients' final scores in all three language modalities covered by the PICA (gestural, $r = -0.73$; verbal, $r = -0.73$; graphic, $r = -0.64$; $P < 0.01$ in each case).

Najenson *et al.* (1978) monitored the recovery of 15 patients with prolonged coma after closed head injury. Six patients remained in a persistent vegetative state with no expressive function and minimal evidence of any comprehension. Six patients showed relatively complete recovery of both receptive and expressive functions over the nine months following their accidents. The comprehension of visual gestures and oral commands returned first of all, followed by reading and writing skills and oral expression. Najenson *et al.* emphasized the good potential for recovery of communicative function even following prolonged coma and the close association between the recovery of communication functions and the recovery of locomotor function. However, the three remaining cases showed persistent communication disorders, and eight of the nine patients who showed at least partial recovery were persistently impaired in terms of the motor aspects of speech and especially in the coordination of respiration, articulation and phonation.

Levin *et al.* (1979a) evaluated language function in 27 patients with severe closed head injury, defined in terms of a score on the Glasgow Coma Scale on admission to hospital of 8 or less. The MAE and three subtests from the Neurosensory Center Comprehensive Examination for Aphasia (NCCEA: Spreen and Benton, 1969) were administered on average one year after injury. By this time, all but the most severely disabled patients exhibited normal conversational speech and comprehension of commands, but many continued to show hesitancy in finding words and especially in naming objects presented either visually or tactually.

Levin and Eisenberg (1979a) used the NCCEA to carry out an assessment of persistent language deficits in 64 children and adolescents with head injuries of varying degrees of severity. Nearly one third of the sample showed some impairment of language function during the first six months following injury, especially in terms of object naming. This study found no relationship between the children's scores on the individual subscales of the Glasgow Coma Scale and the subsequent incidence of language deficits. Nevertheless, Johnston and Mellits (1980) found a negative relationship between the duration of coma in head-injured children and their expressive language ability when tested within the first year of injury. In addition, a more recent study carried out by Winogron *et al.* (1984) involving 51 head-injured children showed significant correlations between their *total* scores on the Glasgow Coma Scale and the *magnitude* of subsequent impairment on both an aphasia screening battery and a test of verbal fluency.

Brooks *et al.* (1980) included a simple assessment of language function in an investigation of cognitive sequelae among 89 patients with severe closed head injury. Comprehension was assessed by one part of the Token Test, while speech production was tested by means of a verbal fluency test. No control group was used in this study and no normative data were presented. Neither task showed any correlation with the duration of coma or with the incidence of skull fracture, but two out of three scores on verbal fluency showed a systematic relationship with the duration of PTA. Sarno (1980) described the performance of 56 patients referred to a rehabilitation centre following severe closed head injury on four subtests of the NCCEA covering object naming, verbal fluency, sentence repetition and the Token Test. Eighteen patients were diagnosed as aphasic on the basis of clinical evaluation of their spontaneous speech production and comprehension, and these individuals were found to be profoundly impaired on all four quantitative tests. The remaining 38 patients were not diagnosed as clinically asphasic, but they too were found to have measurable speech and language deficits on formal testing. Sarno described these deficits as instances of 'subclinical aphasia disorder': that is, 'linguistic processing deficits on testing in the absence of clinical manifestations of linguistic impairment' (p. 687). She concluded that 'all traumatically brain-injured patients who have experienced coma will suffer a significant degree of verbal impairment' (p. 689), but she acknowledged that her sample probably consisted of patients whose injuries were particularly severe.

Levin *et al.* (1981a) studied the progress of 21 patients with severe head injuries who were aphasic on the recovery of consciousness. Their residual language deficits at least six months after their accidents were assessed by means of six subtests of the MAE together with three subtests of the NCCEA. On most of the tests roughly 25 per cent of the sample as a whole produced impaired performance and 40 per cent showed impaired naming of visual or haptic stimuli. Altogether 12 patients proved to have persistent language deficits on formal testing: half of them showed a generalized impairment of both receptive and expressive abilities, whereas the other half showed a language deficit confined to a single function, usually that of object naming. The former patients also showed a persistent deficit in terms of both Verbal IQ and Performance IQ according to the WAIS, whereas the latter patients and the nine patients who had fully recovered from their acute aphasia and who produced normal scores on the tests of linguistic competence also produced normal levels of performance on the WAIS. A persistent generalized language impairment was consistently associated with longer periods of coma and with CT evidence of enlarged ventricles at follow-up. Moreover, across the sample as a whole the duration of coma was found to be significantly correlated with performance on visual naming, word fluency, speech comprehension and reading comprehension. The naming of haptic stimuli was disproportionately impaired in the case of those presented to the left hand, which Levin *et al.* attributed to the disruption of interhemispheric connections as the result of damage to the corpus callosum. These and other results led Levin (1981) to sum up the research findings at the time in the following manner:

> The studies of long-term recovery of language after CHI [closed head injury] show an overall trend of improvement that may eventuate in restoration of language or specific deficits ('subclinical' language disorder) in

naming or word finding in about two-thirds of the patients who are acutely aphasic. Generalized language deficit, which is associated with global cognitive impairment, persists in patients who sustain severe CHI. (p. 441)

As mentioned earlier in this chapter, Sunderland *et al.* (1983) tested 33 patients with severe closed head injuries between two and eight months after their accidents. They showed no sign of any impairment on the Mill Hill Vocabulary test in comparison with 37 orthopaedic control patients. They were also given a simple test of semantic processing which consisted of a series of statements that were either obviously true (e.g., 'Canaries have wings' or 'US Presidents hold political office') or obviously false, the latter statements being constructed by recombining the elements within the true statements (e.g., 'Canaries hold political office' or 'US Presidents have wings'). The subjects were required to read through the statements, marking each one as true or false. The head-injured patients were found to be significantly slower than the control patients, producing barely 70 per cent as many correct responses within the allotted time interval, but they were not significantly impaired in terms of the proportion of errors that they made. The two groups still proved to be significantly different from one another when their speed in a finger-tapping task was used to control for the motor component of the semantic-processing task. These results are consistent with the idea that even patients with severe head injuries are largely intact in terms of their comprehension ability, but have a general impairment in terms of their speed of cognitive processing.

Language and Communication

Although it is clear that patients with closed head injury may show language-processing deficits on formal testing in the absence of clinical manifestations of classical aphasia (Sarno, 1980), the results obtained by Sunderland *et al.* raise the possibility that such deficits when they arise simply reflect a broadly based limitation upon the patients' capacity for complex information processing. Indeed, Halpern *et al.* (1973) found that the language disorders that were caused by head injury were unlikely to represent a specific impairment of the capacity to interpret and formulate linguistic utterances that was disproportionate to any impairment of other intellectual functions. Rather, they were much more likely to be just particular aspects of a condition of 'confused language' in which there was 'reduced recognition and understanding of and responsiveness to the environment, faulty short-term memory, mistaken reasoning, disorientation in time and space, and behavior which is less adaptive and appropriate than normal' (p. 163). Levin *et al.* (1976a) considered the notion that post-traumatic linguistic defects might be viewed as instances of general mental impairment, but rejected it on the somewhat tenuous grounds that head-injured patients were typically unimpaired in the repetition of even relatively lengthy sentences. Though not wholly explicit, their own view seems to have been that such defects were subclinical forms of specific aphasic disorders. This was certainly the position adopted by Sarno (1980) and Levin (1981) in the passages quoted above.

In order to contrast these two viewpoints, Payne-Johnson (1986) tested 20 patients who had sustained head injuries of varying degrees of severity on a broad 'communication competence' test battery designed to assess intelligence, expressive and receptive language, articulation, both auditory and visual short-term memory, oral agility, automatic speech, writing, reading and simple mathematics. The scores of the head-injured patients were very similar to those of 15 other accident victims on a standard audiological evaluation, on a test of articulation, and on five subtests concerned with reading, writing and arithemetic skills. However, they were significantly impaired on the remaining 15 subtests concerned with 'verbal recognition, intelligence, speech, language, and memory' (p. 245). The most pronounced deficit was demonstrated on an Oral Agility subtest, which 'taps subjects' ability to manipulate the articulators for speech upon command and through imitation' (*loc. cit.*), and which Payne-Johnson claimed to be mediated by motor centres in the frontal lobe. However, only an Automatized Sequences subtest that assessed the ability to recall overlearned serial information such as the days of the week and the months of the year was significantly related to the severity of the patients' head injuries, graded according to the centripetal model of Ommaya and Gennarelli (1974; *see* Chapter 2). Payne-Johnson concluded that closed head injury 'has an immediate generalized effect upon the cerebral mechanisms subserving intelligence, speech, language, memory, and specific writing, reading, and arithmetic skills' (p. 237).

Other Disorders of Language

Disorders of reading (dyslexia) and writing (dysgraphia) are often observed in conjunction with post-traumatic aphasia, and occasionally they may be manifested in a selective and perhaps even persistent form (*see* e.g., de Morsier, 1973; Newcombe, 1982). There are also a number of speech disorders which can arise following closed head injury without aphasia. These include: *mutism*, the total abolition of speech following the period of coma, which has already been mentioned; *palilalia*, the automatic repetition of one's own words; and *echolalia*, the automatic repetition of words spoken by others. These are all relatively rare conditions in cases of closed head injury, and normally do not occur as isolated disorders of language processing (Thomsen and Skinhøj, 1976).

Thomsen (1976) suggested that post-traumatic mutism in the absence of any receptive impairment was most likely to be an extreme form of *dysarthria*, an impairment of speech function resulting from a disorder of the neuromuscular mechanism responsible for articulation, probably as the result of brain-stem lesions.

This has frequently been reported in research studies of language and speech following closed head injury (Alajouanine *et al.*, 1957; de Morsier, 1973; Gilchrist and Wilkinson, 1979; Groher, 1977; Sarno, 1980; Thomsen, 1975, 1976), and it may persist following the restoration of language function (Brooks *et al.*, 1986a; Najenson *et al.*, 1978; Thomsen, 1974, 1975, 1984). In particular, it was mentioned by Roberts (1969) as being one feature of the 'relatively stereotyped clinical pattern' of traumatic encephalopathy observed in professional boxers (p. 109). Sarno (1980) identified 21 cases of dysarthria among 50 patients referred to a rehabilitation centre following severe closed head injury, and they were found to be significantly impaired across a broad range of tests concerned with speech production and comprehension. Levin (1981) recommended that the Oral Agility subtest of the Boston Diagnostic Aphasia Examination (Goodglass and Kaplan, 1972) would be useful in evaluating dysarthria, and it was precisely this subtest which showed the best discrimination between the head-injured and control patients in the study by Payne-Johnson (1986). Cases of acquired dysarthria are of some interest to cognitive psychologists who are concerned with language and memory because they appear to be capable of phonological coding and subvocal rehearsal despite the absence of feedback from the peripheral speech musculature (Baddeley and Wilson, 1985).

Verbal Skills and Verbal Memory

Given the prevalence of language disorders and dysarthria following closed head injury, it is important to consider whether they are likely to have a role in determining performance in other cognitive tasks. There at least seems to be an association between the two at a descriptive level; as Levin (1981) noted, 'Patients with closed head injury who become aphasic frequently exhibit concomitant neuropsychological deficits' (p. 460). One possibility, of course, is that both the residual memory impairment and the persistent disturbances of language function which result from closed head injury are the expressions of a common underlying deficit, perhaps resulting from disproportionate injury to the temporal lobes (cf. Levin *et al.*, 1982a, p. 145). Nevertheless, given that most tests of retention and cognition place a primary emphasis upon verbal encoding, processing and performance, it is equally conceivable that observable deficits in these latter areas resulting from closed head injury are the result, at least in part, of impaired language function. An obvious form of direct confounding between the assessment of linguistic abilities and the assessment of recall performance is found in the study carried out by Fodor (1972). She asked her subjects to recall lists of objects which had originally been presented as pictures to be named. At least some of the head-injured patients in this study turned out to be impaired in their object-naming ability. It is thus quite impossible to determine whether the deficit subsequently shown by the head-injured patients in the recall of those same objects was caused by this anomic disorder or by a genuine impairment of memory function.

Confounding of this sort is obviously more likely when the materials presented to the subjects and the responses that are demanded of them are verbal in nature. This would explain why language deficits in head-injured patients have little or no effect upon recognition memory for simple geometrical figures, upon the simultaneous matching of different views of unfamiliar faces, nor upon the performance of sensory or motor tasks (Brooks, 1974b; Levin *et al.*, 1976a, 1977b; cf. Levin *et al.*, 1976b). In contrast to these results, Thomsen (1977) found that the generalized impairment of verbal learning that resulted from severe closed head injury was much more pronounced in aphasic patients. A dissociation between these two forms of memory impairment had been reported earlier by Akbarova (1972). Out of 18 head-injured patients with lesions which were predominantly confined to the left hemisphere, 13 patients had relatively selective deficits of verbal memory, and this group tended to demonstrate concomitant disturbances of language function; the cognitive impairment of the remaining five cases was relatively specific to visuospatial memory.

Groher (1977) administered both the Wechsler Memory Scale (WMS) and the Porch Index of Communicative Ability (PICA) to 14 patients on average nearly five months after they had sustained severe closed head injuries. As mentioned in Chapter 4 and earlier in the present Chapter, serious deficits were apparent on both instruments. Moreover, analysis of the results from individual subjects shown in Groher's Table 4 shows that there were significant relationships between the subjects' Memory Quotients on the WMS and their performance in the different language modalities covered by the PICA (gestural, $r = +0.60$; verbal, $r = +0.60$; graphic, $r = +0.70$; $P < 0.05$ in each case). Of course, these are purely correlational findings, and one cannot be entirely confident in inferring causal relationships. Nevertheless, it is probably fair to say that the contribution of memory factors to performance on the PICA is minimal. It is therefore reasonable to conclude from Groher's results that language deficits, as evaluated by the PICA, are an important determinant of the scores achieved by head-injured patients on memory tasks such as the WMS.

Further evidence has been obtained from the use of intelligence tests such as the WAIS. In assessing patients on average 30 months after they had sustained severe closed head injuries, Thomsen (1974) failed to find any difference in terms of Full Scale IQ between 21 patients who showed aphasic symptoms and 29 patients who did not. Nevertheless, Levin *et al.* (1981a) found that head-injured patients who showed a persistent generalized disturbance of language function were profoundly impaired in terms of both Verbal IQ and Performance IQ on the WAIS, whereas those patients whose language functions had returned to normal showed no sign of any intellectual deficit. Subsequently, Levin and Goldstein (1986) found that Verbal IQ was correlated with performance in free recall, and they concluded that 'verbal intellectual functioning is closely linked with performance on this memory task' (p. 652).

From a practical point of view, it is clear that the disorders of speech and language that follow closed head injury are likely to disrupt performance in a wide variety of cognitive tasks. Such disorders are certainly not the only determinants of post-traumatic neuropsychological dysfunction, since head-injured patients are also impaired in their recognition memory for unfamiliar faces and for random geometrical figures that are difficult to label or encode verbally (Brooks, 1974b; Levin *et al.*, 1976a, 1976b; Sunderland *et al.*, 1983) and even in the simultaneous matching of different views of unfamiliar faces (Levin *et al.*, 1977b). Nevertheless, from a methodological point of view, it is vitally important to avoid or at least to minimize this sort of confounding if researchers are to disentangle the effects of closed head injury on human performance.

Concluding Summary

Patients who have suffered closed head injury manifest a disturbance of cognitive function beyond the period of post-traumatic amnesia across a wide varity of tasks. This impairment is to be attributed to a reduction in their central information-processing capacity rather than to a deficit of selective attention or tonic alertness. While the residual cognitive dysfunction that is exhibited in patients with minor closed head injury tends to resolve within the first few weeks after the accident, severely injured patients may show persistent deficits many months later (*see also* Livingston and Livingston, 1985). These deficits are even more pronounced and widespread, and extend even to fairly simple mental activities such as counting backwards and giving items of general information.

Similar deficits are shown by head-injured patients in terms of their Intelligence Quotients according to standardized psychometric instruments such as the Wechsler Adult Intelligence Scale. Performance IQ and scores on nonverbal tests are typically more vulnerable than Verbal IQ and scores on verbal tests. These two aspects of intellectual function appear to be differentially sensitive to damage within the right and left hemispheres. Both tend to improve to within normal limits over the course of 2–3 years after a closed head injury, although in some studies such improvements are confounded with practice effects.

Pronounced and specific disorders of language function are relatively rare after closed head injury and usually take the form of nominal aphasia or Wernicke's aphasia. However, subclinical disturbances of comprehension and speech production are much more common, especially in severely injured patients. These seem to be manifestations of a more general disruption of cognitive and communicative skills, but it is nevertheless true that some decrements in performance in cognitive tasks following closed head injury appear to be the result of impaired language function.

Chapter 6

Subjective Complaints and Personality Disorders

So far this book has emphasized the consequences of closed head injury for higher intellectual functions, and it is true that these are probably the most obvious features of a patient's clinical condition especially during the early stages of recovery. Nevertheless, head-injured patients exhibit a wide variety of other symptoms, and if these persist they may well prove to be even more debilitating in terms of patients' family relationships or future employment. In this chapter I shall consider the broad pattern of postconcussional symptoms as well as the particular clinical condition of a persistent postconcussional syndrome. I shall then go on to consider in more detail the affective, behavioural and psychiatric disturbances that may result from a closed head injury, and the impact which these have upon the patient's immediate relatives and friends.

Postconcussional Symptoms

Even though a patient may make a good recovery from a clinical point of view, the immediate period following a closed head injury is often marked by a particular set of subjective complaints on the part of the patient. As long ago as 1904 Meyer described the overall symptom picture as 'that of a mental weakness shown by *easy fatigue, slowness of thought, inability to keep impressions, irritability, and a great number of unpleasant sensations, above all headaches and dizziness*' (p. 403). Subsequently, Goldstein (1943) characterized these symptoms in more detail as follows:

> Headache is very common. It is described by the patient as a throbbing, or hammering or a feeling of pressure, etc... The patient may be hyper-sensitive to noise, light, effort, and when exposed headache may increase.... Dizziness occurs spontaneously or upon sudden changes of the position of the body or the head. The patient experiences a sensation either that the world is turning around him or uncertainty as to his own body... Dizziness is usually accompanied by vasomotor disturbances and nausea,

particularly if it occurs during attacks. The emotional instability expresses itself in abnormal irritability, sensitivity upon physical or mental effort, anxiety, depression, etc. (p. 328)

Together with the subjective complaints of poor memory and concentration mentioned in Chapters 4 and 5, these are the features that dominate the symptom picture during the first week or so following closed head injury.

In a detailed study of 200 patients admitted to hospital with closed head injury, Denny-Brown (1945a) classified these symptoms into

complaints derived directly from observed structural injury (symptoms of direct physical disorder), psychiatric complaints (symptoms of the order of fatigue, nervousness, anxiety, depression), symptoms of change in personality (separately coded only when there was evident aggressiveness or irritability or prolonged elation, without other mental symptoms) and complaints of uncertain or variable derivation (headache, dizziness, vertigo). (pp. 430–1)

In Denny-Brown's series, 138 (or 69 per cent) of the patients complained of headache at some time after their injury (Brenner *et al.*, 1944), and 99 (or 50 per cent) complained of dizziness at some time after their injury (Friedman *et al.*, 1945). In both cases the most common precipitating factors were sudden changes in posture, fatigue or effort, and emotional stress. Only 11 (or 6 per cent) complained of true vertigo (that is, the sense that either oneself or one's surroundings are in constant movement). In addition, 110 (or 55 per cent) of the patients complained of one or more symptoms after discharge from hospital, the most frequent combination being that of headache, dizziness and anxiety (Denny-Brown, 1945a). Accurate epidemiological information on the incidence of these symptoms does not exist, but subsequent research has tended to confirm that 50–80 per cent of patients who are admitted to hospital following closed head injury will subsequently complain of one or more of these symptoms (Barth *et al.*, 1989; Cook, 1969, 1972; Hjern and Nylander, 1964; Levin *et al.*, 1987b; Lidvall *et al.*, 1974; MacFlynn *et al.*, 1984; McLean *et al.*, 1983).

Lidvall *et al.* (1974) administered structured interviews on the presence of postconcussional symptoms to patients who had been admitted to hospital following cerebral concussion. Out of a total of 83 patients, 73 per cent reported one or more symptoms when interviewed on the second day after their accidents, and 48 per cent reported one or more symptoms when interviewed on the sixth day afterwards. The most frequently reported symptoms on both occasions were headache, dizziness and fatigue, which also constituted the most frequent cluster of symptoms that were simultaneously reported by the same patients. Nevertheless it can be argued that factor analysis is more appropriate than cluster analysis in evaluating the internal structure of reported symptoms. Levin *et al.* (1987b) carried out such an analysis on the responses given by 155 patients during a structured interview into the occurrence and severity of postconcussional symptoms within the first week after they had sustained a minor head injury sufficient to warrant their hospitalization. The most frequently reported symptoms were headaches, fatigability and dizziness, which were reported by 71.0 per cent, 55.5 per cent, and 50.3 per cent of the sample, respectively. The factor analysis yielded five factors which after oblique rotation took the following form:

1   a 'Cognitive-Depression' factor defined by reports of impaired remote memory, poor concentration, impaired thinking, impaired recent memory and depression;
2   a 'Somatic' factor defined by reports of diplopia (double vision), dizziness, vertigo, poor hearing and blurred vision;
3   a 'Sensory-Sleep' factor defined by reports of hallucinations, sleep difficulties and sensitivity to noise;
4   a 'Gustatory-Olfactory' factor defined by reports of impaired taste, smell and appetite; and
5   an 'Irritability-Anxiety' factor defined by reports of bad temper, impatience, and anxiety (though the factor loadings were less than 0.40 in the case of the two latter symptoms).

Levin *et al.* concluded that these factors represented salient dimensions of postconcussional symptoms which could be used to identify different groups of patients with distinctive patterns of symptomatology. However, these factors were all positively intercorrelated, and it is possible to carry out a second-order factor analysis upon the data contained in Table 18–3 of their paper. This yields just a single factor, which implies that the relevant symptoms define a 'monarchical hierarchy' (*see* Cattell, 1965) in which a set of nonoverlapping first-order factors are tied together by one overarching second-order factor, as one might well expect if they were merely different manifestations of the same underlying clinical condition. Nevertheless, the two symptoms that were most frequently reported in this study (headache and fatigability) did not contribute to the factorial solution at all, and this indicates that the symptom picture during the early phase of recovery from a closed head injury is quite fragmentary.

The symptoms in question are often referred to as 'postconcussional' symptoms, although they are not peculiar to patients who have sustained concussional head injuries: they are in particular common among patients who have sustained mild head injuries that did not give rise to any loss of consciousness and even among patients who have sustained neck injuries without a blow to the head (Jacobson, 1969). In a study by McMillan and Glucksman (1987), a checklist of six postconcussional symptoms was given to 24 patients within seven days of sustaining a closed head injury that gave rise to a period of post-traumatic amnesia (PTA) lasting between 1 and 24 hours. For comparison the same checklist was given to 20 patients who had sustained an orthopaedic injury (usually involving an upper limb fracture or sprain). The results are shown in Table 6.1: the proportion of cases reporting each of the symptoms was significantly different between the two groups. At the same time, however, a relative or close friend was asked to describe each patient's symptoms using a more elaborate checklist. The head-injured patients were more likely than the orthopaedic controls to be described as quieter and more tense since their accidents. Nevertheless, in contrast to their own reports the two groups of patients did not differ in the extent to which they were described by their friends and relatives as being irritable, worried, impatient, angry, violent, childlike, forgetful, depressed, happy, calm, peaceful, relaxed, or 'at ease'. As mentioned in Chapter 4 (p. 95), a similar discrepancy was noted between patients and relatives concerning whether the head-injured cases were impaired relative to the orthopaedic cases in terms of their everyday memory ability. McMillan and Glucksman suggested that these disparities between the perceptions of head-injured patients and their relatives might subsequently lead to the development of marital difficulties and other psychosocial problems.

Table 6.1   Percentage of patients reporting six post-concussional symptoms within the first seven days of sustaining a moderate head injury or an orthopaedic injury

Symptom	Head injury	Orthopaedic injury
Headache	71	10
Dizziness	46	5
Irritability	64	16
Fatigue	75	25
Intolerance to noise	38	0
Intolerance to bright lights	33	0

Source: McMillan, T . M. and Glucksman, E. E. (1987) 'The neuropsychology of moderate head injury', *Journal of Neurology, Neurosurgery, and Psychiatry*, 50, 393–7. Reproduced with permission of the authors, editor, and publisher of the *Journal*.

The Postconcussional Syndrome

In many head-injured patients, these characteristic symptoms of the initial post-concussional phase subside within a matter of days or within at most a few weeks. In such cases, these symptoms are usually regarded as a normal part of the process of recovery from closed head injury, not themselves warranting any clinical attention or treatment. Even though these patients may have been rendered unconscious as the result of their injuries, it is only rarely necessary for them to be absent from work following their discharge from hospital, and any such absences are not prolonged (Cook, 1969, 1972). Nevertheless, a substantial proportion of head-injured patients continue to complain of postconcussional symptoms beyond the initial post-traumatic period, in which case these symptoms may well interfere with their ability to return to their previous employment (Denny-Brown, 1945a; Russell and Smith, 1961). This condition of persistent postconcussional symptoms is referred to as the 'postconcussional syndrome' (or occasionally as the 'post-traumatic syndrome').

Once again, accurate statistics are difficult to obtain on the likely incidence of this condition (*see* Rutherford, 1989). The earliest evidence was obtained by Russell (1932), who described the results of a 6-month follow-up of 141 head-injured patients; 86 (or 61 per cent) of the sample reported one or more persistent postconcussional symptoms. These patients were included in an 18-month follow-up of an extended sample of 200 patients (Russell, 1934), out of whom 120 (or 60 per cent) described such symptoms. The most common symptoms in both studies were: headache, dizziness, loss of memory or mental ability, and nervousness. A similar picture emerged in the case of the 200 head-injured patients described by Denny-Brown (1945a): 63 (or 32 per cent) complained of headaches and 46 (or 23 per cent) complained of dizziness more than two months after their accidents (*see also* Brenner *et al.*, 1944; Friedman *et al.*, 1945). Moreover, Adler (1945) found that 70 of the 200 patients reported persistent psychiatric symptoms, and of these by far the largest group (48 cases) consisted of patients showing fears and anxiety states (*see also* Kozol, 1945).

In a more recent examination of 415 cases roughly five years after their head injuries, Steadman and Graham (1970) found that 50 (or 12 per cent) of the sample had persistent postconcussional symptoms. Lidvall *et al.* (1974) studied 83 cases from a consecutive series of hospital admissions, and found that 24 per cent reported one or more of the relevant set of symptoms when examined 90 days after their accidents. The most common of these were headaches, fatigue and anxiety, each of which was reported by more than 10 per cent of the sample. Klonoff and Paris (1974) interviewed the parents of 196 children one year after they had been admitted to hospital following a head injury and the parents of 163 of them one year later. Postconcussional symptoms were reported among 56 per cent of the children at the first interview and among 44 per cent at the second interview. The most common complaints from the parents tended to be of personality changes, headaches, learning difficulties, fatigue and irritability. Rutherford *et al.* (1977) studied 145 patients with minor head injuries and found that 51 per cent complained of at least one symptom six weeks after their accidents. The most frequently reported symptoms were headache, anxiety, insomnia and dizziness. When 131 of these patients were followed up a year later, 15 per cent still had at least one symptom (Rutherford *et al.*, 1979; *see also* MacFlynn *et al.*, 1984). Wrightson and Gronwall (1981) carried out a prospective study of 66 male patients with minor closed head injuries and found that 13 patients still showed postconcussional symptoms when examined 90 days after their accidents. In ten cases these were mainly impairments of memory and concentration and of coping with difficulties at work; in the three other cases the dominant symptoms were of fatigue and irritability. In a follow-up study two years after their accidents, only eight of these patients could be traced, but four of them still had mild symptoms of the same nature as before.

One fundamental problem in evaluating such findings as these is that the proportion of normal individuals who tend to experience these symptoms is typically unknown. Kozol (1946) carried out an intensive diagnostic interview with 101 head-injured patients on the basis of which he rated 60 'personality traits, tendencies or characteristics' (p. 248) on a 4-point scale with regard to their magnitude or severity prior to the accident and at various occasions after their discharge from hospital. In comparison with their estimated premorbid ratings, more than 25 per cent of Kozol's sample showed an increase in periodic headaches, fatigability, dizziness, anxiety regarding their heads, emotional instability, tension, insomnia, irritability, timorous-ness and abulia (loss of will power). These traits had in most cases simply not been present in any appreciable degree before the head injury: they tended to develop soon after a patient's discharge from hospital, reached a peak about six weeks after the accident, and were often substantially receding at about three months. However, in roughly 50 per cent of these patients such symptoms persisted for at least six months, and in roughly 15 per cent of cases they persisted for a year or more.

In a similar manner, Lidvall *et al.* (1974) asked their patients about the symptoms which they had experienced before their accidents, and they specifically excluded from subsequent consideration 'postconcussional' symptoms which had been present before the injury. Such symptoms were reported by 35 per cent of their total sample: anxiety and fatigue were by far the most common symptoms, but headache was relatively uncommon as a premorbid symptom. McLean *et al.* (1983) administered a 12-item symptom checklist to 20 head-injured patients roughly one month following their accidents and also to 52 normal controls who were friends of head-injured patients in a much larger sample. There were significant differences in the proportions of head-injured patients and control subjects who endorsed particular symptoms, but only in the case of fatigue (which was endorsed by 65 per cent of the head-injured patients), difficulty concentrating (45 per cent), memory difficulties (40 per cent) and blurred vision (20 per cent). The head-injured patients also gave significantly lower self-ratings than the control subjects on a 10-cm analogue scale measuring their perceived overall level of functioning. However, the two groups did not differ significantly in the incidence of headaches, dizziness, hypersensitivity to noise and light, irritability, loss of temper, anxiety and insomnia, nor in their self-ratings along 10-point scales of pain and discomfort, sleepiness and anxiety.

Whereas the postconcussional symptoms that immediately follow the head-injured patient's recovery of consciousness may well have an organic cause, it has typically been assumed that the continued manifestation of these symptoms is psycho-genic in nature. Long and Novack (1986) pointed out two basic reasons for such an assumption. First, the development and exacerbation of such symptoms several weeks or months after the occurrence of a mild or moderate head injury is difficult to explain on an organic basis. Second, some of the symptoms that develop and persist following closed head injury, such as anxiety and depression, are by their nature not easily attributed to actual brain damage. Conversely, as Rutherford (1989) pointed out, some of the more obvious somatic complaints (such as vomiting, nausea, drowsiness and blurred vision) are usually short-lived. There are, however, further arguments that need to be considered relating to the severity of the injury, the role of litigation for compensation, objective performance and the possibility of simulation, and the patient's premorbid personality.

Severity of Injury and Postconcussional Symptoms

It is presumably the case that the incidence of a clinical syndrome that was engendered by organic brain damage would tend to be increased in those patients who had sustained more severe damage. Traditionally, indeed, it was often assumed that the postconcussional syndrome would be associated with more severe damage of the brain (e.g., Meyer, 1904). Nevertheless, Symonds (1940) stated that the severity and duration of postconcussional symptoms had 'no constant relationship to the degree and duration of unconsciousness if it has occurred' (p. 96). Apart from the occurrence and duration of concussion, in subsequent research on postconcussional symptoms 'severity' has also been defined in terms of the duration of PTA. Be that as it may, there is in fact very little evidence using any of these measures that the postconcussional syndrome is more likely following more severe head injuries (*see* e.g., Brenner *et al.*, 1944; Cook, 1969, 1972; Elia, 1974; Friedman *et al.*, 1945; Jacobson, 1969; Kay *et al.*, 1971; Kozol, 1946; Lishman, 1968; McLean *et al.*, 1983; Norrman and Svahn, 1961; Russell and Smith, 1961; Rutherford *et al.*, 1977, 1979; Wrightson and Gronwall, 1981; cf. Livingston and Livingston, 1985).

Indeed, Miller (1961a) presented results which showed an inverse relationship between the incidence of postconcussional symptoms and the severity of the original head injury, whether measured by the occurrence of skull fracture, the duration of unconsciousness, or the duration of PTA. In particular, out of 48 patients in whom PTA had lasted longer than 72 hours, just three cases were said to show 'residual psychoneurosis'; of these Miller claimed that one was a mental defective, one was a lifelong hypochondriac and the third a patient with a long history of recurrent psychiatric disability. On the basis of such results as these Miller and Stern (1965) asserted that postconcussional symptoms were 'conspicuously infrequent' among patients with severe head injury (p. 225). In a series of 100 patients in whom the duration of PTA was longer than 24 hours, they identified just ten patients with 'psychoneurotic symptoms' at an initial examination (on average three years after their accidents) and four patients with such symptoms at a follow-up examination (on average 11 years after their accidents). Such findings contrast directly with the much earlier assertion made by Symonds (1940) that the same pattern of symptoms was 'commonly observed in the course of recovery from moderate or severe brain injury' (p. 97). In this regard, the literature tends to favour Symonds' position rather than Miller's.

Russell (1932) analysed the incidence of postconcussional symptoms in 61 patients with PTA lasting for less than one hour, 45 patients with PTA lasting for between one and 24 hours, and 35 patients with PTA lasting for more than 24 hours. The proportion of patients in each group who reported persistent postconcussional symptoms was 49 per cent, 69 per cent and 71 per cent, respectively, indicating that the frequency of these symptoms varied directly with the severity of injury. Russell then presented a detailed analysis which appeared to indicate that the association between the severity of head injury and the incidence of different symptoms might be positive (memory loss), negative (headache), or nonexistent (dizziness and nervousness); unfortunately, the relevant proportions were expressed only in terms of the patients in each category of severity who reported any symptoms, not in terms of the entire sample. A subsequent study by Lewis (1942) described 64 patients who had been admitted to a psychiatric centre for treatment following head injury. Lewis acknowledged that they had been referred to that centre rather than to a rehabilitation unit because they were considered to have made a full recovery from all the physical effects of the injury. He then added: 'They were, however, very good examples of the [postconcussional] syndrome, clinically, and many of them had had very severe head injuries' (p. 610).

The study of 200 consecutive civilian head injuries that was described by Denny-Brown (1945a) compared the incidence of persistent headache and dizziness with the duration of PTA. Dizziness was more common in those patients in whom PTA had exceeded 12 hours, but headache showed no relationship with the duration of PTA (Brenner *et al.*, 1944; Friedman *et al.*, 1945). Adler (1945) noted that the overall incidence of postconcussional psychiatric symptoms in this series of patients was 31.5 per cent. However, the corresponding figure was 39 per cent in the case of 42 patients in whom coma had lasted for more than 30 minutes and 41 per cent in the case of 22 patients in whom PTA had lasted for more than two days. Conversely, the incidence of postconcussional symptoms was only 15 per cent in the case of 20 patients with no loss of consciousness and 12 per cent in the case of 17 patients with no PTA.

More recently, Landy (1968) compared the duration of PTA and the incidence of postconcussional symptoms in 567 cases who had been referred for a medicolegal assessment after closed head injury. He found that the incidence of persistent post-traumatic headache was highest in the case of the patients who reported no PTA, and it showed a monotonically decreasing relationship with longer periods of PTA. Nevertheless, consistent with the pattern of results presented by Russell (1932), the incidence of complaints of persistent loss of concentration and poor memory showed a positive relationship with the duration of PTA. Bruckner and Randle (1972) found that persistent postconcussional symptoms were associated with a poor occupational outcome in 88 patients with severe head injuries; such symptoms were in particular reported by 65 per cent of those patients who were still unemployed more than three years after their accidents. Kelly (1975) presented data from a prospective study of 152 patients who had sustained severe or minor head injuries. Out of the 56 cases of severe head injury, 26 were judged to have developed the 'post-traumatic syndrome', although out of the 96 cases of minor head injury, 84 were also judged to have developed the syndrome. A somewhat discrepant report was published by Evans *et al.* (1976). These investigators described 121 patients with traumatic brain damage, of whom 103 had suffered injuries that were severe in the sense that they had led to a period of PTA which lasted longer than 24 hours. Evans *et al.* identified just two patients 'in whom the classic syndrome of headaches, dizziness and poor concentration were described' (p. 95), both of whom had suffered minor head injuries. No explanation was offered for the remarkably low incidence of the postconcussional syndrome among this sample. However, many of the patients were members of the UK armed forces, and it is therefore possible that they were not typical of the civilian head-injured population.

To arrive at a clearer idea of the changes in social behaviour that are associated with closed head injury, Oddy *et al.* (1978b) devised a symptom checklist containing 37 items relating to personality changes and somatic, sensory, cognitive and psychiatric symptoms. This was administered to 49 patients with severe head injuries (associated with a period of PTA lasting more than 24 hours) roughly six months after their accidents. Only 23 per cent of the patients claimed that they were free of symptoms, while 35 per cent mentioned six symptoms or more. The three symptoms most frequently cited were 'trouble remembering things', 'often loses temper' and 'becomes tired very easily', and 65 per cent of the patients reported at least one of these. The checklist was also given to a control group of 35 patients who had sustained traumatic limb fractures, but who were then matched with the head-injured subjects for age and socioeconomic status. They produced fewer symptoms and with a different emphasis: 58 per cent were symptom free, and only 20 per cent complained of more than three symptoms. The most frequently mentioned symptoms were those reflecting anxiety and depression. Oddy *et al.* concluded that 'there are indeed subjective complaints that commonly occur after head injury (cf. the 'postconcussional syndrome') but occur less frequently after injuries to other parts of the body' (p. 615).

Minderhoud *et al.* (1980) investigated the incidence of post-traumatic symptoms among 725 patients with minor head injuries in a clinical interview three weeks after their accidents and by means of a postal questionnaire about six months after their accidents. All of the patients were assessed in an accident and emergency department but were referred to their general practitioners without having been admitted to hospital. Nevertheless, 532 of these patients were regarded as having had cerebral concussion on the basis that they had been unconscious for up to half an hour and manifested a period of PTA. The patients who had suffered cerebral concussion were more likely to report sequelae at both three weeks and six months than those who had not. The overall incidence of mental symptoms (i.e., irritability, loss of memory, loss of concentration, fatigue and apathy) and of somatic symptoms (i.e., headache, neck pains and fatigue) was positively correlated with duration of PTA, the time of rest spent in bed and the period of disability. The incidence of sensory symptoms (i.e., loss of hearing, loss of balance and dizziness) was not related to these variables, but was clearly related to external lesions of the vestibular system caused by injuries to the skin and the skull in the parieto-temporal regions.

McKinlay *et al*. (1981) carried out interviews at three, six and 12 months with the relatives of 55 patients who had sustained blunt head injury leading to a PTA lasting at least two days. A wide variety of psychosocial changes in the patients were reported, including emotional disturbances, poor memory and subjective symptoms. In particular, slowness, tiredness and poor memory were each reported in more than two-thirds of the patients and headaches in more than half of the patients 12 months after their accidents. Moreover, in a subsequent report, McKinlay *et al*. (1983) showed that in a substantial proportion of cases these symptoms had been reflected in the accounts of the patients themselves.

Horowitz *et al*. (1983) carried out a follow-up study of children between three and ten years after head injury sustained when they were less than seven years old. There were 154 children who had been admitted to a local paediatric ward and 26 children who had been referred to a district neurosurgical centre because they had received more severe injuries. According to the results of a formal questionnaire administered to the children and their parents, more than 50 per cent of these patients reported persistent symptoms, the most common of which were headache, dizziness, bed-wetting and newly acquired nervous habits such as tics or nail-biting. The latter were significantly more common among the neurosurgical referrals and headaches and bed-wetting showed a trend in the same direction, but dizziness showed no difference between the two samples. However, none of the remaining symptoms showed a significantly higher incidence in the less severely injured patients referred to their local paediatric ward.

A 2-year follow-up of 57 patients with severe closed head injury was reported by van Zomeren and van den Burg (1985). Overall, 84 per cent reported some residual complaint in comparison with their level of functioning before their accidents. In particular, 54 per cent claimed to be more forgetful, 39 per cent claimed to be more irritable, 33 per cent claimed to be slower, and 33 per cent claimed to have more difficulty in concentration. The duration of PTA was significantly correlated with complaints of forgetfulness, slowness and an inability to do two things simultaneously; in each case the correlation was positive, indicating a higher incidence of these complaints among more severely injured patients. More generally, a factor analysis showed that the severity of the original injury was related to the patients' complaints with regard to their 'impairments' rather than their complaints with regard to their 'intolerances' or hypersensitivity to the outside world. A similar pattern emerged from an analysis of the responses produced by relatives of 18 cases when asked about the patients' residual complaints.

Edna and Cappelen (1987) carried out a follow-up of 485 patients between three and five years after head injury, and found that 51 per cent reported new symptoms which they had not experienced before their accidents. Headache, impaired memory, dizziness, fatigue and sensitivity to noise and light were each reported by more than one-sixth of the sample. The incidence of such complaints was significantly higher in the female patients than in the male patients, in those who had sustained a fractured skull, in those who had sustained a subsequent head injury, and in those who had sustained a previous head injury. One problem with this study is that new symptoms were determined with reference to what the patients could remember of the period immediately prior to their accidents, which was of course 3-5 years in retrospect. Nevertheless, an effect of severity of injury was shown indirectly in the increased incidence of a number of symptoms (impaired memory, dizziness, impaired concentration, tinnitus, hearing defect and double vision) in those patients who had sustained a skull fracture. The safest conclusion to be reached on the basis of the evidence available is probably that the relationship between severity of closed head injury and the incidence of postconcussional symptoms is inconsistent both across symptoms and across patient samples.

Compensation Factors

The postconcussional syndrome appears to be relatively rare among those patients who have sustained head injuries in the context of domestic or recreational accidents, but relatively common among those who are involved in industrial or traffic accidents (e.g., Adler, 1945; Brenner *et al.*, 1944; Cook, 1969; but cf. Kelly, 1975). What seems to be the crucial factor in the latter sorts of accident is that they are much more likely to give rise to litigation and to claims for compensation among the parties involved.

During the 1960s, predominantly on the basis of his experience as an expert witness representing insurance companies and other defendants in litigation of this sort, Miller (1961a) had considerable influence among the medical community in maintaining that postconcussional symptoms tended to arise specifically in compensation cases and to subside once any legal claims had been settled. Of course, as McKinlay *et al.* (1983) noted, insofar as Miller's clinical material conisted wholly of medicolegal referrals, his claims were based upon patient samples that were grossly atypical of the broader population of patients with closed head injuries. Initially, at least, Miller was disposed to regard the postconcussional syndrome merely as a form of 'accident neurosis', an emotional reaction to an accident for which blame could be attached to another person or organization against whom or which a legal claim for financial compensation could be made (*see* Miller, 1961b). Subsequently, however, Miller (1966; *see also* Miller and Stern, 1965; Miller and Cartlidge, 1972) came to regard the persistence of postconcussional symptoms as being essentially the product of simulation:

> In my opinion the term neurosis is a misnomer in this context. To claim that motivation in these cases is unconscious is little more than perseveration and in conflict with the facts. Many of the claimants are not only consciously but even frankly and obsessively preoccupied with the question of financial compensation, and the whole situation is one in which only the most naïve would even expect scrupulous honesty or cheerful admission of improvement on the part of the claimant. In my considered opinion these cases are much closer to malingering than to any form of mental illness genuinely outside the patients' control. (p. 258)

Although these views met with a favourable reaction among the general medical community, the response of many researchers was to suggest that Miller had over-emphasized the conscious desire for monetary gain as a causal factor in the development of the postconcussional syndrome (e.g., Cronholm 1972). In particular, Lishman (1973) suggested that the psychological processes associated with compensation and litigation operated at many different levels of consciousness, and that the desire for compensation was merely one possible manifestation of the neurotic conflict that was elicited by the personal crisis of the original injury. In particular, he argued that this sort of emotional impact of a closed head injury would be especially likely in mild cases where there was no post-traumatic amnesia of the accident and its immediate aftermath. This line of thinking would tend to identify the postconcussional syndrome as a form of 'compensation neurosis' which happened to follow injuries to the head (cf. Weighill, 1983).

Nevertheless, other researchers have been led to question whether Miller's premise that the postconcussional syndrome was associated with claims for compensation was even true. Much earlier, indeed, Strauss and Savitsky (1934) had inveighed against 'the implicit confidence and the rigid finality of some observers who assert that most of the persistent complaints of the postconcussion state are psychogenic and result from the subtle suggestions of environment and from unconscious wishes for security' (p. 933). They argued that 'the same complaints (headache, dizziness, fatigability, etc.) are encountered in those unconcerned with the alluring fruits of a favorable decision by a group of experts' (*loc cit.*). They cited in support of this both their own case material and published accounts by physicians themselves of their own experiences following head injuries. Similarly, Symonds (1940) suggested that the development of the syndrome after a latent interval of a few days 'has often been attributed unjustly to the effects of a compensation neurosis, but is in fact observed quite commonly in cases where no such possibility exists' (p. 97). The research evidence once again supports Symonds' position rather than Miller's.

In the study by Russell (1932) mentioned earlier, 86 out of the total of 141 patients reported postconcussional symptoms when examined six months after their accidents. Of these, there were 14 cases in which there were questions of compensation outstanding, and Russell's detailed analysis was based on the remaining 72 cases. Unfortunately he failed to indicate the number of compensation cases that there were among the 55 patients who reported no such symptoms, but it remains true that 51 per cent of the entire sample reported postconcussional symptoms in the absence of any outstanding litigation. Russell (1934) did not provide such detailed information from his 18-month follow-up study of 200 patients. However, he noted that among the 139 cases who were working men and women the 27 patients who had made compensation claims tended to return to work later than the 112 who had made no such claims. This was despite the fact that the former patients had apparently sustained less serious head injuries: Russell reported that 20 (or 74 per cent) of the compensation cases had demonstrated PTA lasting less than an hour, whereas only 41 (or 37 per cent) of the noncompensation cases had shown such relatively brief periods of PTA (*see also* Kozol, 1946; Steadman and Graham, 1970). Nevertheless, he then added: 'In assessing the significance of the compensation factor, however, it must be noted that many of the non-compensation cases returned to work while still suffering from severe postconcussional symptoms' (p. 134).

In the 200 patients who were described by Denny-Brown (1945a) and his colleagues, the incidence of persistent postconcussional headache was 7 per cent in those with no complicating factors, 62 per cent in those with pending litigation, and 60 per cent in those with domestic or occupational difficulties uncomplicated by the possibility of compensation (Brenner *et al.*, 1944). The corresponding figures for persistent postconcussional dizziness were 7 per cent, 41 per cent and 55 per cent (Friedman *et al.*, 1945). These results were interpreted to mean that litigation was merely one of several environmental factors that might increase emotional strain among head-injured patients. Similarly, Adler (1945) found that the incidence of postconcussional symptoms was only 6 per cent in 72 patients in whom there were no factors complicating their psychiatric recovery, but this figure rose to 59 per cent in 34 patients who were involved in litigation and to 93 per cent in 14 cases where litigation was just one of several complicating factors. A recent investigation that was described by Rutherford (1989) also found that the incidence of postconcussional symptoms was far higher in patients referred for medicolegal reports in connection with litigation than in an unselected series. Nevertheless, Rutherford emphasized that head-injured patients may continue to pursue compensation claims even if their postconcussional symptoms have resolved.

Conversely, other studies have tended to confirm that the symptoms in question can be observed where there is no question of litigation. Tooth (1947) evaluated a consecutive series of 100 naval personnel with head injuries. Service regulations determined that any injury sustained on duty was automatically compensable unless it was due to misconduct or negligence on the part of the individual, and there were no instances where an injury had been sustained off duty and there was any question of compensation. Nevertheless, many of these patients complained of postconcussional symptoms, including headache (70 cases), disturbance of memory (61 cases), irritability (50 cases) and dizziness (45 cases). Similarly, Taylor and Bell (1966) described 70 patients who 'had some or all of the symptoms generally recognised in the postconcussional syndrome' (p. 178), despite the fact that they had excluded from their study any patients with a law suit or insurance claim unsettled. Cook (1972) carried out a survey by postal questionnaire of patients with head injuries involving a PTA lasting less than 24 hours. Both the incidence and the persistence of headache, dizziness, irritability and lack of concentration were greater in 27 patients who had entertained claims for compensation than among 36 patients who had not, although there was little difference between the two groups in terms of the severity of their injuries according to the duration of PTA. Cook considered it possible that 'in some instances the occurrence of headache is related to matters of compensation rather than directly to physical injury' (p. 28). However, as McKinlay *et al.* (1983) noted, the fact that Cook's conclusions were based on a response rate to his postal questionnaire of less than 50 per cent detracts considerably from their value.

Merskey and Woodforde (1972) described 27 patients with minor head injury who had been referred for psychiatric assessment: in ten cases no financial claim for compensation was being made, while in the remainder a claim had been made and settled. The two groups showed a very similar pattern of residual symptoms, including headache (23 cases), depressed mood (19 cases), dizziness (14 cases), phobias and anxiety (14 cases), poor memory (12 cases) and lack of energy (nine cases). According to a follow-up examination these symptoms lasted for several years, in ten cases with little or no improvement. Similar results were reported by Kelly (1975), who found that out of 34 patients who were injured in circumstances that involved neither a claim for compensation nor an occupational pension 24 patients subsequently developed a postconcussional syndrome. Conversely, Kelly also reported that out of 110 patients who were involved in litigation 84 returned to work before the settlement of their claims, completely recovered. These results obviously contradict the view that post-concussional symptoms are determined by the possibility of compensation and disappear once any such claims have been settled (Miller, 1979).

Guthkelch (1980) reported a prospective study of 398 head-injured patients who were assessed in connection with claims for compensation. Though this is not entirely clear from the text of his paper, Guthkelch appears to have reserved the phrases 'postconcussional symptoms' and 'postconcussional syndrome' to refer to the experiences of those patients who returned to their previous occupations within an interval of time that was not wholly disproportionate to the severity of their injuries, even if they suffered a serious post-traumatic emotional disturbance in the meantime. He used the expression 'accident neurosis' to refer to 27 patients in whom 'there was no relationship between the duration and severity of their complaints, many of which were bizarre and inconsistent, and the magnitude of the original injury' (p. 98). On the basis of his own assessment of these patients, Guthkelch concluded, like Miller, that this condition 'can only be conceived as a conscious desire for gain, varying in degree from exaggeration and self-pity on the one hand to lying and fraud on the other . . . Accident neurosis is a misnomer and the use of the term should be abandoned in favor of one which expresses the subject's conscious intent to deceive' (p. 101). Nevertheless, it is not at all clear what relation if any the latter condition has to the usual notion of a 'postconcussional syndrome'. One important consideration is that Guthkelch identified accident neurosis in only 6.8 per cent of his series of patients, which (as he himself implied) was remarkably low if the domain of reference of this term is to be regarded as co-extensive with that of 'postconcussional syndrome' in its usual sense.

Rimel *et al.* (1981) reported a 3-month follow-up of 424 patients with minor closed head injuries. Out of the total sample, 84 per cent reported one or more subjective complaints. By far the most frequent symptom (reported by 78 per cent of the sample) was persistent headache, although 59 per cent complained of impaired memory. Nevertheless, only six patients were involved in litigation, which implies that factors having to do with compensation for injury were of very little significance in this group of patients. As mentioned earlier, Wrightson and Gronwall (1981) found postconcussional symptoms persisting for more than 90 days in 13 out of 66 patients admitted to two hospitals in New Zealand with minor head injuries. An important feature of this series was that none of the patients had made any formal legal complaint about their symptoms and none had outstanding claims for compensation, perhaps because of the existence of a no-fault system of compensation for occupational injuries. Despite this, the incidence of persistent symptoms was similar to that found in earlier studies conducted in the UK where there is no such system and where a significant proportion of the patients concerned are likely to have sought compensation (e.g., Cook, 1972; Rutherford *et al.*, 1977, 1979).

In their investigation of postconcussional symptoms among patients with severe head injury, McKinlay *et al.* (1981) selected two subsamples of 21 cases consisting of patients who had consistently maintained that they had grounds to pursue a claim for compensation or that they had no such grounds. There was a tendency for the former patients to have been more severely injured in terms of the duration of PTA, but there were no significant differences between the two groups in the incidence of any of the psychosocial changes reported by their relatives. McKinlay *et al.* (1983) subsequently found that the former group were slightly more likely to report poor concentration, dizziness, or irritability, but that there was little sign of any difference between the two groups in terms of their performance on objective cognitive tests. Once again, these results show that compensation factors have little role in either the development or the persistence of postconcussional symptoms.

Subjective Complaints and Objective Performance

Some researchers have addressed the question of the nature and aetiology of the postconcussional syndrome by measuring patients' performance on objective psychological tests. For instance, Tooth (1947) evaluated his head-injured naval personnel on an abbreviated form of Wechsler's (1941) verbal intelligence test. The sample contained an unspecified number of cases of gunshot wounds, but Tooth considered that they were nevertheless representative of concussional injuries. Poorer levels of performance on the Similarities subtest were achieved by those who complained of memory disturbance or irritability. There were however no such differences in the case of complaints of headaches and dizziness, nor in the case of the other subtests used in this investigation.

Gronwall and Wrightson (1974) administered the paced auditory serial addition task (PASAT) to ten patients who had returned to work following a closed head injury but who had been unable to continue because of poor concentration, fatigue, irritability and headache. When compared with a control group of ten head-injured patients who did not report such symptoms, they were significantly impaired on an initial assessment on the PASAT and took significantly longer to achieve normal levels of performance on repeated testing. Gronwall and Wrightson suggested that the postconcussional syndrome was caused by a reduced rate of information transmission, which manifested itself in subjective complaints of poor concentration in tasks that involved a high information load. All of the subjects who reported postconcussional symptoms achieved a normal level of performance within the first two months after their injuries, although as Miller (1979) noted this may have been merely an artefact of practice effects. Gronwall and Wrightson added: 'There is a strong clinical impression that the symptoms of which the patients . . . complained were associated with a low PASAT score and improved as the score returned to normal' (p. 607). Gronwall (1976) confirmed that the reduction in information-processing rate on the PASAT was correlated significantly with subjective reports of postconcussional symptoms, and that scores on the repeated administration of the PASAT improved in a manner that was roughly commensurate with the resolution of those symptoms.

These two studies confirmed the usefulness of the PASAT in monitoring the course of recovery from closed head injury. Nevertheless, it is also true that the patients who were involved in these studies were no longer complaining of postconcussional symptoms by the third month after their accidents. To that extent, it is not clear how such patients can be seen as examples of a *persistent* postconcussional syndrome. Such a criticism does not apply in the case of the study by MacFlynn *et al.* (1984) in which 45 patients with minor closed head injury carried out a four-choice visual reaction-time task. When assessed within the first 24 hours of admission to hospital, 26 patients reported three or more of the relevant symptoms; when they were assessed six weeks later, 24 of the patients reported one or more symptoms; and when 28 patients were retested six months after the head injury, 15 of them complained of one or more symptoms. In terms of their mean reaction times, however, no significant difference was found between the symptomatic and nonsymptomatic patients at any of the three sessions. Unfortunately, as was mentioned in chapter 5 (p. 141), the head-injured patients tested at six months after their accidents showed no sign of any impairment on the reaction-time task when compared with normal subjects. These results are therefore consistent with the idea that the latter task was simply not a sensitive index of the organic concomitants of persistent postconcussional symptoms.

Waddell and Gronwall (1984) measured the tolerance to light and sound of nine patients with minor head injury who were not admitted to hospital but were referred for assessment. When tested between seven and 19 days after their accidents and compared with a group of matched control subjects drawn from hospital staff and the local community, they were found to be impaired in their objective tolerance to both light and sound. However, there was no relationship between the patients' subjective ratings of hypersensitivity to light and sound and their objective tolerance. The head-injured patients in this study were also given the PASAT, but their scores on this task were not significantly correlated with either their subjective ratings or their objective assessment of hypersensitivity. Waddell and Gronwall took their results to count against the notion of a psychogenic aetiology of the postconcussional syndrome. Nevertheless, for two quite separate reasons their study had simply not addressed this question. First, the study involved an unselected sample of head-injured patients; there was no comparison group of head-injured patients without postconcussional symptoms. The effects of postconcussional symptoms were thus confounded with the effects of head injury *per se*. Second, the only attempt which was made to monitor postconcussional symptoms was to record the patients' complaints of hypersensitivity to light and sound on average just two weeks after their head injuries. This would hardly be sufficient to identify those head-injured patients who would subsequently manifest a persistent postconcussional syndrome.

In this context, it is also interesting to consider a study by Dikmen and Reitan (1977) in which 27 head-injured patients were assessed on the Minnesota Multiphasic Personality Inventory (MMPI: Dahlstrom *et al.*, 1972) initially ('soon after the injury') and again 12 and 18 months later. They were divided into two groups based upon whether their initial performance on the Halstead-Reitan battery revealed (a) moderate or marked neuropsychological deficits or (b) normal function or only mild deficits. Across the three test sessions, significant reductions were found on the Hypo-chondriasis, Depression, Hysteria, Psychasthenia and Schizophrenia scales of the

MMPI; this was taken to suggest that 'head-injured patients in general complain of more depression, anxiety, somatic problems, and strange experiences soon after the injury' (p. 493). Moreover, at both the 12-month and the 18-month sessions the patients with moderate or marked neuropsychological deficits showed significantly greater emotional difficulties on the Hypochondriasis, Depression and Mania scales of the MMPI. Dikmen and Reitan suggested that impairment of neuropsychological functions could be used as an index of the severity of a head injury, and they implied that their data were inconsistent with psychogenic accounts of the difficulties experienced by head-injured patients. One reservation is that a patient's age was apparently a confounded factor associated with both neuropsychological impairment and emotional difficulties on the MMPI in their study.

The broad research strategy in all these investigations was to seek to demonstrate that the subjective complaints which are characteristic of the postconcussional syndrome could be correlated with some objective, measurable deficit. However, a serious criticism of these studies is that such findings would not rule out the possibility that both the subjective complaints and the objective impairment were the product of simulation and malingering. Performance in many psychological tasks is under the control of conscious processing strategies, and it is therefore open to patients to adopt suboptimal strategies if it serves their purposes to do so. Only a few investigators have addressed this issue. First, in the case of the PASAT, Gronwall (1977) suggested that there were certain patterns of test results that indicated either poor motivation or a deliberate attempt at faking low scores, but she acknowledged that not all cases of malingering were clear-cut. Second, Hannay and James (1981) found that students could successfully simulate the pattern of performance on a test of continuous recognition memory which had been produced by head-injured patients in an earlier study (Hannay *et al.*, 1979). There was considerable overlap in the respective distributions of test scores, although extreme false-alarm rates tended to be characteristic of the simulators rather than of the patients. Third, as was mentioned in the previous section, McKinlay *et al.* (1983) found little evidence for any difference in psychometric test performance between head-injured patients who were entertaining claims for financial compensation and those who were not. They concluded that 'claimants did not attempt to fake low scores in order to present as more disabled than they were' (p. 1089). On the basis of their own clinical experience, they considered that faking low scores was rare, and that 'serial testing would uncover it easily in the very few cases where it occurs' (*loc. cit.*). However, in commenting on this assertion, Binder (1986) observed that expert clinicians had sometimes had difficulty in identifying simulation in research studies involving other populations of brain-damaged patients.

More generally, it is now well established in laboratory research that both the uncertainty of the experimental subjects and the hypotheses of the researcher may significantly affect the outcome of an experiment (Rosenthal, 1976; Silverman, 1977).

In other areas of clinical research, such as investigations of the psychological effects of drugs, it is now customary to try to avoid these problems by using 'double-blind' methods whereby neither the subject nor the experimenter knows which treatment or pharmacological compound has been administered. In research on the effects of closed head injury, as in most areas of clinical neuropsychology, it is difficult to ensure this degree of ignorance in the two parties involved. It would be difficult (though perhaps not totally impossible) for research psychologists to avoid any awareness of the diagnosis of their subjects; and it would certainly be expected of clinical psychologists that they familarize themselves with the detailed history of individual patients referred for testing. In either case, it would be entirely natural for the psychologists involved to anticipate some degree of impairment on the part of their patients. Conversely, virtually all head-injured patients are aware at least of having suffered brain injury, and most are perfectly ready to attribute any cognitive failures to that event, even those which previously they would have regarded as normal and natural. As a result, both head-injured patients and psychologists with whom they are involved have strong prior expectations which might well tend to produce objective results that are indicative of cognitive deficits, quite independently of any conscious simulation or malingering. Research is urgently needed to clarify the influence of these expectations upon the outcome of testing, both in formal research programmes on the effects of closed head injury and in the practice of clinical assessment with individual patients.

Psychogenic Aspects of Postconcussional Symptoms

The possibility that persistent postconcussional symptoms constitute a functional reaction to closed head injury and its immediate consequences has led to an interest in factors that might be involved in the aetiology of the syndrome other than the physiological aspects of the injury itself: both endogenous, constitutional properties of the patient prior to the injury and exogenous, circumstantial properties of the injury and its clinical management (Lishman, 1973).

The role of endogenous factors in the aetiology of postconcussional symptoms was first emphasised by Symonds (1928), who recommended that 'it should be a rule in such cases to inquire for a family history of mental instability and to ascertain the patient's previous biological record, with especial reference to nervous breakdowns' (p. 831). Russell (1934) pointed out that 'identical injuries to the head in two individuals may produce quite different after-effects' (p. 139). Subsequently, Symonds (1937) reiterated his earlier recommendation in an often-quoted passage:

> The later effects of head injury can only be properly understood in the light of a full psychiatric study of the individual patient, and in particular, his constitution. In other words, it is not only the kind of injury that matters, but the kind of head. (p. 1092)

Symonds and Russell (1943) presented some preliminary data to support the notion that 'the mental constitution before injury plays an important part in the prognosis of head injuries' (p. 8). Nevertheless, just as there are problems in estimating a patient's premorbid cognitive abilities (*see* pp. 117–9), it may well be extremely difficult to arrive at an accurate assessment of a particular patient's premorbid personality. Indeed, Kozol (1945) maintained that 'no personality test . . . can be depended on to give an evaluation of a patient's personality before injury to the head when the test is given after the injury' (p. 359). In a subsequent paper (Kozol, 1946), he emphasized that 'as none of these patients had ever been given any formal personality tests . . . before the head injury, there was no logic in giving such tests after the injury because there was no basis for comparison' (p. 248). Lidvall *et al.* (1974) administered such a test to head-injured patients three days after their accidents 'with instructions that they should only give an account of their habitual state before the present accident and that they should ignore troubles and symptoms appearing for the first time after the trauma' (p. 73). However, it is simply not at all clear whether patients who have recently undergone a major trauma are able to discriminate between their habitual premorbid state and their current symptomatology.

The latter consideration supports the view expressed by Symonds and Russell (1943) and by Kozol (1945, 1946) that information concerning a patient's pretraumatic personality could normally only be inferred from a detailed enquiry into their family and personal history. Nevertheless, this information may prove to be very important in determining both effective management and the likely prognosis (Cronholm, 1972). The fact that there is no clear relationship between the severity of the original head injury and the persistence of postconcussional symptoms is usually taken to imply that the latter condition affects only those patients with a constitutional vulnerability or susceptibility (e.g., Behrman, 1977). Specifically, it would be expected that the incidence of postconcussional syndrome would be higher in patients with a premorbid anxiety or neurotic instability (Cronholm 1972; Lishman, 1973).

An early study by Lewis (1942) compared 64 head-injured patients with postconcussional symptoms who had been admitted to a psychiatric unit for assessment with 64 neurotic patients from the same hospital. The former group was somewhat more likely to include individuals who had been of a stable, well-organized premorbid personality, and more likely to complain of severe headache, fainting and irritability. However, in most other respects the two groups were remarkably similar in terms of their family and personal history, intelligence, symptoms, response to treatment and outcome. Lewis concluded that 'the long-standing, relatively intractable post-contusional syndrome is apt to occur in much the same person as develops a psychiatric syndrome in other circumstances without any brain injury at all' (p. 610).

Ruesch and Bowman (1945) described 125 patients who had developed postconcussional symptoms, and they suggested that this was associated with a high premorbid level of neuroticism (*see also* Brenner *et al.*, 1944; Friedman *et al.*, 1945).

However, they provided little information about the precise nature of the psychiatric assessment on which this conclusion was based. In a separate study of 128 cases of head injury, Ruesch *et al.* (1945) found that post-traumatic personality changes were typified by complaints of increased fatigability, lowered tolerance to alcohol, unstable work history, decrease of interests and occasional impotency. Moreover, these patients produced higher scores than normal on the neuroticism scales of the Minnesota Multiphasic Personality Inventory, and the latter showed a correlation of +0.80 with the number of post-traumatic complaints. Ruesch *et al.* concluded that pre-existing neurotic tendencies seemed to prolong the duration of post-traumatic syndromes.

Working with the same population of patients as Ruesch and Bowman (1945), Kozol (1945) determined that 32 per cent of the 200 cases had developed postconcussional symptoms; for those patients with previously normal personality, with premorbid neurotic personality, with premorbid psychopathic personality, and with other premorbid personality variants the corresponding figures were 30 per cent, 26 per cent, 35 per cent and 30 per cent, respectively. From these figures, Kozol concluded that 'the pretraumatic personality is not a dominant factor in the production of post-traumatic symptoms' (p. 361). However, on the basis of her own work with these patients Adler (1945) noted that the incidence of such symptoms rose to 57 per cent among those patients who had a history of pre-existing anxiety, hypochondriasis, or depression. She also found that the symptom which predominated in those patients with normal premorbid personalities was almost always anxiety, whereas the symptoms which developed in those patients with pre-existing psychiatric abnormalities tended to reflect their previous clinical condition.

Kozol (1946) presented a more detailed account of the relationship between pretraumatic personality and postconcussional symptoms in 101 of the patients in his original sample. He maintained that 'as none of these patients had ever been given any formal personality tests . . . before the head injury, there was no logic in giving such tests after the injury because there was no basis for comparison' (p. 248). As mentioned earlier, instead of such tests Kozol developed a detailed schedule of 60 individual characteristics that were assessed in diagnostic interviews with regard to their magnitude or severity prior to the accident and at various occasions after the patients' discharge from hospital. He noted that a substantial number of patients showed certain characteristics after their head injury that had not been present previously, and that this was true in particular of specific psychoneurotic traits such as anxiety and fatigability. Kozol commented that this 'refutes the oft expressed view that post-traumatic psychiatric symptoms represent a pretraumatic psychiatric liability to such symptoms' (p. 256). Those patients with premorbid psychoneurotic personality tended to show little change on those characteristics which were associated with that personality, but this was because they were already at or approaching a ceiling on those traits in terms of their pretraumatic ratings. Conversely, however, these patients tended to show a greater post-traumatic reaction on other characteristics than those with normal premorbid personality or with other abnormalities. The net result was that the occurrence of sequelae of any kind and the occurence of the most severe sequelae was more likely in the patients with psychoneurotic personalities than in the other patient groups. Nevertheless, Kozol also emphasized that 'some of the patients in this series who were heavily burdened with neurotic traits recovered from the acute head injury without sequelae' (p. 273).

Some of the most interesting evidence on the role of the patient's premorbid personality has come from the comparison of pairs of twins in whom one member has suffered a closed head injury. Dencker (1958, 1960) assessed 117 such pairs, consisting of 36 monozygotic or identical pairs and 81 same-sexed dizygotic or fraternal twins. At a long-term follow-up examination on average ten years after their accidents, the incidence of headache, vertigo or dizziness, impaired memory, increased sensitivity to noise and light, and decreased tolerance of alcohol were assessed in both the head-injured patients and their co-twins. There was no significant difference between the head-injured monozygotic twins and their co-twins in terms of the incidence of these symptoms. Moreover, the monozygotic pairs were found to be more alike or concordant than the dizygotic pairs in this respect. Those patients who showed these symptoms more than their co-twins appeared to be more accident-prone and in particular were more likely to have suffered additional head injuries in the past. Dencker concluded that these late 'postconcussional' symptoms were largely of constitutional origin rather than the result of the head injury itself.

Dencker's results also imply that those patients who subsequently demonstrate the postconcussional syndrome are a distinctive sub-group of patients with closed head injury. In line with the observations of Lewis (1942), other clinicians have noted that patients who manifest this sort of post-traumatic reaction are in many respects much more similar to other neurotics than to other head-injured patients (Editorial, 1973). On the basis of a 6-month follow-up of 162 children, Hjern and Nylander (1964) claimed that persistent mental sequelae were seen only 'in children who came from an insecure home environment or who had already shown symptoms of mental illness previously' (p. 35). To some extent, the study of Merskey and Woodforde (1972) supported this view, in that a number of their patients referred for assessment with persistent postconcussional symptoms had evidence of neurotic problems that predated their accidents. However, these researchers also remarked that several patients 'showed quite convincing past evidence of stable personalities and successful adjustment at home and at work' (p. 523). In other words, in a substantial proportion of cases, the relevant symptomatology could not be related to a poor premorbid psychiatric history (Newcombe, 1982). The subsequent study by Lidvall *et al.* (1974) failed to demonstrate such an association between the premorbid level of neuroticism and persistent postconcussional symptoms. Nevertheless, apart from the methodological problem over retrospective self-assessment that was mentioned above, the index of neuroticism that was used in this study was somewhat different from the standard personality measures that are in general clinical use and lacked adequate validation.

To the extent that persistent postconcussional symptoms constitute a variety of neurotic conflict that arises out of a closed head injury, they would be expected to depend to a large extent on the circumstances of the accident itself. The putative relationship between the postconcussional syndrome and legal claims for compensation implies that the possibility of ascribing blame for the accident to a separate individual or organization is an important factor in this regard. Indeed, Rutherford *et al.* (1977) confirmed specifically that the persistence of postconcussional symptoms among patients with minor closed head injury was significantly greater in those who blamed their employers or a large impersonal organization for their accidents. Guthkelch (1980) also cited the role of circumstantial factors in order to explain his own finding that the postconcussional syndrome was more common among semiskilled or unskilled manual workers who had been involved in industrial accidents than among members of the same occupational group who had been involved in vehicular accidents or among nonmanual workers who had been involved in industrial accidents.

Even if the persistence of postconcussional symptoms is determined to a large extent by the patient's premorbid personality, this would not mean that the condition was beyond clinical treatment. Indeed, Gronwall and Wrightson (1974) suggested that the postconcussional syndrome would require continued monitoring and management, and the precise form which that management takes is likely to determine whether those symptoms are satisfactorily resolved. A more extreme point of view was expressed by Gruneberg (1970) and by Kelly (1975), who argued that the condition is often the result of an unsupportive attitude on the part of the patient's doctor. Evans (1987) noted that the patient's involvement in litigation may exert a similar influence upon the persistence of postconcussional symptoms through the attitudes adopted by insurance companies and their representatives. He cited a highly pertinent remark made more than 50 years before by Strauss and Savitsky (1934):

> The harshness, injustice and brutal disregard of complaints shown by the physicians and representatives of insurance companies and their ready assumption for intent to swindle do not foster wholesome patterns of reaction in injured persons. The frequent expression of unjustifiable skepticism on the part of examiners engenders resentment, discouragement and hopelessness and too often forces these people to resort to more primitive modes of response (hysterical). The repeated psychic traumas bring out the worst that there is in them and makes manifest all their frailties and constitutional insufficiencies. (p. 949)

Organic Aspects of Postconcussional Symptoms

The contrary view was put more than 60 years ago by Symonds (1928): 'My impression is that the frequency of traumatic neuroses following head injury is a good deal exaggerated and that the minor mental symptoms so often encountered are mainly due to organic damage' (p. 831). More recent accounts have suggested that Miller (1961a) may have overemphasized the importance of psychoneurotic influences upon postconcussional symptoms, and that a number of physiological mechanisms may be responsible (e.g., Taylor, 1967). It is however only during the last twenty-five years that the data to support this claim have been available.

The earliest data were obtained from arteriographic investigations which tended to show persistent disturbances of cerebral circulation even following relatively minor closed head injuries (*see* Taylor, 1969). For instance, Taylor and Bell (1966) found a reduction in cerebral blood flow (as evidenced by a significant decrease in blood flow amplitude and a significant increase in mean circulation time) among 70 patients with postconcussional symptoms tested typically 4–8 weeks after concussional head injuries when compared with 70 cases with minor injuries elsewhere than to the neck or head. They argued that this was the result of increased arteriolar vasomotor tone. When individual patients were tested repeatedly during the course of their recovery, postconcussional symptoms and an increased cerebral circulation time tended to come and go together. In particular, normal circulation time roughly 2–3 weeks after concussion was said to 'carry a good prognosis for the non-occurrence or early disappearance of post-concussional symptoms' (p. 180). However, these were presented as informal findings with no supporting data, and the authors acknowledged that the causal relationship between the two remained to be determined. A similar global reduction in cerebral blood flow has been demonstrated in cases of migraine, and it has therefore been suggested that cerebral vasoconstriction may be the mechanism responsible for postconcussional headache, which can in extreme cases take the form of a classic migraine (Behrman, 1977).

However, an alternative causal mechanism has been suggested for the occurrence of postconcussional headache. Similar subjective complaints may be made by patients with superficial injuries to the neck and scalp, especially in 'whiplash' injuries which do not involve actual head impact (Jacobson, 1969; Lishman, 1973). (Of course, in more severe cases of head injury, headache may also be produced by increased intracranial pressure as a result either of disturbances to the flow of cerebrospinal fluid or else of intracranial bleeding.) Similarly, postconcussional dizziness appears to be caused by vestibular pathology rather than by damage to the brain stem, and this disturbance too may occur both with actual head impact and with 'whiplash' injury (Jacobson, 1969; Toglia, 1969). Indeed, Guthkelch (1980) established that injuries to the neck and vestibular disturbances were the major factors preventing patients with relatively minor head injuries from returning to their normal occupations. This would explain why the incidence of postconcussional symptoms does not appear to be related to the severity of the head injury, as measured by the duration of coma or of PTA: postconcussional symptoms result from injury to the superficial structures of the head and neck, whereas coma and PTA result from shearing damage within the brain (cf. Jacobson, 1969).

The study by Rutherford *et al.* (1977) compared the persistence of postconcussional symptoms in 145 patients who had sustained minor head injuries with the incidence of various signs at neurological examination roughly 24 hours after the original accidents. The signs in question were headache, diplopia (double vision), anosmia (loss of the sense of smell) and the presence of other abnormalities of the central nervous system. In each case there proved to be a positive correlation with the incidence of postconcussional symptoms at a follow-up examination six weeks later, which Rutherford *et al.* took to confirm the involvement of organic factors in the aetiology of such symptoms. When 131 of these patients were followed up a year after their accidents, these neurological signs were no longer associated with a higher symptom rate, although the incidence of other positive neurological signs did show such an association (Rutherford *et al.*, 1979).

One might have anticipated that direct evidence on the involvement of organic factors in such symptoms would come from the use of computerized tomography (CT), and CT scans typically prove to be normal in patients with postconcussional syndrome (Weisberg, 1979). However, the relative insensitivity of CT scans in detecting parenchymal lesions was noted in Chapter 2 (pp. 46, 54). It is certainly recognized that during the early stages of recovery patients with closed head injury may show normal CT scans in the face of clinical evidence of brain damage (Stevens, 1982). Electroencephalographic (EEG) recordings too are often normal after closed head injury, even when there is neurological evidence of cerebral dysfunction; nevertheless, even a relatively mild head injury can on occasion result in the findings of an abnormal EEG (Binder, 1986). Similarly, Noseworthy *et al.* (1981) and Montgomery *et al.* (1984) have shown that evoked potentials to auditory stimuli recorded in the brainstem tend to be significantly delayed in head-injured patients. MacFlynn *et al.* (1984) recorded EEG and brainstem evoked potentials in 24 cases of minor closed head injury within 48 hours of their accidents and again six weeks later. When these patients were compared with normal-hearing controls, it was found that 33 per cent had an excess of theta power and nearly half showed evidence of delayed brain-stem conduction time. Once again, however, none of these studies distinguished between the effects of postconcussional symptoms and those of head injury *per se,* although MacFlynn *et al.* found that the changes which they observed were maximal in those patients (12 in all) who had suffered vomiting, vertigo or diplopia at the time of their injury.

A Postconcussional Syndrome?

During the 1960s, Miller's (1961a, 1966) pronouncements encouraged the idea that the persistence of postconcussional symptoms following minor closed head injury was purely functional in nature. As Newcombe (1982) summarized the position, the constellation of subjective symptoms that defined the postconcussional syndrome (that is, headache, dizziness, hypersensitivity to light and sound, difficulty in concentrating, anxiety and irritability) was 'thought to be related to predisposing psychogenic influences and aggravated by the lure of compensation' (p. 122). However, the evidence that was described in the previous sections suggests that any such conclusion would be wholly inadequate. Contemporary opinion has it rather that the postconcussional syndrome represents a long-term neurotic reaction to the short-term organic consequences of a closed head injury (Binder, 1986; Editorial, 1973; Elia, 1974; Evans, 1987; Gronwall and Wrightson, 1974; Long and Novack, 1986; Minderhoud et al., 1980; Richardson, 1979c; Rutherford et al., 1977).

However, many authors have been led to question whether it is really appropriate to refer to the condition of persistent postconcussional symptoms as a cliniclal 'syndrome'. Symonds (1940) considered that it was convenient to do so because the symptoms of headache, giddiness and 'nervous instability' did very often occur together (*see also* Brenner et al., 1944: Friedman et al., 1945). Lewin (1970) argued that the individual symptoms which were supposed to be characteristic of the postconcussional syndrome had distinct aetiologies, and should be assessed and treated separately from each other. On the basis of a detailed statistical analysis of postconcussional symptoms, Lidvall et al. (1974) considered that the symptom picture during the later phase of recovery was polymorphous and varied over time in an irregular manner, although anxiety appeared to constitute the nucleus of that picture. Similarly, Rutherford et al. (1977, 1979) suggested that the various individual symptoms might recur over an indefinite period, but that they constituted part of the normal pattern of recovery from a closed head injury and did not deserve to be regarded as a specific clinical syndrome. Minderhoud et al. (1980) classified postconcussional symptoms on an a priori basis into three syndromes reflecting mental sequelae, sensory sequelae and somatic sequelae. These syndromes showed different patterns of correlations with biographical and clinical characteristics of the patients.

One should also consider whether the relevant symptoms are in any way peculiar to the aftermath of concussional head injury. The specific set of symptoms which appears during the early phase of recovery does appear to be characteristic of closed head injury and a direct result of cerebral trauma. However, the persistence of these symptoms beyond the initial post-traumatic period does not seem to be dependent upon the actual occurrence of concussion (Elia, 1974). Indeed, Miller (1966) claimed that 'the syndrome occurs in its most florid and enduring form after trivial knocks on the head where consciousness was never impaired' (p. 258), although the incidence of persistent postconcussional symptoms in such cases appears to be relatively low (e.g., Brenner *et al.*, 1944; Casey *et al.*, 1986; Friedman *et al.*, 1945). Several writers have pointed out that exactly the same symptoms may occur in other clinical conditions (Dencker, 1958; Lidvall *et al.*, 1974); as was noted earlier in this chapter these include injuries to the back, the neck, or the hand where there is little possibility of direct cerebral damage (*see* Jacobson, 1969; Miller, 1966).

Lewis (1942) pointed out that the postconcussional syndrome was 'apt to occur in much the same person as develops a psychiatric condition in other circumstances without any brain injury at all'. The evidence that is currently available suggests that it is less useful to regard persistent postconcussional symptoms as a clinical syndrome than as more indefinite characteristics of a post-traumatic neurosis (*see* e.g., Lidvall *et al.*, 1974; Long and Webb, 1983). Reference was indeed made earlier to Miller's (1961a, 1961b) notion that the postconcussional syndrome was merely a special case of 'accident neurosis' which happened to be associated with injuries to the head. However, even this concept has been criticized as being of little clinical value (Gruneberg, 1970), and more recently it has been supplanted by that of a 'post-traumatic stress disorder' (American Psychiatric Association, 1980). It is certainly true that the symptoms of a post-traumatic stress disorder may emerge during the course of recovery from any form of trauma, regardless of whether the victim has sustained a closed head injury. This condition typically involves emotional episodes of over-whelming fearfulness, anxiety, rage, or helplessness, contrasting with a lack of interest and initiative regarding everyday matters. Such patients may tend to complain of sleep disturbance, memory impairment and difficulty in concentrating, and they may also show exaggerated startle responses and a generalized hyperalertness (Peterson, 1986).

Nevertheless, this account falls to explain why the early organic aspects of closed head injury should have psychogenic consequences in some patients but not in others. Goldstein (1942, 1952) argued that 'neurotic' sysmptoms following head injury reflected not merely actual damage to the brain, but also the organism's efforts to cope with the resulting deficits while attempting to meet the demands of the environment (cf. Tooth, 1947). Hillbom (1960) stressed that chronic compensatory effort of this sort would be more likely among patients with relatively mild head injuries, because the disabilities of those with more severe head injuries would be immediately apparent and there would be little or no social pressure upon such patients to resume their former responsibilities. A similar account was offered by Gronwall and Wrightson (1974) on the basis of their finding of a reduced information-processing capacity in patients with minor closed head injury:

> The occurrence of symptoms when channel capacity has been reduced is not difficult to understand. A patient who has made a good physical recovery after concussion feels well enough to return to work. His intelligence appears to be unaffected and he will indeed score normally on standard

psychometric tests. However, jobs which he could previously have done easily now require his whole attention, and therefore soon tire him. Tasks which require simultaneous attention to a number of factors are quite beyond his capacity, and this he interprets by saying that he cannot concentrate. Stress mounts, and with it headache and irritability . . .

The development of this group of symptoms into a disease in its own right depends on several factors. There is first the patient's reaction to a disabling condition that he cannot understand. How he responds will depend on his personality and on the explanation and support that he receives. He may work patiently within his limitations, calm in the assurance of his therapist that the situation will improve with time and that he will regain his old powers . . . On the other hand, his personality may lead him to react with excessive alarm, precipitated by financial or other external stress, and he may become inaccessible to counsel. Resentment of his plight contributes to the situation, and may be transferred to the establishment or the physician who will not acknowledge a disability which is very real to him. A fixed neurotic reaction develops and the state is perpetuated as a post-concussion syndrome. (p. 608)

In accordance with this account, it was noted by Rimel *et al.* (1981) that the difficulties which head-injured patients experienced in coping with cognitive deficits were the source of considerable stress and tended to exacerbate such symptoms as headache and dizziness in the acute phase.

Subsequently, van Zomeren *et al.* (1984) developed the hypothesis that persistent postconcussional symptoms reflected a coping response to the impact of a reduction in information-processing capacity upon the demands of everyday life. Van Zomeren and van den Burg (1985) explained this hypothesis in the following manner:

The coping hypothesis . . . states that 'neurotic' symptoms may result from chronic effort by the patients to compensate for their cognitive deficits. This effort is an answer to the demands made by the social environment and the patient's own standards. Such demands are made specifically to those patients who are not visibly handicapped and whose injuries are not considered to be so severe as to prevent a complete resumption of previous activities. When the cognitive functions are not yet completely recovered, the resulting stress may lead to intolerances as secondary symptoms, especially in the less severely injured patients. (p. 27)

On the basis of these discussions, Long and Novack (1986) concluded that the potential for the development and persistence of postconcussional symptoms would exist whenever the environmental demands made upon the head-injured patient exceeded his or her residual cognitive capacities that were available for dealing effectively with those demands.

Personality Disorders

A wide variety of other affective disturbances which may result from a closed head injury have also been described in the clinical literature. The early investigation by Meyer (1904) distinguished between two major varieties of post-traumatic disorder. First, a patient might remain in the state of 'partial consciousness or actual delirium' after awakening from coma. This condition of protracted mental derangement, which Meyer described as 'primary traumatic insanity', was generally typified by 'an absence of manic-depressive symptoms, *a certain tendency to dream-states, fabrications of whole situations and great inconsistency of statement*, but no hallucinosis' (p. 401). Second, the patient might make a good recovery but subsequently develop 'secondary traumatic insanity' in any of a wide variety of forms. The latter included 'imbecility, change of character, epileptiform psychoses, catatonic deterioration . . . , circular insanity, in some cases with more or less somatic symptoms referable to the trauma or its consequences' (p. 405). In most cases, these conditions would be marked by an increasing defect of intelligence, memory and judgement. Meyer estimated that 'traumatic insanity' was responsible for about 1 per cent of all admissions to psychiatric hospitals, and his own case material indicated that it was more likely in cases of more severe concussion and in cases with skull fracture.

In a subsequent report, Schilder (1934) described the broader changes in consciousness and mood that were characteristic of the acute phase of recovery among 35 severely injured cases, and he commented that 'emotional disturbances and changes towards schizoid, psychopathic and epileptoid trends may be the final outcome of the organic disturbance' (p. 186). It is true that persistent psychiatric disturbances following closed head injury are potentially the most serious sequelae for both relatives and prospective employers; yet, as Newcombe and Artiola i Fortuny (1979) pointed out, they are perhaps the least well studied and understood. There have indeed been few major developments in the field since an authoritative and influential review was published by Lishman (1973), who considered four main categories of post-traumatic psychiatric disorder: intellectual impairment; change of personality and temperament; psychotic illness; and neurotic disability. With regard to the first of these, he felt that organic brain damage was undoubtedly the principal aetiological factor, but he emphasized that cognitive performance might be impaired by reduced motivation or by disturbances of affect. Other researchers have similarly argued that the cognitive impairment shown by patients with head injury is at least partly attributable to depression (e.g., Daniel, 1987). Conversely, Lishman asserted that post-traumtic personality changes were typically associated with cognitive impairment, but were not incompatible with intact performance on formal psychometric testing.

Personality Change

In the survey by Steadman and Graham (1970), 42 out of a total of 415 head-injured patients complained of personality change when interviewed five years after their accidents, and this was supported in 35 cases by the testimony of a relative. There was also a positive relationship between the incidence of personality change and the severity of the original head injury as measured by the duration of PTA. This would explain why an earlier study involving relatively minor cases of closed head injury had identified personality change in just 3.5 per cent of a series of 200 patients (Adler, 1945). Conversely, personality change is far more likely in cases of severe closed head injury. Thomsen (1974) described 50 such patients on average 30 months after head injuries which in many instances had given rise to coma lasting several weeks. At interview, the relatives of 42 (or 84 per cent) of the patients complained of changes in personality, often marked by irritability, hot temper, lack of spontaneity, restlessness, emotional regression, emotional lability and stubbornness. These changes were still evident in 65 per cent of cases when 40 patients out of the original sample were followed up between 10 and 15 years after their accidents (Thomsen, 1984). In a similar study reported by Roberts (1976; 1979, pp. 57–62), personality changes were noted in 117 (or 40 per cent) of 291 patients assessed between 10 and 24 years after they had sustained severe head injuries.

In a 2-year follow-up study of 44 patients with very severe head injuries (Weddell *et al.*, 1980), 34 cases (or 70 per cent) of the sample had suffered a personality change, and this was associated with poorer scores on the Progressive Matrices test and an increased probability of memory impairment according to the testimony of a close relative. Timming *et al.* (1982) noted 'personality abnormalities including irritability, inability to concentrate, temper tantrums, aggressive behavior, and depression to varying degrees' (p. 155) in the discharge notes of all but one of 30 patients with very severe head injuries. Finally, Livingston and Livingston (1985) found that subjective reports of personality change were far higher in patients with severe head injury than in patients with mild head injury and exhibited no sign of any improvement during the first 12 months after injury, despite the fact that they had been corroborated by a close relative.

The pattern of disturbance seen in cases of personality change after severe closed head injury is often typical of the syndrome associated with lesions from other causes of the frontal lobes, involving impaired social judgement, euphoria and disinhibition (e.g., Brown *et al.*, 1981). Rutter (1981) cautioned that 'even in studies of adults with localized injuries there is far from a one-to-one association between these disinhibited behaviors and frontal lobe lesions' (p. 1541), while Stuss and Benson (1984) concluded that 'the concept of frontal lobe personality alteration remains vague' (p. 21). Nevertheless, this is an interesting notion in the light of the effects of closed head injury upon higher executive function, which as mentioned in the previous chapter have also been associated with damage to the frontal lobes (*see* pp. 143–6). Malkmus (1983) speculated that behavioural disturbances following closed head injury were 'directly related to impaired cognitive function and the individual's attempts to function in an environment beyond his processing capacity'. She argued more specifically that:

> [the disruption of brain function] results in a concomitant disruption of the internal cognitive structure necessary for bringing organization and stability to the individual's internal and external environments. Such a breakdown in internal structuring mechanisms, or cognitive function, results in the individual's inability to effect and maintain an appropriate balance or relationship between self and environment . . . The behavioral chaos reflects the head-injured individual's neurologically inadequate attempts to abate the cognitive chaos . . . Ultimately, these behaviors become ingrained patterns of inappropriate behavior. (p. 1953)

This is of course very reminiscent of the sort of account that was offered by van Zomeren *et al.* (1984) in the case of the postconcussional syndrome but in this model the functional aetiology is linked specifically to 'internal structuring mechanisms' and not simply to information-processing capacity.

In children, and especially in those who have sustained very severe head injuries, disinhibited behaviours may take the form of outbursts of temper, disobedience and hyperactivity (Brink *et al.*, 1970), which given the poor judgement of head-injured patients tends to increase the risk of subsequent injury (*see* Barin *et al.*, 1985). However, similar behaviours may be identified as having occurred in children with moderate head injuries before their accidents (Brown *et al.*, 1981; Oddy, 1984b). In adults, they may also take the form of hypersexuality, and this poses additional problems for rehabilitative efforts (Price, 1987). Thomsen (1974) noted that the emotional lability of patients with severe head injuries tended to lead their relatives to isolate them from social situations; as a result, the main problem for 60 per cent of the patients in her sample was loneliness. Thomsen commented: 'Most patients had lost contact with premorbid friends and they had very few possibilities of establishing new contacts, because they spent nearly all [of their] time at home' (p. 182). Social isolation was also noted in 37 per cent of a sample of 27 severely injured patients studied by Levin *et al.* (1979a).

An early report by Hooper *et al.* (1945) had been concerned with adult head-injured patients who regularly showed outbursts of explosive and uncontrollable rage. Similar disturbances were described in subsequent research (e.g., Fahy *et al.*, 1967; Panting and Merry, 1972; Thomsen, 1984). In the follow-up study of severely head-injured patients described by Roberts (1979), these tended to occur in those patients (50 cases, or 17 per cent of the total sample) in whom the 'frontal' signs of euphoria, disinhibition and irresponsibility were combined with irritability and intellectual impairment. Roberts commented that in many of these patients it was their aggression rather than their dementia, euphoria, disinhibition, or apathy which was the principal cause of domestic misery and which in some cases had led to their commitment to long-term psychiatric institutions. He added that 'it was striking how often the main target and victim of ill-tempered and violent outbursts was the spouse' (p. 57). As Newcombe (1982) observed, such aggressiveness 'can be a source of distress to the patient, who may have some insight into the anguish it causes but has little control over its manifestation' (p. 122). Moreover, Gans (1983) argued that rage should be distinguished from feelings of hatred, which he claimed were an intrinsic part of the process of recovery and rehabilitation from a disabling condition.

Psychiatric Disorders

Meyer (1904) had emphasized that it might often be very difficult to say whether post-traumatic psychiatric symptoms were to be attributed to the trauma itself or to the 'mental shock' and its consequences. However, Ruesch *et al.* (1945) administered the Minnesota Multiphasic Personality Inventory to 128 head-injured patients, and concluded that 'the post-traumatic personality is more dependent on the pre-traumatic personality than on factors related to the injury' (p. 539). Lishman (1973) suggested that affective psychoses and neurotic disorders in cases of head injury were largely psychogenic in origin, having been precipitated by the trauma in those individuals who were constitutionally predisposed towards such conditions. Meyer also commented that the nature of these disorders 'hardly allows us to use the traditional terms mania, melancholia, etc. These terms would obscure the characteristic traits, since, indeed, the attacks deviate quite a little from non-traumatic mental disorders, notwithstanding superficial resemblances' (p. 430). Essentially the same point was subsequently made by Kozol (1946), who suggested that the comprehensive personality classification employed in psychiatry, general medicine and neurology 'might be inadequate in contributing information regarding the etiologic factors in the psychiatric sequelae of head injury' (p. 246). Similarly, Newcombe (1982) more recently observed that the emotional changes seen after closed head injury did not conform to the conventional patterns of psychiatric illness, and that the psychologist could not rely on techniques based solely on the psychiatric categories of neurosis and psychosis.

Nevertheless, under the broad heading of 'post-traumatic neuroses' Lishman (1973) included 'depressive reactions, anxiety states often with phobic symptomatology, neurasthenic reactions with fatigue, irritability and sensitivity to noise; cases of conversion hysteria and of obsessional neurosis; and, most common of all, a variety of somatic complaints, including headache and dizziness, which may become the subject of anxious introspection and hypochondriacal concern' (p. 314). The latter category obviously relates to the postconcussional syndrome; the issue of whether this condition should be characterized as a variety of 'anxiety neurosis' was discussed earlier in this chapter (p. 199). Lishman went on to conclude that on the balance of evidence post-traumatic schizophrenia was at least in some instances the direct result of organic damage. A similar conclusion had been reached by de Morsier (1972). There is even at least one report of Capgras' syndrome following head injury in a patient with no previous history of psychiatric disturbance (Weston and Whitlock, 1971): this is a state marked by the delusion that one's close relatives and friends have been replaced by imposters of identical physical appearance.

Shaffer *et al.* (1975) studied the psychiatric outcome in 98 children at least two years after a unilateral compound depressed fracture of the skull that was associated with a dural tear and visible damage to the underlying cortex. On the basis of a structured interview with each child's parents, the degree of psychiatric handicap was rated on a 5-point scale separately for the child, the mother, and the father, and a separate assessment was obtained from each child's teacher concerning behavioural problems. There was no significant relationship at all between the presence of psychiatric disorder (either according to a rating in the three highest points on the global interview or according to the teacher's overall assessment) and the child's age at injury, the anatomical locus of the skull fracture, or the severity of the injury as measured by the duration of coma. Nevertheless, the incidence of psychiatric disorder from the global interview rating was extraordinarily high (62 per cent), and Shaffer *et al.* found that it was significantly related to a number of adverse social and family variables: a broken or unhappy marriage between the parents, contact with two or more social agencies, psychiatric disorder on the part of the mother or father, and having four or more siblings. Indeed, the likelihood of psychiatric disorder varied directly with the total number of these factors to which each child had been exposed. Shaffer *et al.* concluded that these children might well require continuing support of a kind that was not customarily provided by a purely neurological or neurosurgical follow-up service.

In his follow-up study of 291 patients with severe head injuries, Roberts (1979, pp. 62–5) identified just nine cases of 'schizophreniform psychosis', though he also noted that many other patients had experienced paranoid delusional symptoms either transiently during the initial period of post-traumatic confusion or else more persistently during the first year or so following the injury. All of the cases with schizophreniform psychoses had been well before their accidents and none had any family history of schizophrenia. Seven of these patients were demented to varying degrees, while the two cases who were not demented did not develop their illnesses until many years after the injury. Roberts (pp. 85, 182) suggested that the latter illnesses were basically affective disorders which had not been precipitated by the trauma itself, and that the psychotic symptomatology displayed after head injury was more appropriately described as 'traumatic paranoid dementia' (*see also* Lewin *et al.*, 1979). Thomsen (1984) also identified eight cases of 'post-traumatic psychosis' among

40 patients who had sustained very severe closed head injury, including one schizophreniform patient. White *et al.* (1987) described a patient who developed a paranoid condition nearly four years after sustaining a minor closed head injury. Since the patient's delusions centred around his preoccupation with the litigation that was in progress, White *et al.* coined the expression 'compensation psychosis' to describe his condition.

Premorbid Personality

It is of course true that negative social behaviour following closed head injury may reflect the patient's premorbid personality rather than organic brain damage (Hayden and Hart, 1986; Jennett, 1984; Miller and Stern, 1965). In the study of head-injured twins reported by Dencker (1958, 1960), nine monozygotic and eleven dizygotic twins were said (either by themselves or their close relatives) to have undergone a change in personality following the head injury. Even so, the monozygotic patients still closely resembled their co-twins, and in 15 out of the 16 cases in which there was evidence of the patient's pretraumatic personality it appeared that any such 'change' actually predated the head injury. More specifically, although both the monozygotic twins and the dizygotic twins who had sustained head injuries were judged to be significantly more antisocial in their behaviour than their co-twins (as evidenced by alcohol abuse or committing criminal offences), in most cases these traits predated the head injury and could not therefore be regarded as being the result of that injury. Dencker concluded that people whose behaviour was more antisocial were simply more disposed to suffering head injuries. It should however be recognized that fewer than 10 per cent of the patients in this study had sustained severe head injuries, and that they were being assessed on average ten years after their accidents.

Black *et al.* (1971) presented findings from a consecutive series of 105 head-injured children of up to 14 years of age. Although there was a considerable increase in the incidence of behavioural disorders such as eating problems, hyperkinesis and impaired attention, the reports of their parents and guardians suggested that one-third of the children had suffered from at least one of these symptoms before their injury. Nevertheless, roughly 20 per cent of the children who had shown no such symptoms previously became symptomatic after their injury, and the same proportion of children who had shown premorbid behavioural problems showed symptoms that were different in kind or degree after their injury. Black *et al.* concluded as follows: 'Although premorbid personality may influence the nature of post-traumatic sequelae, the injury itself appears to be responsible for the development or aggravation of symptoms. Whether this effect of injury has an organic basis or represents a psychological reaction to trauma cannot be determined from these data' (p. 133)

Further evidence on this matter was obtained by Levin and Grossman (1978) from

70 patients recovering from closed head injuries of varying degrees of severity who had no history of psychiatric illness. Each patient was assessed along a 7-point scale on the severity of 18 symptoms taken from the Brief Psychiatric Rating Scale (BPRS: Overall and Gorham, 1962). The scores on selected clusters of symptoms were used to generate composite scores on four factors reflecting Thinking Disturbance, Hostile-Suspiciousness, Withdrawal-Retardation and Anxiety Depression, and the total score across all 18 symptoms was used as a global index of psychopathology. The patients who had been conscious on their admission to hospital and who had shown no neurological deficits produced little or no sign of any behavioural disturbance except in terms of somatic concern and anxiety. More severely injured patients showed a distinct pattern of behavioural sequelae that was characterized by cognitive disorganization, motor retardation, emotional withdrawal and blunted affect. The degree of behavioural disturbance shown by individual patients was positively related to the duration of coma, the incidence of hemiplegia and aphasia, and the incidence of abnormalities according to electroencephalography and computerized tomography (CT). However, the incidence of mesencephalic damage, skull fracture and intracranial haematoma and the intracerebral lateralization and localization of the predominant lesion had little or no effect. A detailed comparison of patients with specific CT abnormalities led Levin and Grossman to conclude:

> Our findings suggest that early compression of the ventricular system by edematous brain is predictive of substantial behavioral disturbance and that persistent CT abnormalities such as ventricular enlargement without signs of obstructive hydrocephalus are accompanied by prolonged psychiatric manifestations. (p. 726)

Agitated behaviour during the acute stage of recovery was also found to have prognostic value in this connection.

Levin *et al.* (1979a) identified a similar pattern of disturbance among 27 patients with severe closed head injuries to whom the BPRS was administered on average more than one year after their accidents. It was noted that patients who manifested moderate or marked Thinking Disturbance tended not to appreciate the severity of their cognitive deficit, but instead tended to complain about relatively minor residual symptoms or else to deny any sequelae at all. Moreover, ratings on this factor 'reflected tangential, fragmented speech not attributable to aphasia and deficient cognitive filtering of irrelevant material' (p. 417). In contrast, ratings of Withdrawal-Retardation were influenced by motor signs such as slowing or aspontaneity of movement and speech.

Brown *et al.* (1981) carried out a comparative investigation of three groups of children: 28 had suffered severe head injuries, resulting in PTA lasting for at least seven days, 29 had suffered mild head injuries, resulting in PTA lasting for less than seven days, and 28 had suffered orthopaedic injuries not involving the head. In order to obtain an assessment of these children's behaviour before the injury, interviews were carried out with their parents as soon as possible after the accident, on the assumption that they would not yet know how the children would be affected. The children who had sustained severe head injuries were very similar to the orthopaedic control patients in terms of their previous behaviour; however, within four months of their accidents they showed a substantial increase in their level of behavioural disturbance, and this was still apparent at a follow-up assessment carried out two years later. In contrast, the children who had sustained mild head injuries manifested a premorbid rate of behavioural disturbance which was markedly higher that that of the orthopaedic control patients, but which showed no increase as a result of the accident. In other words, children with mild head injuries seemed to be behaviourally different before their accidents, but the head injuries did not themselves appear to increase the risk of subsequent psychiatric disorder. Nevertheless, severe head injuries did appear to exert a causal influence upon personality and social behaviour, and this followed a 'dose-response' relationship insofar as the incidence of post-traumatic behavioural disturbance was correlated with the severity of the injury as measured by the duration of PTA (*see also* Rutter, 1981).

In short, some psychiatric disturbances manifested after closed head injury are merely manifestations of pre-existing behavioral disorders, whereas others are genuinely the result of organic damage incurred as a direct result of the injury. Fuld and Fisher (1977) reported the case of a child who exhibited serious behavioural problems at school following a relatively mild head injury; they suggested that these had arisen from the stress of coping with temporary intellectual impairments in addition to previously borderline functioning. Malkmus (1983) similarly argued that behavioural disorders might be related to and mediated by various aspects of impaired cognitive function in head-injured patients:

> Diffuse craniocerebral trauma disrupts the neural structures that subserve cognitive-behavioral functions. This disruption results in a concomitant disruption of the internal cognitive structure necessary for bringing organization and stability to the individual's internal and external environments . . . .
>
> Once the brain is no longer able to initiate, direct, suppress, and redirect mental activity adequately, the behavioral display of impaired cognition may include confusion; disorientation; impairment of attention, memory, and learning; disorganization of verbal and nonverbal activity; and incompleteness of thought and action . . . . Thus, the behavioral chaos demonstrated after craniocerebral trauma is the result of cognitive chaos. (p. 1953)

This is an interesting analysis of the functional basis of post-traumatic psychiatric disturbances that serves to integrate current understanding of the cognitive and behavioural consequences of closed head injury. Though it is far from clear whether this sort of account is empirically testable, it does serve to direct the attention of professionals concerned with the treatment of behavioural disorders in head-injured patients towards their concomitant neuropsychological deficits.

Family Relationships

The Burden on Relatives

During the 1950s it was demonstrated that prompt treatment of respiratory insufficiency could substantially reduce the level of mortality following severe head injury. In reporting this finding Maciver *et al.* (1958) also claimed that the prospects for the survivors were relatively good:

> With the regime described, the majority of patients who recovered have developed little in the way of intellectual deterioration or severe mental symptoms. Most of the patients will be fit to return to productive work and will not remain a burden on their family or the community. (p. 550)

Subsequently, however, London (1967) argued that these statements obscured the 'crushing magnitude' of the burden that permanently disabled survivors imposed upon their close relatives by virtue of the changes in their moods and behaviour:

> One of the most distressing effects of severe cerebral injury has been on the patient's personality, and this lays a much heavier burden on the family than on the community. Physical injury is fairly easily handled, but emotional and intellectual damage can be disastrous. One can only marvel at the patience and understanding shown by the relatives, and particularly the wives, of some of these violent and handicapped persons. (p. 469)

In a study of 46 children with severe head injuries, Brink *et al.* (1970) similarly noted that 'the aggressive, impulsive, and sometimes destructive behaviour exhibited by our patients was very often more difficult for the families to manage than the residual physical disability' (p. 570).

This impression was born out by the results of interviews carried out by Thomsen (1974) with relatives of 50 patients between 12 and 70 months after the latter had sustained severe closed head injuries. Most of the patients still had some physical impairment, but none of their relatives complained of the difficulties involved in coping with limited mobility. The patients' intellectual impairment often created problems, especially their disorders of memory, but the most serious difficulties in everyday life for their relatives were the result of their changes in personality. As

Thomsen (1984) commented, 'while lack of social contact . . . was the greatest subjective burden to the patients, changes in personality and emotion represented the severest problem to the families' (p. 264; *see also* Lewin *et al.*, 1979). Jennett (1976d) pointed out that it was this particular combination of mental impairment with physical handicap that made brain damage so devastating in its consequences, and so different from the 'heroic and happy survival' of mentally intact patients which typified spinal paralysis (p. 597).

As Livingston and Brooks (1988) commented, most studies that attempt to assess the burden on families after head injury measure the relatives' perceptions of their burden rather than its objective effects. The former (that is, the 'subjective' burden) can be studied by means of a variety of self-report methods, but even the latter (that is, the 'objective' burden) tend to be measured in terms of the changes that are reported by relatives in comparison with the patients' premorbid behaviour (e.g., Brooks *et al.*, 1986a; McKinlay *et al.*, 1981). Moreover, these investigations are usually confined to family members who live with the patient in question. For example, in the investigation by Oddy *et al.* (1978b) that was described earlier (p. 182), the checklist concerning personality changes and somatic, sensory, cognitive and psychiatric symptoms was also given to a close relative (usually a parent or the spouse) of 49 patients with severe head injury. The symptoms that were mentioned most frequently by the relatives were 'trouble remembering things', 'becomes tired very easily', 'often impatient', 'often loses temper' and 'often irritable'. The patients and their relatives gave broadly similar accounts of the symptoms experienced, although there were some marked discrepancies in individual cases which Oddy *et al.* took to 'underline the hazards of accepting the patient's report as definitive' (p. 615).

The relatives in this study also received a detailed interview and a depression questionnaire within one month of the accident and at roughly six and 12 months afterwards (Humphrey and Oddy, 1978; Oddy *et al.*, 1978a; *see also* Oddy, 1984a). The results indicated that there was overt disturbance in roughly 25 per cent of the patients' families, whether measured by the depression scale or the relatives' reports. The level of reported stress was highest during the first month following the head injury and appeared to reach a plateau between six and 12 months later. More than half of the physical illnesses that were reported by the relatives could be regarded as stress-related, including asthma, migraine and duodenal ulcer. Many had received support and medication from their general practitioners, but none had received psychiatric treatment. The principal sources of stress were anxieties arising from the patient's condition (including the risk of epilepsy, loss of self-control and the effort of coping with disability) and concern about the patient's future.

Not surprisingly, family relationships appeared to be significantly poorer in the case of patients who had suffered adverse personality changes (Oddy and Humphrey, 1980). The frequency of arguments and disagreements and problems in communication increased markedly between six and 12 months after the injury; as in the study by

Thomsen (1974) these difficulties were more apparent between the married patients and their partners than between the single patients and their parents (*see also* Livingston *et al.*, 1985a). Lezak (1978) discussed the special problems faced by the spouse of a head-injured patient. The same general problems were seen in a more pronounced form in a 2-year follow-up study carried out by Weddell *et al.* (1980). This involved 44 patients from a regional rehabilitation centre who constituted some of the most severely injured survivors of closed head injury. Once again, increased irritability among the patients was a common problem leading to higher levels of friction within their families.

A similar investigation was carried out by Brooks and Aughton (1979) in the case of relatives of 35 patients with severe blunt head injuries. They received a subjective assessment in which they were asked to rate the extent of their experienced burden or stress along a 7-point scale, plus an objective questionnaire concerned with observable changes in the family routine, health, or housing resulting from the patient's head injury and with the patient's post-traumatic symptoms and changes in behaviour and personality. The most frequently reported items of objective burden when relatives were assessed roughly six months after the head injuries proved to be related to the patient's mental impairment, and more specifically to changes in the level of irritability, slowness, tiredness and tension or anxiety; conversely, the least frequently cited items of objective burden were concerned with physical and sensory change. The items of objective burden that best predicted the relatives' perceived subjective burden were the patient's childish behaviour, loss of interest, change in sex life, depression, and tension or anxiety. A similar pattern had been found by Rosenbaum and Najenson (1976) among the wives of 16 head-injured soldiers, though in half of these cases the injuries in question had been caused by penetrating missiles. In accordance with the view of London (1967) which was quoted at the beginning of this section, Brooks and Aughton concluded that 'families are apparently well able to deal with physical impairment, but find emotional and personality change in the patient a source of great burden' (p. 164).

McKinlay *et al.* (1981) used the same procedures to interview close relatives of 55 patients with severe closed head injury at 3, 6 and 12 months after their accidents. Once again, the symptoms in the patients that were most frequently reported as problems by their relatives were emotional changes, memory impairment and subjective changes such as slowness and tiredness. There was no change in the amount of stress reported in terms of the perceived subjective burden across the three sessions, although there was a tendency for emotional difficulties to be reported in the patients more frequently at the later sessions. It was suggested that the latter might be either consequences of the injury which had not been acknowledged during the earlier phase of recovery or else the patients' reactions to their developing awareness of disability. Increased levels of reported stress in the relatives were associated with mental and behavioural changes in the patients rather than with problems in the areas of perception, speech and mobility, although McKinlay *et al.* cautioned against the assumption of any direct causal relationship between reported changes in the patients and the stress that relatives attributed to those changes.

The relatives in this study were also asked to complete an adjective checklist containing 18 analogue scales that were labelled with pairs of bipolar adjectives (e.g., 'talkative-quiet') chosen to reflect the sorts of changes in personality and behaviour that follow severe head injuries. At each session the relative completed the checklist, first, with regard to the patient's personality before the closed head injury and, second, with regard to the present time. The results were reported by Brooks and McKinlay (1983). Not surprisingly, the ratings produced by the relatives on the current and retrospective checklists showed significant changes in the anticipated direction on many of the constituent scales. These were mainly confined to those cases where the relatives judged that there had indeed been some change in the patients' overall personality, though even in the cases where there was no such change the patients were reported to be significantly more quick-tempered, irritable, lifeless and listless by the 12-month session. Brooks and McKinlay suggested that the latter were characteristics of all head-injured patients rather than specific features of those who had suffered personality change.

In this study, the relatives tended to be more likely to judge that there had been a personality change in patients with more severe injuries according to the duration of PTA, although the latter was not a good predictor of the scores on the individual scales of the adjective checklist. The perceived subjective burden showed little or no relationship to the adjective checklist scores at the 3-month session; however, the association between the stress experienced by the relatives and the patients' personality increased over time, so that the subjective burden was significantly related to 12 of the 18 scales by the time of the 12-month session. Since the relatives had clearly acknowledged changes in the patients' personality even at the 3-month session, these results were taken to reflect a progressively decreasing ability to accept or cope with the negative changes in the patients' personality. A major consideration here is probably that the generalized social isolation that affects patients following severe closed head injures entails an equally significant degree of social isolation for their partners and families (Newcombe, 1982; Thomsen, 1984). This may be exacerbated by physical or verbal abuse from the patients themselves and by the withdrawal of support from members of their extended families as the patients' disabilities and prognosis become apparent (Lezak, 1978; *see also* Roberts, 1979, p. 57).

Brooks *et al.* (1986a) repeated the above procedures at a 5-year follow-up assessment of 42 of their original sample of head-injured patients. The symptoms that were reported as problems by their relatives were broadly the same as those that had been reported at the 12-month assessment. Two items (irritability and tiredness) showed marginal reductions in the intervening period but two other items (personality change and threats of violence) showed marked increases. The perceived subjective burden showed a highly significant increase in this period according to a single rating on a 7-point scale, although once again this was primarily associated with mental and behavioural changes in the patients. Brooks *et al.* concluded that for the relatives the situation had deteriorated markedly over the 5-year period. In particular, 'Frank violence against relatives had risen dramatically, and a number of relatives reported feeling afraid of the patient. Others reported constant anxiety as they tried to avoid provoking aggressive outbursts, and many felt that the patient could not be left alone' (p. 769).

A detailed assessment of the psychiatric and social impact of severe head injury upon the patient's relatives was carried out by Livingston *et al.* (1985a, 1985b). They studied a female relative (wife, mother, or daughter) of each of 57 male patients who had sustained a head injury that had led to a period of PTA longer than 48 hours. Out of this total sample the relatives of 42 patients were evaluated at three months after the injury, those of 47 patients were evaluated at six months, and those of 50 patients were evaluated at 12 months. Their psychiatric morbidity was compared with that of similarly defined relatives of 41 other patients who were assessed three months after mild head injury which had required admission to hospital for less than 48 hours. The relatives of the severely injured patients produced higher scores on both the General Health Questionnaire (Goldberg, 1978) and the Leeds Anxiety Scale (Snaith *et al.*, 1976) which persisted throughout the first year. Indeed, on both measures 30–40 per cent of these relatives produced scores that were within the clinical 'caseness' range at each of the follow-up sessions. However, no such pattern was demonstrated on the Leeds Depression Scale or the somatic complaints or depression subscales of the General Health Questionnaire. As Livingston *et al.* (1985b) concluded, psychiatric disturbance among the relatives of patients with severe head injuries 'is affective and indeed is anxiety based rather than depressive' (p. 872).

In comparison with the relatives of patients with mild head injuries, the relatives of the severely injured patients in this study also reported a much higher incidence of problems on a formal questionnaire concerned with the perceived burden of living with the patient, and this if anything manifested a slight increase throughout the year. On a Social Adjustment Scale (Weissman *et al.*, 1978), the latter group of relatives showed lower subjective levels of functioning within their marital and familial roles. In other words, they rated themselves as being less well adjusted in their social relationships in the family home, whereas their relationships within their extended family, at work, and in their social and leisure activities were largely unaffected. Their scores on global social adjustment became significantly worse between the 3-month and 6-month assessments and remained poor for the remainder of the year. Finally, the various measures of the relatives' psychosocial functioning were better predicted by the level of subjective complaints on the part of the patient than by other clinical characteristics, and in particular they showed no relation with measures of the severity of the original injury. The implication of these results, as Livingston *et al.* noted, is that 'it is the patients' functioning at the time of assessment, which is critical for the relatives' wellbeing' (p. 880). More precisely, as Livingston (1985) pointed out, insofar as the relatives of head-injured patients sometimes complain that they receive inadequate information from clinicians, it is the relative's perception of the burden imposed by the patient rather than the objective outcome that is important.

Livingston (1987) carried out a further regression analysis in order to determine the biographical characteristics of the relatives of severely head-injured patients which predicted the various measures of psychosocial functioning. The most important determinant of the latter was found to be the relatives' previous experience of illness, as determined from their psychiatric and physical health records. Taken together, these findings led Livingston to suggest a two-stage model of psychosocial breakdown in the families of head-injured patients, based upon accounts of individual vulnerability towards other psychiatric conditions: 'Firstly, relatives are "sensitized" by previous illness experience themselves. Secondly, a maladaptive coping strategy is provoked by the current life stress of the head injury patient's symptoms display' (pp. 37–8). Livingston concluded that therapeutic programmes for relatives of head-injured patients might usefully focus on conflicts which they had encountered during their own previous experiences of illness, while Livingston and Brooks (1988) also suggested that vulnerable relatives could be identified during the early stages of the patients' recovery and helped accordingly.

Discrepancies between Patients' and Relatives' Reports

A fundamental problem in evaluating the reports given by the relatives of head-injured patients is that they may differ in important respects from the patients' own accounts. This was first noted in a 6-year follow-up study by Fahy *et al.* (1967) involving patients who had undergone surgical treatment of severe head injury. These researchers carried out standard psychiatric interviews with patients in their own homes in the presence of 'suitable informants':

> There were interesting discrepancies between disability as recounted by relatives and as perceived by the patients themselves. Spontaneous complaints by the patients were rare, and motor disabilities were lightly dismissed by patients and relatives alike. Witnessing a standard interview, however, often provoked informants to supply details of abnormal behaviour which would otherwise have been missed because of lack of insight in demented survivors. Sensible of their difficulties in the fields of intellect, memory, and speech, patients seldom acknowledged temperamental changes, which in turn distressed their families most. (p. 477)

Thomsen (1974) also noted that patients with severe head injuries seldom seemed to be aware of the changes in their personality that constituted a major problem for their families. Nevertheless, in evaluating the effects of closed head injury on intellectual ability in children, Fuld and Fisher (1977) concluded that 'neither the child's mother nor the physician can be relied upon to be an accurate judge of the child's mental status; some tend to deny and others to exaggerate changes in the child's abilities' (p. 497). In particular, they described a child who was reported to be 'back to normal' by both his mother and his paediatrician, and yet who on examination was found to be obviously lethargic and withdrawn and to be so impaired in attention and comprehension that conventional tests of verbal intelligence could simply not be administered.

McKinlay and Brooks (1984) addressed this issue in a more systematic fashion by comparing the subjective complaints of 55 patients assessed six months after severe closed head injury with the accounts of their close relatives as described in previous publications from their research group (i.e., Brooks and Aughton, 1979; Brooks and McKinlay, 1983; McKinlay *et al.*, 1981). They reported a relatively high agreement between the patients' and the relatives' accounts with regard to the incidence of sensory or motor impairment, only a moderate level of agreement with regard to the incidence of cognitive impairment, and very poor agreement with regard to the incidence of emotional and behavioural changes. In particular, there was agreement in only 60 per cent of these cases as to whether or not the patient had become more bad tempered and in only 52 per cent of the cases as to whether or not the patient had become more anxious since the injury. As in the case of the earlier studies by Fahy *et al.* (1967) and by Thomsen (1974), instances of disagreement over emotional and behavioural changes tended predominantly to arise from patients failing to admit to changes that were reported by their relatives.

Obviously, in such cases the patients' reports and their relatives' reports cannot both be accurate. In the passage quoted above, Fahy *et al.* (1967) ascribed these discrepancies to a lack of insight amongst demented survivors, and the account given by Thomsen (1974) appeared to extend this explanation to a lack of awareness of personality changes even in the case of head-injured patients who had recovered a normal level of orientation. McKinlay and Brooks (1984) noted that this left open the question whether the putative lack of insight was to be attributed to cognitive deficits or to some other mechanism. To explore this possibility further, McKinlay and Books compared the number of aspects of behaviour for which each of their patients denied a change which had been reported by a relative with their scores on a variety of psychometric tests. They found no consistent pattern of correlations, even when the effects of premorbid intelligence were statistically controlled by partialling out the effects of Verbal IQ. They concluded that 'where patients deny problems which relatives report them to have (i.e., when patients "lack insight"), this is not related to cognitive deficit' (p. 92).

The alternative possibility is that the perceptions and reports of the relatives of head-injured patients are coloured in a systematic way, perhaps as a coping response to the stress of caring for a disabled and characterologically altered member of the family. It was noted earlier that stress among the relatives of head-injured patients was associated with post-traumatic changes in personality (*see* Lezak, 1978; McKinlay *et al.*, 1981; Oddy *et al.*, 1978a; Rosenbaum and Najenson, 1976), and it has also been suggested that relatives' stress levels tend to be especially pronounced in those cases where the patients deny problems which their relatives report them to have (e.g., Fahy *et al.*, 1967; Thomsen, 1974). Nevertheless, McKinlay and Brooks (1984) advocated caution in postulating a direct causal link between the reported sequelae of head injury and the degree of family disruption, and they suggested that the levels of stress experienced by the relatives of head-injured patients might be modulated by certain personality characteristics (for instance, emotional stability) that led them to cope more or less easily with their altered situation.

To evaluate this notion, McKinlay and Brooks administered the Eysenck Personality Questionnaire (Eysenck and Eysenck, 1975) to the relatives of the 55 severely head-injured patients in their investigation. They found that the relatives' scores on the Neuroticism scale of this inventory were significantly correlated both with their subjective reports of changes in the head-injured patient, especially of emotional and behavioural changes, and their levels of perceived stress. McKinlay and Brooks commented that emotional and behavioural changes were still more frequently reported by the relatives of head-injured patients and more closely related to their levels of perceived stress than physical or intellectual changes even when the influence of

Figure 6.1   Possible relationships between relatives' reports, stress in relatives, and personality

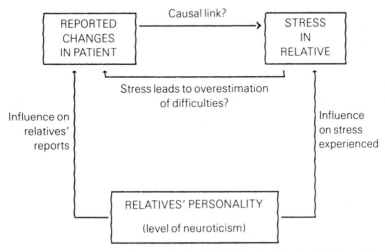

Source: McKinlay, W. W. and Brooks, D. N. (1984) 'Methodological problems in assessing psychosocial recovery following severe head injury', *Journal of Clinical Neuropsychology*, 6, pp. 87–99. Adapted with permission.

personality characteristics was statistically controlled. Nevertheless, they took the fact that Neuroticism was related both to the nature and incidence of the reported changes in head-injured patients and to the level of perceived stress amongst their relatives to mean that the psychosocial outcome was dependent on a complex set of interrelationships rather than a single causal connection (*see* Figure 6.1).

Concluding Summary

In addition to subjective complaints of poor memory and concentration, the initial period of recovery following closed head injury is associated with reports of headache, dizziness, fatigue, anxiety and irritability. These symptoms subside within a matter of days or weeks in many patients, while in others they persist beyond the immediate post-traumatic period. This 'postconcussional syndrome' may occur both following minor head injuries and following severe head injuries, but it may be more common in patients with a premorbid neurotic personality. This condition also affects both patients who are involved in litigation arising out of their injuries and those who have no possibility of making claims for compensation, but seems to be more common in those who blame their employers or a large impersonal organization for their accidents. Persistent postconcussional symptoms may be associated with poorer performance on psychometric testing, though this is obviously under the strategic control of the patients themselves, and they may result from an unsympathetic attitude on the part of doctors. Such a condition probably represents a long-term neurotic reaction to the short-term organic consequences of head injury. From a cognitive point of view it can be seen as a coping response to the impact of a reduction in central information-processing capacity upon the demands of everyday life.

Apart from intellectual impairment, the main types of post-traumatic psychiatric disturbance are personality changes, psychotic illnesses and neurotic disability. Personality changes are more common in patients who have suffered severe head injury; indeed, behavioural disorders following minor head injury may simply reflect the patients' premorbid personality. Post-traumatic personality changes are often reminiscent of the pattern of disturbance that is commonly associated with lesions of the frontal lobes, and have been attributed to a disruption of internal cognitive structure. They involve impaired social judgement, euphoria and disinhibition, but in extreme cases may include outbursts of uncontrollable rage. Psychoses and neuroses are less common following closed head injury; they do not conform to conventional patterns of psychopathology and may occur in patients with no history of psychiatric illness. Such conditions impose a severe burden upon the families of head-injured patients, though relatives' descriptions of the patients' behaviour will not necessarily tally with the accounts of the patients' themselves. These discrepancies are attributable sometimes to a lack of insight on the patients' part and sometimes to the relatives' stress in caring for a disabled and characterologically altered member of the family.

Chapter 7

Outcome, Recovery and Rehabilitation

The preceding chapters have been concerned with the short-term impact of closed head injury upon psychological functioning, both during the period of the patient's hospitalization and following his or her discharge into the community. This chapter is concerned with the patient's subsequent progress, with the likely nature of the long-term outcome, the recovery processes which lead to that outcome, and the scope for facilitating those processes by means of formal rehabilitative intervention. London (1967) pointed out that strictly speaking 'to rehabilitate' means 'to restore to a former position of power and influence', and he observed that following severe head injury

> discharge from hospital is all too often the prelude to the longest and most frustrating period of all; a period in which the prospect of truly rehabilitating the patient sometimes gives way to the hope that he will be able to do something to earn a living and finally to resigned acceptance that a once productive and creative member of the community has become a heavy and lifelong burden upon his family. (pp. 475–6)

In contrast to this gloomy picture, many head-injured patients are said to make an excellent recovery. However, Newcombe (1982) commented that such a description is variously used in different accounts of the consequences of a closed head injury to refer to patients' vegetative functions, their superficial conversation, and their capacity to return to work. As Miller (1979) noted, in each case what is considered to be a 'good' outcome could nevertheless encompass patients with definite residual impairments. Such comments as these illustrate the many different ways of characterizing the long-term outcome following closed head injury and the variety of possible goals of rehabilitation (*see also* Aitken *et al.*, 1982; Oddy *et al.*, 1978b). However, the rigorous definition of different categories of outcome is a prerequisite for the systematic analysis of the prognostic significance of patient characteristics and other clinical variables (*see* Jennett, 1976b; Jennett *et al.*, 1975a).

Measures of Outcome

Mortality

Epidemiological information concerning the incidence of fatal head injury was presented and discussed in Chapter 1 (pp. 28–32). As a measure of the outcome of closed head injury, death might seem relatively unproblematic, but Jennett and Bond (1975) emphasized that it might be difficult to agree on the criteria for specifically attributing the causal responsibility to the head injury itself. Those patients who fail to survive closed head injury have often sustained other major traumatic lesions, and they may well go on to develop extracranial complications or fatal systemic disease that is complicated by coma. Most deaths following head injury occur within the first two or three days, and the vast majority of these can be ascribed to the primary brain damage. However, extracranial lesions and complications have an increasing importance after this time and may be responsible for 40 per cent of all deaths occurring during and after the third week; acute renal insufficiency and bronchopulmonary infections seem to be especially important secondary causes of death following closed head injury (Bricolo *et al.*, 1980; Carlsson *et al.*, 1968; Jennett and Teasdale, 1981, p. 41; Pazzaglia *et al.*, 1975).

A number of studies have shown that mortality following severe head injury is inversely related to the patient's score on the Glasgow Coma Scale during the first 24 hours after the accident and directly related to the subsequent duration of coma (e.g., Alexandre *et al.*, 1983; Bowers & Marshall, 1980; Bricolo *et al.*, 1980; Gennarelli *et al.*, 1982; Marshall *et al.*, 1983a). It was noted in Chapter 1 that the total score on the Glasgow Coma Scale during the early phase of recovery from severe closed head injury was largely a function of the patient's motor responses (p. 10), and it is therefore not surprising that the latter element has been found to be the best predictor of mortality (Makela *et al.*, 1982). Some studies have found an increased risk of mortality among patients in whom intracranial mass lesions had been visualized by means of angiography or computerized tomography (CT) (e.g., Bricolo *et al.*, 1980; Gennarelli *et al.*, 1982; Pazzaglia *et al.*, 1975). Nevertheless, severely injured patients with normal CT scans still show a high mortality rate (Snoek *et al.*, 1979), suggesting that CT may often fail to detect life-threatening cerebral lesions (cf. Chapter 2, pp. 46, 54–5). The risk of mortality also seems to be increased among those head-injured patients who produce abnormal electroencephalograms or oculomotor responses that are suggestive of mesencephalic damage during the early stages of recovery (Alexandre *et al.*, 1983).

Finally, the mortality rate is higher among older patients (e.g., Bricolo *et al.*, 1980; Heiskanen and Sipponen, 1970; Jennett, 1976c; Jennett *et al.*, 1976; Pazzaglia *et al.*, 1975; Teasdale *et al.*, 1979b). Indeed, in a study of the outcome of severe head injury, Heiden *et al.* (1983) found that not one of 26 patients aged 60 or more survived the subsequent 12 months. Carlsson *et al.* (1968) found that this trend could be attributed entirely to the occurrence of extracranial complications rather than to primary cerebral injury, except in the case of children aged up to ten years whose mortality rate was only half that of older patients. In contrast, Jennett (1976c; Jennett *et al.*, 1979b) found a higher mortality among children under the age of five than in those aged between five and 20; he suggested that previous studies of paediatric head injury had included a disproportionate number of patients with less severe injuries. However, this cannot apply to the analysis of Carlsson *et al.*, which excluded any patients who emerged from coma within 12 hours of their accidents, and was thus restricted to those who had 'received a brain concussion of critical magnitude' (p. 242).

Jennett and Plum (1972) observed that some patients with severe head injuries never regain recognizable mental functioning, but

> recover from sleep-like coma in that they have periods of wakefulness when their eyes are open and move; their responsiveness is limited to primitive postural and reflex movements of the limbs, and they never speak. Such patients are best described as in a persistent vegetative state... (p. 734)

Graham *et al.* (1983) studied 28 patients with fatal head injury who had survived for at least a month after their accidents in a vegetative state together with seven patients who had been assessed as severely disabled. Apart from cerebral contusions, the most common findings at *post mortem* were diffuse axonal injury and extensive hypoxic necrosis. Only three patients showed both types of pathology, indicating that either of these processes might cause a vegetative state or severe disability after head injury. In three cases the hypoxic brain damage was severe and diffuse of the type associated with resuscitation following cardiac arrest or status epilepticus (*see* Jennett and Teasdale, 1981, pp. 39, 85–6.) Within the first three months of a head injury there is limited scope for improvement from this condition. In a prospective study of 213 severely injured patients carried out by Heiden *et al.* (1983), 16 per cent were in a vegetative state when assessed one month after their accidents. More than a quarter of these patients were found to be conscious (although severely disabled) when followed up 11 months later. On the other hand, more than half had died of infections during the intervening interval. The overall proportion of patients with severe closed head injuries who survive in a persistent vegetative state beyond the first three months appears to be less than 5 per cent (e.g., Alexandre *et al.*, 1983; Bowers & Marshall, 1980; Bricolo *et al.*, 1980; Bruce *et al.*, 1978; Gennarelli *et al.*, 1982; Heiden *et al.*, 1983; Heiskanen & Sipponen, 1970; Rimel & Jane, 1983; Roberts, 1979, p. 33), although this may be somewhat more likely in the case of patients who prove to have enlarged ventricles on CT scans (Timming *et al.*, 1982). While this is a 'persistent' condition, such patients rarely survive more than ten years after the injury (Higashi *et al.*, 1977; Roberts, 1979, pp. 41, 151). Jennett and Bond (1975) commented that their deaths might be technically attributed to complications such as pneumonia, but that 'it would be deception to deny that they are due to the original brain damage' (p. 482).

Considerable public and professional interest has been expressed in the notion that programmes of intense sensory stimulation might help the recovery of such patients. Malkmus (1983) explained the rationale for this approach by saying that it 'provides an organized presentation of heightened sensory input to prevent further sensory deprivation, to encourage responsiveness to external input, and to monitor and to assess cognitive status' (p. 1954). Nevertheless, Hayden and Hart (1986) argued that there was no evidence that these programmes of 'sensory bombardment' had any beneficial effect at all on the survival of comatose patients, and they concluded that 'the medical community would do well to treat sensory bombardment programs with a healthy skepticism' (p. 206). They also noted that Luria *et al.* (1969) had specifically advised that patients with closed head injury 'should be protected against strong and excessively strong stimuli' during the acute phase of recovery so as to facilitate the gradual reactivation of temporarily inhibited nerve cells (p. 370). Instead, Luria and his colleagues suggested that this process might be successfully accomplished by the use of pharmacological agents. As Hayden and Hart observed, it follows from this that scope for direct intervention in these cases will largely be restricted to their medical management, and that the functions of the rehabilitation specialist will be confined to monitoring their responsivity and providing support for their families and carers.

Alternatively, some patients may apparently regain consciousness soon after a closed head injury, but subsequently deteriorate rapidly. Reilly *et al.* (1975) noted that some such patients appear sufficiently lucid that they are not admitted to hospital at first and might not even seek medical advice themselves; in others, their speech during this 'lucid interval' is confined to a few muttered words. Adams *et al.* (1985) identified 134 such cases among 434 patients who died of closed head injury. On investigation many cases of this sort are found to have raised intracranial pressure and a midline shift on CT, both of which contribute to the risk of fatality (Marshall *et al.*, 1983b; but cf. Graham *et al.*, 1987). Bricolo *et al.* (1980) found that the occurrence of a lucid interval had no influence upon the likelihood of subsequent survival.

Neurological Outcome

Nevertheless, most closed head injuries are not fatal, and it was noted above that most deaths which are attributable to closed head injury occur within the first few days. It follows that most head-injured patients who survive this period will subsequently have a normal life expectancy, and that with regard to the outcome of treatment for these patients 'success should be measured less by the fact of survival and more by the quality of survival' (Jennett and Bond, 1975, p. 481). London (1967) considered that insufficient prominence had been given to the plight of those victims of head injury who suffered permanent disablement:

Unfortunately, survival is not synonymous with recovery and we are liable to find ourselves looking after living creatures that for all their obvious human form show none of the features of the human personality and no sign of ever recovering it. This is the extreme example, and mercifully rare, but severely and permanently handicapped persons — lamebrains — are more numerous. (p. 462)

On the basis of his experience at the Birmingham Accident Hospital, London estimated that head injuries were giving rise to 1000 new 'lamebrains' in the United Kingdom each year, roughly half of whom would never work again. This figure is of course cumulative over the years and more recent reports have suggested that the *prevalence* of chronic disability following closed head injury (that is, the total number of permanently disabled survivors) is between 100 and 150 per 100 000 population or between 55 000 and 80 000 across the UK as a whole (Aitken *et al.*, 1982; Bryden, 1989).

Motor impairment is the most conspicuous form of residual disability. Brink *et al.* (1970) studied the motor function of 46 children with severe head injuries, and found that 93 per cent of the sample manifested varying degrees of spasticity (defined as hyperactive deep tendon stretch reflexes and increased resistance to passive movement). In half of the sample this was moderate to severe and associated with limited control of fine manual movements, while in the most severe cases only gross flexion and extension of the extremities were possible. Bilateral spasticity was more common in patients who had been in coma for more than four weeks. In addition, 60 per cent of the sample showed unsteady movements and gait (ataxia), which in some cases inhibited even simple activities such as eating or walking. Johnston and Mellits (1980) subsequently found that the duration of coma was highly correlated with the degree of impairment in walking in the case of 19 children with traumatic coma and 21 children with nontraumatic coma. In a prospective study of 150 adult survivors of severe head injury Jennett *et al.* (1981) found that the most frequent neurological sequelae were hemiparesis (paralysis of one side of the body), dysphasia, cranial nerve palsy, post-traumatic epilepsy, and ataxia, although no neurological disability was detected in 26 per cent of the sample.

Lewin *et al.* (1979) carried out a follow-up study of 291 patients of all ages between 10 and 24 years after they had sustained head injuries leading to post-traumatic amnesia (PTA) lasting at least one week (*see also* Roberts, 1979, chap. 5). These researchers devised an 11-point scale of central neural disability that was based upon the degree of akinesia (loss of normal muscular responsiveness), ataxia, paresis (muscular weakness), and sensory deficit. However, they suggested that their patients could be grouped into four different patterns of residual neurological disability:

In *decerebrate dementia* decerebrate reflexes were the principal response to stimulation, though semi-purposive movement developed on one side of the body in a few cases many months after injury. There was usually no detectable intellectual function. In the consecutive series no patient in this category was still alive more than ten years after injury.

In the *athetoid pseudobulbar* pattern of lesion (5% of the consecutive series) there was severe bilateral pyramidal damage with postural dystonia and often bradykinesia and fragmentary athetosis. A few patients showed remarkable discrepancy between the severity of the physical disability and the relative presevation of personality and intellectual function, suggesting that focal injury by secondary ischaemic effects caused this pattern as well as primary traumatic damage.

In the *brain-stem cerebellar* pattern (20% of the consecutive series) the most striking feature was the evidence of asymmetrical cerebellar and pyramidal lesions. Damage was clearly not confined to the brain stem, especially since frontal personality changes were often apparent, but this condition reflects the lesions found extensively throughout the brain stem either directly because of trauma or indirectly because of compression from brain swelling.

The *hemiparetic* was the commonest residual pattern (40% of the consecutive series) but signs of unilateral pyramidal injury were usually slight. Severe hemiparesis was usually associated with the preceding three patterns, and only then was cortical sensory loss commonly encountered. About 21% of the consecutive series had no detectable neural lesion, and 14% did not fall into any of these categories. (p. 1534)

Roberts (loc. cit) argued that these patterns of cerebral dysfunction reflected different clinical syndromes with distinct, though overlapping underlying pathologies.

Lewin *et al.* noted that patients with decerebrate dementia or the athetoid pseudobulbar syndrome required continuing care in institutions or from relatives, although most patients who had survived in a state of decerebrate dementia had died within a year of the head injury. Roberts (op. cit., pp. 173–4) suggested that this was especially true of older patients, whereas head-injured children could survive decerebration with only slight to moderate mental or physical disability in later life. The ominous prognostic significance of decerebrate rigidity had been noted much earlier by Maciver *et al.* (1958), although they suggested that it could be successfully treated by proper control of respiratory function. In contrast, many of those with the brain-stem cerebellar pattern appeared to enjoy a tolerable domestic or social life despite severe ataxia. The persistent disabilities of the remaining patients were determined more by personality change and intellectual impairment than by neural disorders.

Finally, Lewin *et al.* showed that the long-term outcome in terms of the level of residual neurological disability could be predicted in most cases on the basis of knowing the patient's age at injury, the worst state of central neural disability after injury, and the duration of PTA. Evans *et al.* (1975) had also shown that the severity of residual handicap was a direct function of both the duration of unconsciousness and that of PTA. Similarly, Livingston and Livingston (1985) found that the overall incidence of neurological signs was significantly greater among patients with severe head injuries (defined by a Glasgow Coma Scale score of 8 or less on admission and a PTA lasting longer than 48 hours) than in patients with mild head injuries. Any improvement in the former group was confined to the first six months after their accidents, while the latter group showed virtually no residual signs when assessed three months after injury.

Timming *et al.* (1982) studied 28 victims of very severe head injury who had received CT and undergone an in-hospital rehabilitation programme. They were assessed at the time of their discharge from hospital in terms of the number of areas (out of four: walking, self-care, communication, and bladder continence) in which they had achieved independence. Most of the patients who had normal CT scans or small ventricles (consistent with brain swelling) attained independence in all four areas within 13 weeks of the head injury, as did about half of those with focal lesions (consistent with intracranial haematomas). However, none of the patients who showed enlarged ventricles (consistent with diffuse axonal injury) had attained independence in walking or self-care, and most of them remained dependent in their communication ability and lacking in bladder control. Patients' overall ratings of independence were significantly related to the duration of coma, the presence or absence of skull fracture (those with a fracture having the *better* outcome), and the occurrence of post-traumatic epilepsy.

Thomsen (1984) described the long-term residual disabilities of 40 patients who had sustained very severe closed head injuries. When they were initially assessed on average 4.5 months after their accidents, all of these patients showed at least some signs of motor impairment. At a first follow-up examination on average 30 months after their accidents, three-quarters of the patients still showed such signs, often associated with cerebellar dysfunction. In 17 cases these signs of motor impairment were moderate or severe, although no patient was actually bedridden. At a second follow-up examination 10–15 years after their accidents, there was little change in the patients' physical status, and indeed in one case the cerebellar signs had become more pronounced; seven patients were confined to wheelchairs and six had severe ataxia. There was however some change in the patients' degree of dependence. At the time of the first follow-up examination, information from relatives as well as clinical observations had indicated that 24 of the 40 patients were dependent in some way on the presence of other people; by the time of the second follow-up examination, 12 of these patients were able to take care of themselves. Thomsen argued on the basis of these findings that, 'though the patient with very severe head trauma may remain disabled, improvement in psychosocial functions can continue for several years' (p. 267).

The Glasgow Outcome Scale

Although the studies mentioned above were mainly concerned with residual neurological disability, it was quite inevitable that many of them would relate this to the patients' degree of social dependence or independence. Jennett and Bond (1975) emphasized that the outcome of any serious illness had important implications for the provision and deployment of resources within the health services as well as for the patients and their families. They therefore argued that the measurement of outcome in cases of severe brain damage should take into account the degree of permanent disablement which required continuing social support. They also criticized previous schemes for classifying outcome in survivors of severe head injury because they used vague and ambiguous terms to characterize a somewhat restricted number of exclusive categories which inevitably included patients with a wide range of residual disabilities. Instead, Jennett and Bond offered the following scheme, which became known as the Glasgow Outcome Scale:

1 *Death*. This might seem to require no further definition, but agreement must be reached on what conditions should be met before ascribing death to brain damage . . .

2 *Persistent vegetative state*. This is the least ambiguous term to describe patients who remain unresponsive and speechless for weeks or months until death after acute brain damage . . .

3 *Severe disability (conscious but disabled)*. This is used to describe patients who are dependent for daily support by reason of mental or physical disability, usually a combination of both . . .

4 *Moderate disability (disabled but independent)*. Such patients can travel by public transport and can work in a sheltered environment, and are therefore independent in so far as daily life is concerned . . .

5 *Good recovery*. This implies resumption of normal life even though there may be minor neurological and psychological deficits. (pp. 482–3)

Jennett and Bond commented that the Scale had already been in use for some time and shown a good measure of agreement between different observers. Jennett *et al.* (1981) examined the interobserver reliability of the Scale more formally in the case of 150 patients seen six months and (in 122 cases) 12 months after severe head injuries; at both sessions there was agreement between two independent judges in more than 95 per cent of the patients. However, Jennett *et al.* also pointed out that the original Glasgow Outcome Scale would be insensitive to degrees of improvement occurring within one of its categories, and they therefore divided the categories corresponding to severe disability, moderate disability, and good recovery into a better and worse level of outcome. Brooks *et al.* (1986b) found that, in assessing 51 patients with severe head injuries, two experienced users of the Outcome Scale were agreed to within one outcome category in 100 per cent of cases on the original Outcome Scale and in 92 per cent of cases on the extended Outcome Scale. Most cases of disagreement were not substantial and had to do with the use of the 'moderate disability' category. Among survivors of severe head injury, poor ratings on the Glasgow Outcome Scale are related to neurological sequelae, clinically assessed personality changes and to impaired performance on formal cognitive tests (*see* Brooks *et al.*, 1986b; Jennett *et al.*, 1981).

An important question is whether patients who have survived a closed head injury continue to improve indefinitely or whether there is a point during the process of recovery at which the final outcome is established. With regard to the Glasgow Outcome Scale, Teasdale and Jennett (1976) suggested that the outcome became stable at six months in most survivors of head injury: that is, any subsequent improvement was rarely sufficient for the survivor to move into a better category on the Scale. Bond and Brooks (1976) presented findings from 212 patients who had suffered head injuries leading to a period of PTA lasting longer than 24 hours, and were assessed on the Glasgow Outcome Scale at three months, six months, and one year after their accidents. Of the patients who had made a good recovery by the time of the 1-year assessment, 67 per cent had reached this level within the first three months and 91 per cent had done so within the first six months. Of the patients who were moderately disabled at the 1-year assessment, 66 per cent had been similarly disabled at three months and 95 per cent had been so at six months. Finally, all of the patients who were vegetative or severely disabled at the 1-year assessment were in the same state at three months and at six months. Jennett *et al.* (1977b) supplemented this sample with another 100 cases and confirmed the general conclusion that only a small number of head-injured patients exhibit a change of category on the Glasgow Outcome Scale more than six months after their accidents (*see also* Heiden *et al.*, 1983; Jennett *et al.*, 1981).

In a major series of papers Jennett and his colleagues explored the possibility of predicting the category on the Glasgow Outcome Scale to which a patient was assigned six months after suffering a severe head injury on the basis of clinical features determined within the first week of the accident. This was achieved by means of a collaborative programme between 1968 and 1976 which involved clinicians in Glasgow, Rotterdam, Groningen, and Los Angeles and which eventually included 1000 patients who had spent at least six hours in coma following their accidents (Jennett, 1976b, 1976c; Jennett *et al.*, 1975a, 1976, 1977b, 1979b, 1981). Six months later 49 per cent of these patients were dead, 3 per cent were vegetative, 10 per cent were severely disabled, 17 per cent were moderately disabled, while 22 per cent had made a good recovery. Thus, while nearly half of all severe head injuries are fatal, nearly half of the survivors who regain consciousness make a good recovery in terms of their ability to live independently (cf. Bond, 1986). Not surprisingly, the overall picture is considerably better when the Glasgow Outcome Scale is applied to the full range of hospital admissions after head injury (that is, including cases of both minor and severe injury). Rimel and Jane (1983) studied 1248 patients admitted during a 20-month period to a single regional centre, and found that 69 per cent had already made a good recovery by the time of their discharge.

The Glasgow Outcome Scale was designed to complement the Glasgow Coma Scale, in order to provide the basis for a predictive system (Jennett and Bond, 1975). The central finding from this collaborative investigation was that a patient's category on the Glasgow Outcome Scale six months after a severe head injury was strongly associated with the depth of coma noted during the immediate period of hospitalization on the Glasgow Coma Scale. This has been replicated in similar studies in the United States (Bowers and Marshall, 1980; Bruce *et al.*, 1982; Gennarelli *et al.*, 1982; Heiden *et al.*, 1983) and extended to patients with minor or moderate head injuries (Levin *et al.*, 1987a) and to patients with coma resulting from nontraumatic causes (Levy *et al.*, 1981). In addition, the rate of improvement on the Glasgow Coma Scale during the first few days of hospitalization (Jennett *et al.*, 1975a) and the overall duration of coma (Bricolo *et al.*, 1983; Jennett, 1976c; Levin and Eisenberg, 1986) appear to be related to the subsequent outcome. The latter is also associated:

1   with age, such that a poor outcome is more likely in older patients (Bricolo *et al.*, 1983; Heiden *et al.*, 1983; Jennett and Teasdale, 1981, p. 321; Jennett *et al.*, 1976, 1979b; Teasdale *et al.*, 1982);

2   with the duration of PTA, whether assessed informally by clinical questioning (Brooks *et al.*, 1986b; Jennett *et al.*, 1981; Livingston *et al.*, 1985b) or by means of formal devices such as the Galveston Orientation and Amnesia Test (Levin and Eisenberg, 1986; Levin *et al.*, 1979b);

3   with disturbances of spontaneous eye movements and the pupillary, oculocephalic and oculovestibular reflexes (Heiden *et al.*, 1983; Jennett, 1976c; Jennett *et al.*, 1976); and

4   with the presence or absence of focal lesions such as intracranial haematomas (Bricolo *et al.*, 1983; Gennarelli *et al.*, 1982; Jennett *et al.*, 1976; Snoek *et al.*, 1979; but cf. Levin *et al.*, 1979a).

However, autonomic abnormalities affecting respiration, blood pressure and circulation, and body temperature, the cause of the head injury, the lateralization of damage to one cerebral hemisphere, and extracranial injuries seem to have little influence on the final outcome when other factors are statistically controlled (Jennett *et al.*, 1979b). Moreover, the results obtained from the Scottish and Dutch centres involved in the collaborative study were very similar, despite the major differences in their policies for the disposal and management of head-injured patients (Jennett *et al.*, 1975a, 1977b; Teasdale and Jennett, 1976).

The approach adopted by Jennett and his colleagues was to devise a statistical model by which newly occurring cases of head injury could be compared with the existing data bank to predict the likely outcome on the basis of certain combinations of critical clinical features (Jennett *et al.*, 1975a). The predictive system was to be based solely upon clinical data, because it was intended for use in situations where no laboratory investigations or computer facilities were available (Jennett, 1976c). Even so, over 300 items of data were available for each patient, though in most cases where an outcome could be predicted with 97 per cent confidence this could be achieved on the basis of only 17 items of data, of which the most important were the depth of coma according to the Glasgow Coma Scale, the motor response pattern, the pattern of eye movements (both spontaneous and reflex), the pupil reactions to light, and the patient's age (Jennett *et al.*, 1979b). The predictions proved to be fairly accurate, especially when based upon clinical information available on the third day following the head injury; however, the accuracy of prediction was not substantially improved by additional information available at the end of the first week. Errors tended to be optimistic ones, in that the system failed to predict deterioration in the outcome as a result of complications (Jennett, 1976b; Jennett *et al.*, 1976, 1979b; Teasdale and Jennett, 1976).

This methodology aimed to provide clinicians with a basis for making rational decisions about the management of head-injured patients and in particular with a way of testing whether new forms of treatment improved the subsequent outcome (Jennett, 1976b; Teasdale and Jennett, 1976). It might also be of value in allocating limited resources and in counselling the families of head-injured patients. However, the particular model used by Jennett and his colleagues was the Bayesian discriminant method, which assumes that the various prognostic factors are statistically independent of one another (Jennett, 1976b; Jennett *et al.*, 1979b). This assumption is acknowledged to be false by virtue of 'the undoubted inter-dependence between certain predictive features' (Jennett *et al.*, 1976, p. 1034), and this in principle might leave the predictive model prone to making errors. An alternative model based upon logistic regression analysis was described by Stablein *et al.* (1980), and this seems equally successful in predicting the outcome of severe head injury on the basis of early clinical data.

Return to Work

The Glasgow Outcome Scale was intended to provide a measure of a patient's 'social reintegration' (Jennett and Bond, 1975, p. 481) in addition to his or her recovery in purely neurological terms, and Jennett (1976a) stated explicitly that the Scale was designed to enable surviving patients to be classified 'according to the overall social outcome' (p. 653). However, the traditional indicator of social recovery following closed head injury has been the patient's capacity for resuming normal employment. Humphrey and Oddy (1980; Oddy *et al.*, 1978b) noted that this was a crucial concern for most head-injured patients, psychologically if not financially, and especially so in the case of the young adults who were most likely to be involved as the victims of closed head injury. It might be expected that a patient's earning capacity would prove to be a useful index of outcome. Nevertheless, Miller and Stern (1965) found that this was contaminated by irrelevant financial variables such as differential increases in earnings amongst different trades and professions during the follow-up period, and they concluded that the *nature* of the patient's subsequent employment was a more reliable guide to functional recovery.

The earliest study to consider this aspect of outcome in head-injured patients was reported by Symonds (1928), who presented findings from the 1-year follow-up of 80 patients referred with persistent postconcussional symptoms. Of the 71 patients who were dependent for their livelihood on regular employment, 33 had been able to return to full work, 31 had been able to return to light work, while seven were totally incapacitated. PTA had lasted less that 24 hours in the case of 54 of these patients, of whom 52 per cent had been able to return to full work, and only 4 per cent were totally incapacitated. Of the remaining 17 cases in whom PTA had exceeded 24 hours, 29 per cent had been able to return to full work and 29 per cent were totally incapacitated. Russell (1934) presented similar results from an 18-month follow-up of 139 head-injured patients who had previously been in employment. However, while the patients with the most severe injuries (according to the duration of PTA) were more likely to suffer a prolonged incapacity, Russell noted that a relatively high proportion of them were nevertheless able to return to work within six months of their accidents. He suggested instead that the age of the patient was 'the most important single factor in estimating the prospects of recovery' (p. 129). In his sample the proportion of patients who had not returned to full employment within 18 months of the injury was 6 per cent in those aged between 15 and 30, 21 per cent in those aged between 30 and 50, and 46 per cent in those over the age of 50. Despite the fact that 96 of these cases had undergone radiography, the presence or absence of a skull fracture was not important in determining the ultimate prognosis.

During the Second World War this research was extended by considering whether or not head-injured service personnel were able to return to duty. Symonds (1942) tabulated data from 871 cases, showing that the duration of PTA was inversely related to the likelihood that the patient would return to active duty, and directly related to the likelihood that a patient who was returned to duty would subsequently relapse and have to be invalided after all. Similar findings were presented by Symonds and Russell (1943) based upon a consecutive series of 237 acute cases, of whom 80 per cent returned successfully to active duty within a few months of their injury. The final outcome in these patients was also related to the incidence of complications such as intracranial haematoma and post-traumatic epilepsy. Symonds and Russell supplemented this series with 718 cases of chronic head injury, and showed that the proportion of patients in the combined sample who were finally invalided was nearly twice as high in those that appeared to be predisposed to mental disorder according to their personal and family histories (cf. Lewis, 1942). Conversely, the prognosis for return to active duty was four times as good in 111 head-injured flying personnel from the Royal Air Force, who were assumed to have been selected by virtue of their lack of any such predisposition.

A large number of subsequent studies have considered a wide variety of possible predictors of return to work after closed head injury in the civilian population (e.g., Brooks *et al.*, 1987; Bruckner and Randle, 1972; Carlsson *et al.*, 1968; Denny-Brown, 1945a; Gilchrist and Wilkinson, 1979; Guthkelch, 1980; Heiskanen and Sipponen, 1970; Levin *et al.*, 1979a; Lewin *et al.*, 1979; McKinlay *et al.*, 1983; Oddy and Humphrey, 1980; Rimel *et al.*, 1981; Steadman and Graham, 1970; van Zomeren and van den Burg, 1985; Weddell *et al.*, 1980; Wrightson and Gronwall, 1981). Humphrey and Oddy (1980) concluded from a review of many of these studies that, apart from the severity of the injury as measured by the duration of coma or of PTA, occupational resettlement after head injury was influenced by the age of the patient, his or her previous personality and occupational level and the occurrence of post-traumatic personality changes, but that much less importance attached to gross physical handicap or specific disabilities. There is some evidence that return to work tends to be later in the case of patients injured in industrial accidents (Guthkelch, 1980) or traffic accidents (Wrightson and Gronwall, 1981), though the time taken to return to work does not seem to depend on whether or not the patient is pursuing a claim for financial compensation (McKinlay *et al.*, 1983).

Generally speaking, residual neurological deficits are not important determinants of occupational resettlement following closed head injury. One exception to this is post-traumatic epilepsy: Evans (1989) suggested that this had had a 'devastating' effect on whether patients with severe injuries had been able to resume their original or equivalent employment, although it is unclear to what extent this was because his data had been obtained from patients who were originally in military service. Another interesting exception is the loss of the sense of smell (anosmia). This disorder is associated with orbitofrontal damage contiguous to the site of the olfactory bulbs; its incidence seems to vary with the duration of PTA (e.g., Guthkelch, 1980). Varney (1988) described 40 patients with total anosmia as the result of closed head injury, almost all of whom had had major employment problems despite having been medically cleared for work and despite having no significant cognitive, motor, or sensory deficits. Interviews carried out with their relatives and employers nevertheless revealed psychosocial dysfunction in the areas of planning, decision making, and judgement of the sort that are associated with lesions of the frontal lobes (cf. Lezak, 1982; Stuss and Benson, 1984). Varney concluded that these patients' employment problems were caused by subtle cognitive deficits which affected their reliability as productive employees.

Occupational resettlement is related to a number of other measures of outcome following closed head injury, including the category achieved on the Glasgow Outcome Scale (Levin *et al.*, 1979a), the persistence of postconcussional symptoms

(Brenner *et al.*, 1944; Friedman *et al.*, 1945; Guthkelch, 1980), and disturbances of cognition, memory, and personality (Evans, 1989; Weddell *et al.*, 1980). In a prospective study of 538 patients who had sustained minor head injuries, Rimel *et al.* (1981) found that 34 per cent of those who had been gainfully employed before their accidents were still unemployed three months afterwards; this outcome was attributed to subtle organic deficits of attention, concentration, memory or judgement and the emotional stress that was involved in coping with these problems. In the case of victims of severe head injury, Brooks *et al.* (1987) found that the relatives of patients who had returned to work within seven years of an injury reported fewer residual deficits in memory and communication than the relatives of those who had not, and these reports were confirmed in terms of the patients' performance on objective psychometric tests. A multiple regression analysis demonstrated that the patient's occupational status was predicted mainly by their scores on the Logical Memory subtest of the Wechsler Memory Scale and a paced auditory serial addition task. As the former team of investigators subsequently acknowledged, however (Barth *et al.*, 1983), it is difficult to make firm causal inferences from such findings without detailed information on the premorbid employability of the patients concerned.

The attitudes of employers and working colleagues will be important determinants of successful occupational resettlement. In this context, Bruckner and Randle (1972) suggested that the lower likelihood of older patients returning to work was 'due to a combination of diminishing powers of adaptation on the part of the patient and a reluctance of employers to take on employees with only a limited working lifespan ahead' (p. 346). On the other hand, Jennett and Bond (1975) suggested that patients may be permitted to return to full employment despite persisting impairments or symptoms, either because the nature of the work was compatible with their particular disabilities or because their employers were providing what was essentially sheltered employment (*see also* Oddy *et al.*, 1978b). However, there is very little hard evidence on the attitudes of employers towards the re-employment of head-injured patients (cf. Humphrey and Oddy, 1980). Oddy and Humphrey (1980) assessed 45 patients who had been in full-time employment when they sustained severe head injuries. They found that 30 had resumed work within the first six months, while a further eight had done so within the next 18 months. None had been downgraded or required to take on less demanding work, but some were restricted in their activities and believed that they had still not regained their full working capacity two years after the injury. In addition, there was some evidence of 'subtle alterations in the expectations of employers. For example, a policeman and a marine engineer had been confined to office duties, [and] skilled workers were no longer required to work at heights and were working under closer supervision' (p. 799). Oddy and Humphrey concluded that return to work was not a sensitive index of outcome after head injury.

Similarly, in a subsequent investigation involving 66 patients with minor head injuries, Wrightson and Gronwall (1981) found that roughly half were still experiencing postconcussional symptoms on their return to work on average 4.7 calendar days after their accidents; in some cases, these symptoms persisted for as long as two years. Wrightson and Gronwall argued that the time of return to work might be a useful index of the severity of a head injury but that returning to work did not itself indicate recovery. Brooks *et al.* (1987) interviewed the relatives of 134 patients during the course of a 7-year follow-up study of severe closed head injury. In some cases, it was suggested that despite having returned to work the patients were unable to work at their full capacity, and even that their colleagues were 'covering' for them in this regard. Such a situation was apparently much more likely to be found in middle-class employees than working-class employees, and Brooks *et al.* suggested that the employers of managerial or similar workers were rather more prepared to accept back patients who were not strictly ready to return to work.

Humphrey and Oddy (1980) noted that the occupational resettlement of head-injured patients would depend on such factors as their intelligence, education, and professional training because of the range of personal and cognitive skills which these entail, but this can hardly be a peculiarity of the victims of head injuries. Dresser *et al.* (1973) reported the main results of a 15-year follow-up study of 864 head-injured veterans from the Korean War (roughly one-quarter of whom had sustained blunt head wounds), together with 121 control subjects drawn from the same units. Individuals in *both* groups who on their induction had obtained low scores on the Armed Forces Qualification Test were found to be more likely to be unemployed at the follow-up assessment. Similar considerations apply in the case of the patient's age and the nature of his or her original employment as possible predictors of occupational resettlement. Moreover, the likelihood that a head-injured patient will subsequently return to work obviously depends upon local socioeconomic circumstances and unemployment levels (Baddeley *et al.*, 1980; Jennett and Bond, 1975).

A more fundamental problem is that strictly speaking this criterion can only be used in assessing the recovery of patients who have previously been in gainful employment. Brooks *et al.* (1987) found that 14 per cent of employable individuals who sustained a severe closed head injury in the west of Scotland had in fact been unemployed at the time. Apart from the fact that the notion of *return* to work is in principle inappropriate in such cases, it is highly improbable that their prospects for occupational resettlement would be the same as those of patients who were previously in employment. Moreover, this criterion of recovery is of even less value in the case of children, those who are near or in retirement, and those who devote themselves to housekeeping or the care of dependants (Baddeley *et al.*, 1980). Steadman and Graham (1970) suggested that recovery from head injury among housewives could be judged against the ability to perform their former routine of housework, while children could be judged against their previous school performance. Of course, as was pointed out by Levin and Eisenberg (1979a), the capability of children merely to attend school does not necessarily imply a good recovery, since they might still exhibit learning problems. Indeed, most children of school age who have sustained severe closed head injuries show impaired academic performance (Brink *et al.*, 1970), and in particular Heiskanen and Kaste (1974) concluded that 'children who remain unconscious for two weeks or more will only rarely be able to manage well at school' (p. 13).

Nevertheless, because of the above considerations recent commentators have tended to denigrate return to work as a somewhat crude criterion of recovery following head injury (e.g., Baddeley *et al.*, 1980). Moreover, it ignores the leisure activities and personal relationships that may be of more importance to the patient (Humphrey and Oddy, 1980; Jennett and Bond, 1975; Oddy *et al.*, 1978b). Oddy and Humphrey concluded that a much more searching, qualitative appraisal was needed of the problems faced by patients with head injuries in their return to working life.

Social Outcome

Until the mid-1970s researchers devoted very little attention to broader aspects of recovery following closed head injury, and the few references to social outcome were apparently based merely upon clinical impression (*see* e.g., Hpay, 1971). Two studies were published in which patients with severe closed head injuries were classified at follow-up according to the degree of social independence or reintegration (Lundholm *et al.*, 1975; Pazzaglia *et al.*, 1975); these found that the quality of survival was much poorer among older patients, but was not related to the duration of coma. Pazzaglia *et al.* noted that social reintegration was inversely related to the severity of physical sequelae, but that approximately one-third out of 96 patients who had achieved full recovery in their social activities had done so in spite of such sequelae, which in some cases were marked.

Bond (1975) sought to quantify the outcome of severe brain damage in terms of its impact upon a patient's daily life. Many different scales of 'activities of daily living' have been devised by geriatric specialists to assess social independence in terms of basic functions of self-care after stroke (Aitken *et al.*, 1982). Instruments of this sort show continuing improvement during the first year of recovery following severe head injury (Livingston and Livingston, 1985). Deficits in self-care are important predictors of long-term employment problems among adult patients (Brooks *et al.*, 1987) and can also have a devastating impact on the capacity of children to participate in a conventional school setting (Deaton, 1987). However, persistent difficulties of this sort are relatively rare even in severely injured patients (Brooks *et al.*, 1986a). Although such scales may be useful in planning community support for elderly patients following closed head injury (Wilson *et al.*, 1987), they are often considered to be too restricted for evaluating recovery in young head-injured adults (e.g., Jennett, 1984; Jennett *et al.*, 1981).

Instead, Bond constructed three separate rating scales for the assessment of physical disability, mental handicap, and social reintegration among patients with severe head injury. The components of these subscales are shown in Table 7.1. Relevant data were obtained from a standard clinical interview and were supplemented by information from a close relative or friend. The procedures for scoring individual patients are contained in an appendix to Bond's report; these yield ratings increasing from zero on each scale reflecting the degree of disability or impairment relative to the patient's premorbid state. These scales were then evaluated in a pilot study involving 56 patients examined between three months and more than two years after head injuries which had given rise to a PTA lasting longer than 24 hours (*see also* Bond, 1976).

The overall ratings of physical and mental disability were found to be significantly

Table 7.1   Scales for the assessment of severe brain damage

Neurophysical scale
Motor deficit
Sensory deficit
Aphasia
Ataxia
Cranial nerves
Physical deficits

Mental scale

1	Intellect	(a)	Memory
		(b)	Distractability
2	Personality	(a)	Apathy to euphoria
		(b)	Irritability to aggression
3	Mental symptoms	(a)	Free anxiety
		(b)	Phobic anxiety
		(c)	Obsessional symptoms
		(d)	Hysterical symptoms
		(e)	Depressive symptoms

Social scale
1   Work
2   Family cohesion
3   Leisure
4   Criminality
5   Sexual activity
6   Alcohol consumption

Source: Bond, M. R. (1975) 'Assessment of the psychosocial outcome after severe head injury', in *Outcome of Severe Damage to the Central Nervous System*, Ciba Foundation Symposium No. 34 (new series), Amsterdam, Elsevier/Excerpta Medica/North-Holland. Reprinted with permission.

correlated with the ratings of social disability, but not with each other. Bond explained this by suggesting that 'the neurological scale is primarily a measure of focal brain damage whereas the aspects of mental function assessed are probably affected more by diffuse brain dysfunction' (p. 147). Nevertheless, he noted that the overall degree of physical disability was specifically associated with the degree of memory impairment and a loss of work capacity; that the overall degree of mental disability was associated with a loss of work capacity, leisure pursuits, and family cohesion; and that the overall degree of social impairment was associated with disorders of memory and personality but not with symptoms of mental illness. The duration of PTA was significantly associated with the degree of impairment on all three scales, although with regard to the mental and social scales it was mainly related to memory impairment, loss of work capacity, and disruption of leisure pursuits. Additional results from this study were presented by Bond and Brooks (1976) relating scores on the three scales to the time after injury when the assessment had been conducted; there was no sign of any improvement on the neurophysical scale between patients tested six months and two years after their accidents, which was taken to suggest that 'the greater part of recovery must have taken place within six months of injury' (p. 130). The mental and social scales showed modest improvements beyond six months of the injury, but in neither case was the trend statistically significant.

Weddell *et al.* (1980) used Bond's neurophysical scale as part of the clinical assessment of 44 young adults admitted to a rehabilitation centre after very severe head injury. These patients demonstrated a substantial improvement on this scale between six months and two years after the injury, although only eight were totally free from neurophysical deficits at the time of the latter examination. Poor neurophysical status was correlated with a number of aspects of social recovery according to interviews with the patients' relatives, including a failure to resume work, an increased dependency on the family, and a tendency to participate more in activities with parents. However, there was no significant association with overall frequency of social contact or with the relatives' assessment of memory impairment or personality change. These findings were taken to confirm Bond's (1975) suggestion that the ability to return to work after head injury was determined by two relatively independent factors reflecting physical recovery and mental recovery, respectively.

A more elaborated scale, the Glasgow Assessment Schedule, was devised by Livingston and Livingston (1985) for use in clinical and research settings where longer-term management and rehabilitation of head-injured patients is envisaged. It focuses upon the practical implications of particular forms of impairment rather than their aetiology, and is based on clinical examination, self-report measures, and simple objective tests. It yields a comprehensive assessment of neurophysical signs, subjective complaints, personality change, cognitive functioning, activities of daily living, and occupational status. In evaluative studies, the Schedule was found to demonstrate acceptable inter-rater reliability, a high level of discrimination between cases of mild and severe head injury, and a strong association with patients' global ratings on the Glasgow Outcome Scale. It is also sensitive to changes in patients' clinical status during the course of recovery, though mainly in the areas of occupational status and activities of daily living. (It should be noted that in Table 2 of the published report, the mean ratings obtained three and six months after severe head injury were transposed in error, so that the changes in question are indeed improvements: M. G. Livingston, personal communication.) It is interesting that subjective reports of physical symptoms and personality change failed to show any significant improvement from three to six months and from six to 12 months after injury, even though they were corroborated by the patients' relatives. Nevertheless, the Glasgow Assessment Schedule has been specifically criticized because of its inadequate coverage of post-traumatic complaints, especially those relating to fatigability, slowness of thinking, depressive symptoms, anxiety, and flattening of affect (Editorial, 1986).

Recovery of Function

Subjective Reports

A fundamental problem in measuring psychosocial recovery following closed head injury is the paucity of objective measures of psychological function which are sensitive indicators of mental processing and at the same time valid predictors of the ability to cope with the problems of daily life. As Baddeley *et al.* (1980) observed, this means that information regarding the quality of outcome must come in the first instance from the reports of head-injured patients and their relatives. Some of the concerns involved in the evaluation of these reports were discussed in the previous chapter (pp. 215–8). In particular, the patients may lack awareness of the true extent of their disabilities, perhaps because of their cognitive deficits, whereas the perceptions of their families may be coloured in a systematic way, possibly as a coping response to the stress of caring for a disabled relative. Not surprisingly, these considerations proved to be especially important when evaluating emotional and behavioural changes, which tended to be reported by the relatives of head-injured patients but denied by the patients themselves. Nevertheless, with regard to persistent cognitive impairment following closed head injury, the reports of the patients seem to be somewhat more concordant with those of their relatives, and there is no evidence that the frequency of such complaints is systematically either increased, as would reflect the maintenance of a 'sick role', or reduced, as would reflect a lack of 'insight' (*see* McKinlay and Brooks, 1984).

Oddy *et al.* (1978b) constructed a checklist of 37 items that related to personality changes and somatic, sensory, cognitive, and psychiatric symptoms. This was administered to 48 patients roughly six months after they had received head injuries leading to a period of PTA lasting longer than 24 hours. In each case the checklist was also completed by a close relative (normally the patient's parent or spouse) with reference to the patient's current condition. The duration of PTA was positively related to the number of reported symptoms, and the patients and their relatives produced similar distributions of symptom frequency. In both, cognitive and personality changes were predominant, and the most commonly reported symptom was 'trouble remembering things'. Similar results were obtained by Levin *et al.* (1979a) in the case of 27 patients with severe closed head injuries assessed on average one year after their accidents (the incidence of subjective cognitive impairment being inversely related to the degree of recovery on the Glasgow Outcome Scale) and also by Thomsen (1984) in the case of 40 patients with very severe closed head injuries who were assessed roughly 30 months and 10–15 years after their accidents.

Kapur and Pearson (1983) devised a Memory Symptoms Test on the basis of the everyday memory difficulties that had been previously reported by a large hetero-geneous group of patients with established cerebral pathology. This test was then administered to 14 head-injured patients in whom the duration of PTA had varied from a few minutes to a year during a routine assessment carried out between seven and 60 months after their injuries. The test took the form of a questionnaire in which the patient was to indicate whether his or her memory was unimpaired, slightly impaired, or very much impaired in ten different functions compared with its capacity before the head injury. For nine of these patients the test was also completed by a close relative or acquaintance with regard to the patient's current condition. The correlation coefficient between the patients' reports and the relatives' reports was substantial and highly significant ($r = +0.92$). However, for neither the patients' reports nor the relatives' reports was there any sign of a relationship between memory symptoms and the patient's objective performance on a number of clinical tests of memory function.

Sunderland *et al.* (1983) compared the everyday memory performance of 32 patients with severe closed head injuries interviewed between two and eight years after their accidents and that of a control group of orthopaedic patients with no history of head injury. The patients were given a questionnaire in which they reported the frequency with which they suffered from each of 35 different types of memory failure; they were then asked to keep a daily check list for seven consecutive days, indicating which of these memory failures they had experienced during each day. Both tasks were also carried out by a close relative living in daily contact with the patient with reference to the patient's recent condition. There was a reasonable consistency among the four measures, and three of the four showed a higher incidence of memory failures amongst the patients with closed head injuries than amongst the orthopaedic controls. However, the responses given to the patients' questionnaire did not differ between the two groups and failed to correlate with objective performance on a battery of memory tests. In contrast, the relatives' questionnaire did correlate with the patients' objective memory performance and showed the anticipated pattern of a higher frequency of memory failures amongst the head-injured patients than amongst the controls.

Sunderland *et al.* (1984b) devised a new questionnaire containing 27 items, which was based on those items that had most clearly discriminated between the head-injured and control patients in their first study. This was used in a postal survey of 78 patients between 18 months and six years after they had sustained a severe closed head injury (defined by a PTA lasting longer than 24 hours) and a comparison group of 78 patients with minor closed head injury (in whom the maximum duration of PTA was 10 min). A second version of the questionnaire was to be completed by a close friend or relative with reference to the patient's recent condition. Unfortunately, 30 of the patients had died or could not be traced, only 83 (or 66 per cent) of the remainder returned completed questionnaires, and four of these did not return a completed relative's questionnaire. In the instances where both versions of the questionnaire had been completed, the number of memory failures reported by the patients with minor head injury was significantly higher than the number of memory failures ascribed to the same patients by their relatives. Nevertheless, the latter patients produced overall scores that were similar to those generated by members of a large subject panel, and it was concluded that patients with minor head injuries did not differ greatly from normal subjects in the incidence of memory failures in everyday life.

The patients with severe head injuries did not differ from those with minor head injuries in terms of the reported frequency of memory failures, but the relatives reported a higher incidence of memory failures among the severely injured patients. Similar results were obtained when the respondents were asked to provide a single rating on a 4-point scale of the overall severity of the patients' memory and concentration difficulties; although two-thirds of the patients reported that these were to some extent a nuisance, only half of their relatives did so. There was however no difference between the patients with 'very severe' injuries (in whom the duration of PTA was longer than seven days) and those with 'severe' injuries (in whom the duration of PTA was between one and seven days) in either their own or their relatives' reports of memory failures. Finally, 21 of the severely injured cases for whom there was clinical evidence of major cerebral lesions produced a significantly higher incidence of memory failures than the remaining cases on their relatives' questionnaires but not on their own questionnaires.

The findings of the two latter studies suggest that self-reports have little validity as measures of memory failure, perhaps because forgetful patients tend to forget their own memory lapses. Somewhat more promising results were obtained by Bennett-Levy (1984) using a similar Subjective Memory Questionnaire in which subjects rated their memories on a 5-point scale with regard to 43 everyday situations (Bennett-Levy and Powell, 1980). This study compared 39 severely head-injured patients with 32 orthopaedic controls: the patients in whom PTA had lasted for between one and three weeks rated their own memories if anything more favourably than did the control group, while significantly poorer ratings were given by the patients in whom PTA had lasted for more than three weeks. Moreover, while the findings described by Sunderland and his colleagues indicate that the reports of a close observer (e.g., a relative) may be of some clinical value, these may well be biased by how easily different classes of memory failure can be observed. As Sunderland *et al.* (1984a) noted, deficits in aspects of verbal behaviour will be immediately obvious in everyday conversation, whereas failures in face recognition will only be apparent if patients comment on them or behave inappropriately towards individuals whom they should recognize. Nevertheless, under constant test conditions the reports of close observers may be useful in monitoring both the progress of spontaneous recovery and the effectiveness of rehabilitative interventions, and to this end Wilson (1984; 1987a, p. 101) reported that the checklist devised by Sunderland *et al.* (1983) had been successfully adapted for use by the therapists at a rehabilitation centre.

Finally, Brooks *et al.* (1986a) asked the relatives of 42 patients with severe closed head injury to report on the changes that were apparent in the patient one year and five years after the accident. Apart from reports of continuing personality change, the most frequent symptoms were concerned with slowness, memory, irritability, and bad temper. Increases were noted in reports of concentration and memory problems, particularly in terms of the patient forgetting what he or she was doing in the middle of an action sequence, repeating or double-checking actions, or losing track of what he or she was saying. One reason for such increases may be that impairments of memory function become more significant once patients have returned to work. However, the incidence of these problems at the 5-year assessment did not show a significant correlation with the severity of the original injury according to the duration of PTA.

Memory Function

Situations that demand learning and remembering are clearly a source of concern for head-injured patients and their relatives. Nevertheless, the question arises whether these subjective complaints of persistent memory impairment are confirmed by the results of objective testing.

In the case of minor closed head injury, the empirical research that was described in chapter 4 (pp. 92–100) suggested that patients suffer an impairment of memory function which persists beyond the period of PTA but which is a purely transient phenomenon that resolves during the weeks and months after the injury. Evidence on the long-term consequences of minor closed head injury was obtained in a study by Dencker and Löfving (1958), who compared 28 head-injured monozygotic twins with the uninjured co-twins as controls. From a clinical point of view, the former group constituted an unselected sample of head-injured patients, and the duration of PTA had exceeded 24 hours in only four cases (Dencker, 1958). When the twins were tested on average ten years after the accidents, the head-injured patients showed no sign of any impairment on tests of digit span, serial learning, and the retention of narrative. Of course, the failure of this or other research to detect permanent psychological dysfunction might be attributed to an insensitivity on the part of the tests or procedures that were used. Nevertheless, these results are entirely consistent with the view that the observable deficits in learning and remembering which are consequent upon minor closed head injury are largely transient in nature.

In contrast to this optimistic picture, other research described in Chapter 4 indicated that a severe closed head injury gives rise to a more global and persistent impairment of memory function (pp. 100–26). There is some evidence of improvement in performance on repeated testing (e.g., Groher, 1977; Lezak, 1979), but if comparisons are made between patients tested at different follow-up intervals there is usually no sign that the impairment becomes less pronounced with the passage of time (e.g., Brooks, 1972, 1974a, 1974b, 1975, 1976; Levin *et al.*, 1976b; Sunderland *et al.*, 1983; cf. Parker and Serrats, 1976). This apparent lack of improvement can often be ascribed to a need to delay the testing of the most severely injured patients, and it does not therefore necessarily indicate a lack of spontaneous recovery (cf. Levin and Eisenberg, 1979a). Nevertheless, the impairment in question can be readily demonstrated on formal psychometric testing several years after the original accident (Norrman and Svahn, 1961; Sunderland *et al.*, 1983; Thomsen, 1984).

The magnitude of this impairment varies directly with the severity of the head injury, as measured by the duration of coma or PTA (Dailey, 1956; Norrman and Svahn, 1961; Parker and Serrats, 1976). Indeed, Bennett-Levy (1984) compared 29 patients between two and five years after they had sustained a severe head injury with 32 orthopaedic cases, and found that significant deficits on memory tasks were confined to those patients in whom PTA had lasted for longer than three weeks. He suggested that a 'threshold' of brain damage in terms of PTA operated at about three weeks: 'patients above this threshold are likely to exhibit persistent cognitive impairment, while patients below this threshold are unimpaired in the long term' (p. 294). Smith (1974) tested patients between 10 and 20 years after severe closed head injury, and found that the degree of verbal memory impairment tended to be more pronounced in patients who had suffered an impact to the right side of the head than in those who had suffered a left-sided impact. She attributed this finding to the effects of contrecoup lesions of the left temporal lobe, but in Chapter 2 (pp. 43–6) it was noted that the notion of contrecoup damage following closed head injury has been discredited by recent *post-mortem* evidence (*see also* Adams, 1988).

Levin *et al.* (1979a) compared 27 severely head-injured patients with 50 intact control subjects in terms of their recall of a word list using the selective reminding procedure. Both the incidence and the magnitude of impairment were related to the quality of recovery according to the Glasgow Outcome Scale. In particular, roughly one-third of the patients and all of those rated as severely disabled fell below the 4th percentile of the normal control sample in terms of both storage into and retrieval from long-term memory. Moreover, roughly one-half of the patients and all of those rated as severely disabled fell above the 96th percentile of the normal control sample in terms of the number of intrusion errors that they produced. Other researchers have confirmed that the memory performance of severely head-injured patients is related to their recovery on the Glasgow Outcome Scale, mainly because of the poor performance of the patients who are classified as severely disabled (Brooks *et al.*, 1986b; Jennett *et al.*, 1981). In evaluating the outcome of a neuropsychological rehabilitation programme, Prigatano *et al.* (1984) found that those severely head-injured patients who returned to gainful employment or study were significantly different from those who did not in their Memory Quotients on the Wechsler Memory Scale, and especially in terms of their performance on the Visual Reproduction and Associate Learning subtests. Although these results are purely correlational in nature, they do suggest that memory skills may be important determinants of occupational resettlement.

In Chapter 4, post-traumatic memory impairment was attributed to a deficit in the use of relational organization (p. 126), but a case study reported by Zatorre and McEntee (1983) indicates that in severely head-injured patients other aspects of memory processing may be affected. When evaluated on the Wechsler Adult Intelligence Scale 19 years after his head injury, this patient was found to have a Verbal IQ of 101 and a Performance IQ of 89, achieving his worst performance on the Digit Symbol subtest. On the Wechsler Memory Scale he achieved a Memory Quotient of only 66, mainly because of his poor performance on the Logical Memory, Visual Reproduction, and Associate Learning subtests, and he displayed only limited retention of daily events. From a theoretical point of view the most interesting finding is that on a variety of formal memory tasks he showed very little evidence of the use of semantic processing (cf. Brooks, 1975). Zatorre and McEntee remarked that the pattern of encoding deficits which they had found in their patient resembled that observed in cases of alcoholic Korsakoff's syndrome.

Cognitive Function

The empirical research reviewed in Chapter 5 suggested that a minor closed head injury gives rise to a transient and relatively slight impairment of cognitive function. Indeed, the clinical literature is fairly consistent in suggesting that performance returns to broadly normal levels during the month or so after a minor head injury. In their long-term follow-up study of head-injured identical twins and their uninjured co-twins, Dencker and Löfving (1958) found statistically significant deficits on tests of mirror drawing, sorting and tachistoscopic figure/ground discrimination, and also on a paced choice reaction-time task. However, these effects were fairly small in magnitude, and they were not regarded as being of any practical importance; in particular, as Dencker (1960) subsequently observed, 'they seemed to make no difference to the occupation the twins chose and did not handicap them in their work' (p. 571). Nevertheless, more recent work has indicated that a significant proportion of patients with minor head injury may encounter problems in returning to work (Rimel *et al.*, 1981), and this does appear to be linked to persistent cognitive impairment (Barth *et al.*, 1983). In particular, Gentilini *et al.* (1989) found that patients with mild head injury (defined as a loss of consciousness lasting less than 20 min) exhibited significantly slower response latencies in visual search and choice reaction-time tasks three months after their accidents.

Be that as it may, other research has identified a more substantial, persistent, and global impairment of cognitive functioning among those patients who have sustained severe closed head injury (e.g., Klonoff *et al.*, 1977; Norrman and Svahn, 1961; but cf. Chadwick *et al.*, 1981b). This impairment is associated with a poor recovery on the Glasgow Outcome Scale (Brooks *et al.*, 1986b; Jennett *et al.*, 1981), and several early studies suggested that it was the most important indicator of problems with social and vocational rehabilitation (e.g., Heiskanen and Sipponen, 1970; Lundholm *et al.*, 1975; cf. Najenson *et al.*, 1975).

In the follow-up study which Smith (1974) carried out with patients between 10 and 20 years after they had suffered severe closed head injury, she found that those patients who had received an impact to the right side of the head generally performed less well on verbal tasks than those with a left-sided impact, which she again ascribed to the effects of contrecoup lesions of the left hemisphere. In the case of visuospatial tasks, the poorest performance was demonstrated by the patients with a left frontal or a right parietal site of impact. Such tasks as these might normally be regarded as vulnerable to damage to the right parietal cortex (e.g., Walsh, 1978, chap. 6), but on the basis of Courville's (1942) research, Smith also entertained the possibility that they were susceptible to the use of verbal labelling and thus vulnerable to left-hemisphere lesions. It is true that Courville's results indicated that damage to the left fronto-temporal cortex might be consequent upon left frontal or right parietal impact, but recent *post mortem* evidence shows that cerebral contusions following closed head injury are bilateral and independent of the original site of impact (Adams *et al.*, 1980b, 1985). In addition, Smith's study did not include any control subjects, and she provided no independent data from her patients concerning either the locus of organic damage or the coding strategies used by patients to carry out her tasks. Her results are therefore quite uninformative about the neuroanatomical structures that are responsible for performance in visuospatial tasks.

The magnitude of the cognitive impairment following severe head injury appears to be directly related to the duration of coma (Klonoff *et al.*, 1977; van Zomeren and Deelman, 1976; but cf. Lundholm *et al.*, 1975). Using a four-choice visual reaction-time task, van Zomeren and Deelman (1978) found that patients who had been unconscious for seven days or less performed within the normal range by the end of the first year. However, the patients who had been unconscious for longer than seven days showed a persistent deficit on this task, although they showed a slight continuing improvement that extended through the second and third year following injury. Similarly, Klonoff *et al.* (1977) found that children with severe head injuries continued to improve on the Halstead-Reitan battery even up to five years after their accidents. Nevertheless, these data were obtained using serial assessment of the same subjects, and it is not clear whether such improvements were not merely the result of practice (cf. van Zomeren, 1981, pp. 64–7). Livingston and Livingston (1985) found that significant improvement using serial assessment on a simple battery of cognitive tests was confined to the first six months following severe head injury.

In this regard the results of a study by Miller (1980) of a group of eight patients with severe head injury are especially interesting. These patients demonstrated a substantial impairment on a timed psychomotor task (the Minnesota Spatial Relations Test). However, they then received daily practice sessions on the task, which led to an impressive increase in the level of performance and good transfer to alternative versions of the same task. Nevertheless, Sunderland *et al.* (1983) found that the performance of severely injured patients tested on a four-choice reaction-time task between two and eight years after their accidents was significantly better than that of other severely injured patients assessed between two and eight months after their accidents (and, indeed, was not significantly different from that of orthopaedic control patients). This finding suggests that there is continuing scope for recovery of cognitive function after severe head injury.

In the study mentioned earlier by Bennett-Levy (1984), 39 patients with severe closed head injury were assessed between two and five years after their accidents and were asked to carry out a timed test of information processing that involved cancelling the largest number in each of a series of rows. Once again, the patients in whom PTA had lasted for more than three weeks were significantly impaired in comparison with a control group of 32 orthopaedic cases, but the patients in whom PTA had lasted for between one and three weeks showed no sign of any impairment on this task. This was taken to confirm the concept of a 'threshold' of brain damage that corresponded roughly to a period of PTA lasting three weeks. Neither group of patients showed a deficit on unpaced tests of nonverbal skills, which suggested that a reduced speed of information processing was a salient feature of the long-term sequelae of severe closed head injury.

Of course, these findings were obtained in research using artificial tasks, and it does not necessarily follow that they would be replicated in real-life situations that demanded rapid information processing, of which driving would be an excellent example and one that is especially familiar to most young adults. Stokx and Gaillard (1986) studied 13 patients who had sustained closed head injuries sufficiently serious to give rise to coma lasting at least a week. They were tested at least two years after their accidents and compared with healthy volunteers matched individually for age, sex, education, and driving experience. The performance of the head-injured patients was much slower than that of the controls, both in laboratory tests of choice reaction time and in realistic tests of driving skills in a specially instrumented car, although there was no difference between the two groups of subjects in the numbers of errors they produced. The magnitude of an individual patient's impairment in response time was related to the duration of coma, and was especially pronounced in the case of patients in whom coma had lasted three weeks or longer. Van Zomeren *et al.* (1987) provided an interesting discussion of the implications of these and other findings for the fitness of patients with brain damage to drive.

Intellectual Function

Research on the effects of closed head injury which has used standardized intelligence tests has yielded similar conclusions to those obtained with other cognitive tasks. In particular, patients who have sustained minor closed head injury typically show no persistent impairment of intelligence (e.g., Barth *et al.*, 1983; Dencker and Löfving, 1958; Rimel *et al.*, 1981). Patients who have sustained severe closed head injury often do show such an impairment (e.g., Alexandre *et al.*, 1980, 1983; Klonoff *et al.*, 1977; Levin *et al.*, 1979a), though some studies have not confirmed this general pattern (Norrman and Svahn, 1961; Shaffer *et al.*, 1975; Sunderland *et al.*, 1983). This has led some commentators to question the sensitivity of standard psychometric tests as indicators of subtle cognitive dysfunction (Baddeley *et al.*, 1980; Barth *et al.*, 1983; Miller, 1979).

The magnitude of this intellectual impairment is directly related to the duration of coma (Chadwick *et al.*, 1981c; Dailey, 1956; Johnston and Mellits, 1980; Klonoff *et al.*, 1977; but cf. Levin *et al.*, 1979a), and to the depth of coma on admission according to the Glasgow Coma Scale (Alexandre *et al.*, 1983; cf. Brooks *et al.*, 1980). Indeed, in research with severely head-injured children Levin and Eisenberg (1979a, 1979b) found that any persistent intellectual deficit was essentially confined to patients who had been in coma for more than 24 hours. In a $2\frac{1}{4}$-year follow-up study of 48 head-injured children, Chadwick *et al.* (1981a) found that the duration of PTA was related to the likelihood of subsequent impairment on the Wechsler Intelligence Scale for Children. This 'dose-response' effect of the severity of the head injury upon intellectual function was taken to provide evidence for the idea that the resulting intellectual disabilities were due to brain damage (*see also* Rutter, 1981). Unfortunately, it must be added that many other investigators have failed to find any significant relationship between the impairment of head-injured patients on standard psychometric tests and the duration of PTA (e.g., Alexandre *et al.*, 1983; Brooks *et al.*, 1980; Klonoff *et al.*, 1977; Mandleberg, 1976; Mandleberg and Brooks, 1975; Smith, 1974; cf. Bond, 1975, 1976).

In reviewing research concerning the effects of closed head injury on intellectual function in Chapter 5, it was noted that tests of nonverbal intelligence demonstrate a more pronounced impairment than tests of verbal intelligence. Levin *et al.* (1979a) assessed 27 patients on average one year after they had sustained severe head injuries, and found that Verbal IQ on the Wechsler Adult Intelligence Scale (WAIS) was significantly correlated with the patients' educational level, while Performance IQ was not. They therefore concluded that 'Performance IQ more specifically characterized long-term recovery from CHI [closed head injury] as distinguished from premorbid educational background' (p. 415). In this regard, it should also be remembered that head-injured patients show a characteristically poor premorbid academic attainment (Haas *et al.*, 1987; Rutter *et al.*, 1980); one should not therefore assume that such patients would match the general population in terms of their long-term post-traumatic level of intellectual function. Be that as it may, research involving the serial assessment of severely head-injured patients has shown that Verbal IQ returns to normal levels before Performance IQ (Chadwick *et al.*, 1981a, 1981b; Mandleberg, 1976; Mandleberg and Brooks, 1976; *see also* Mandleberg, 1975), although Bond and Brooks (1976) found very similar rates of recovery between the Mill Hill Vocabulary Test and the Progressive Matrices test.

One study is often cited as an illustration of these phenomena. Bond (1975, 1976) presented data which had been obtained by administering the WAIS to patients with severe head injury at intervals between three and more than 24 months after their accidents. Those patients who had been tested within the first six months showed a pronounced decrement in Full Scale IQ that varied with the duration of PTA. Subsequently, those patients whose PTA had lasted for less than 12 weeks achieved mean IQs that were within the normal range; however, those in whom PTA had lasted for longer than 12 weeks continued to demonstrate impaired performance with little sign of any restitution of intellectual function. Across the entire sample, there were significant negative correlations between Full Scale IQ and clinical ratings of the degree of neurophysical, social and mental disability using the scales shown in Table 7.1, although not surprisingly the last of these three scales showed the strongest association with IQ scores.

Unfortunately, the results of Bond's study are extremely difficult to interpret because of a serious lack of clarity in the basic description of the methodology. The impression given in his original accounts is that 56 patients participated in the study, each of whom was assessed once during the course of recovery:

> Fifty-six patients (47 men and 9 women) took part in the study . . . The past psychiatric history and current mental state of the patients was assessed by the same psychiatrist during a standard interview which was supplemented by information from a close relative or friend. On the day of the interview, the patient was also examined neurologically and psychometrically tested on the Wechsler Adult Intelligence Scale . . . The time from accident to inter-view varied from 3 to 24 months or more but the distribution of intervals

was not unduly weighted at any point ... Different groups of subjects were assessed psychometrically 3, 6, 9, 12, 18 or 24 months after their injury. (Bond, 1975, pp. 142, 143, 149).

A population of 56 patients (47 men and 9 women entered the study ... All patients and a relative were interviewed by a psychiatrist and their past history and current mental state were assessed during the course of a standard interview. On the same day they were examined neurologically and psychometrically tested using the Wechsler Adult Intelligence Scale ... Patients were assessed psychometrically at 3, 6, 9, 12, 18 or 24 months following injury. (Bond, 1976, pp. 59, 64).

Had this study employed a between-subjects design, as is clearly implied in these extracts, it would naturally have been uncontaminated by practice effects, to which the WAIS is known to be vulnerable (*see* Chapter 5, pp. 153–4), and it would therefore have been very informative about the recovery of intellectual function in severely head-injured patients.

However, identical findings were presented in a separate report by Bond and Brooks (1976), where they were described as having been produced by *40* patients who were 'assessed using the test-retest method [i.e., a *within*-subjects design] at intervals of less than 3 months, 4–6 months, 7–12 months and more than 13 months after injury' (p. 129). In addition, these data were identified as those that had been obtained by Mandleberg and Brooks (1975) in a study which was discussed in detail in chapter 5 (pp. 155–7). It will be recalled that the latter researchers tested patients with severe head injuries on average six weeks, five months, ten months, and three years after their accidents, but that for different subgroups of patients the testing programme began at different points in this sequence. The account of this study that was given earlier came to the conclusion that the research protocol had not satisfactorily excluded practice effects from the resulting data (*see* p. 157), and the same must therefore be said of the findings that were presented by Bond. He himself failed to provide any data to evaluate possible practice effects from appropriate comparison groups that had received a similar programme of repeated psychometric testing. As was implied elsewhere (*see* p. 154), this unfortunately means that Bond's findings are quite uninformative about the nature or the extent of recovery of intellectual function following closed head injury.

Finally, some researchers have considered the relationship between intellectual impairment and other aspects of the outcome following closed head injury. For instance, in commenting upon the modest reduction in IQ that he had found in a follow-up study of severely head-injured children, Richardson (1963) presaged more recent criticisms of the sensitivity of psychometric tests as indicators of the likely outcome following close head injury: 'The moderate loss of points on formal intelligence tests in no way represents the long-term crippling effects of the injury on the patient and his family' (p. 481). Despite this, some studies have found significant relationships between the residual intellectual function after closed head injury and the patient's rating on the Glasgow Outcome Scale, largely because of a particularly pronounced deficit in patients who are rated as 'severely disabled' (Brooks *et al.*, 1986b; Jennett *et al.*, 1981; Levin *et al.*, 1979a). Prigatano *et al.* (1984) found no difference in Full Scale IQ between severely head-injured patients who did and did not return to gainful employment or study, but out of a variety of psychometric tests the most powerful in discriminating between the two groups was the Digit Symbol subtest from the WAIS. Once again the data in question were purely correlational, but this finding is of considerable practical interest. As Prigatano *et al.* commented:

> This test measures, among other things, the ability to learn with practice and speed of new learning. It does not sample higher abstract reasoning or problem solving skills. If the patient is within the lower limits of normal on this test by the end of rehabilitation, it suggests that he/she has the basic cognitive capacities to be taught work skills and to be competitive, in terms of efficiency of functioning (at least for some jobs). (p. 511)

Language Function

The research literature that was reviewed in Chapter 5 concerning language disorders in the immediate period after a closed head injury (pp. 161–73) indicated that classical aphasia was a relatively rare consequence. Acute disturbances of comprehension and repetition may result from damage to the left temporal lobe (Heilman *et al.*, 1971; Thomsen, 1976), but often show rapid recovery (e.g., Arseni *et al.*, 1970; Stone *et al.*, 1978), and the prognosis for traumatic aphasia is considered to be much better than for language deficits resulting from other causes, such as vascular disease (Alajouanine *et al.*, 1957). Levin *et al.* (1979a) found that any obvious and persistent impairments of comprehension and conversational speech were confined to those patients who were rated as severely disabled on the Glasgow Outcome Scale.

Nevertheless, subclinical disturbances of language function and of communication in general are much more common, especially in patients who have sustained severe head injuries. As Milton and Wertz (1986) observed, the persistent cognitive and communicative problems of these patients have a potentially devastating impact upon their everyday activities:

> The symptoms that characterize this population include difficulty in (1) being concise or specific when expressing thoughts; (2) staying on topic; (3) selecting appropriate words or phrases to convey information; (4) using pronouns with an unambiguous referent; (5) selecting topics to talk about; (6) maintaining a mature presence when interacting with others; (7)

assimilating and using contextual cues; (8) paying attention to what is said; (9) remembering information; (10) understanding abstract or implied information; (11) integrating information across sentences to come up with an understanding of the whole; (12) reading information accurately; and (13) writing thoughts completely and accurately. (pp. 225–7)

In studying recovery from severe head injury in 46 children, Brink *et al.* (1970) remarked that 'the relearning of intelligible speech paralleled the recovery of motor function' (p. 567). Najenson *et al.* (1978) made a similar observation regarding nine patients with prolonged traumatic coma, even though in some patients neither communicative function nor locomotor function exhibited any recovery at all until 5–7 months after the injury. Paradoxically, however, Najenson *et al.* noted that it was the motor aspect of speech impairment that showed the slowest and least complete recovery. In a more recent study Brooks *et al.* (1986a) confirmed that dysarthria was a common outcome of severe head injury and one which showed little sign of restitution even over the course of five years after the injury. The other predominant form of residual language disturbance after closed head injury is in the area of word finding; Levin (1981) noted that such an impairment could be demonstrated by appropriate formal testing even in those patients who had relatively intact spontaneous speech.

Thomsen (1974, 1975, 1976) described the results of a follow-up study of 50 patients with severe closed head injuries. There had not been any complications in 26 of these cases, but in the remainder focal lesions had resulted from intracranial haematoma or depressed skull fracture. When initially examined roughly four months after their injuries, 12 of the former cases and 15 of the latter cases were described as 'aphasic'; and at a subsequent examination on average 30 months after their accidents, eight of the former cases and 13 of the latter cases were still regarded as 'aphasic'. However, Thomsen seems to have used this term to encompass a variety of mild symptoms, and it would appear that only five patients (all of whom had focal lesions) were aphasic in a strict clinical sense at the time of the second examination. Thomsen (1984) presented a long-term follow-up of 40 patients from her original sample, including 19 of those who had been described as 'aphasic' at their initial examination. When re-examined 10–15 years later, only four patients presented with aphasic symptoms, all of whom had sustained focal lesions in the left cerebral hemisphere. In contrast to this, dysarthria remained a serious problem, and at the time of follow-up was still evident in all 15 of the patients who had been dysarthric at the initial examination. In addition, many patients, regardless of whether or not they had originally been described as 'aphasic', showed some residual problems in their spontaneous speech: 'Subnormal rate of speaking, impaired word finding and sporadic verbal paraphasia of the semantic type, frequent pauses, the use of many set phrases, and perseveration on words and sentences were common' (p. 263).

In their 7-year follow-up study of 134 cases of severe head injury, Brooks *et al.*

(1987) found that communication deficits were significant predictors of a failure to return to work. In particular, 34 per cent of the patients who had been previously employable were said by relatives to have difficulty in carrying on a conversation, and 31 per cent were said to have difficulty in understanding a conversation; either problem seemed to preclude any gainful employment. Nevertheless, Brooks *et al.* suggested that these problems were not the result of any single specific impairment such as dysphasia or dyslexia, but were 'rather subtle and multifactorial' and reflected a wide range of deficits including attentional difficulties, slowness in thinking, and memory problems (p.17).

Social Interaction

It was noted earlier in this chapter that some of the measures of outcome following closed head injury were supposed to reflect the degree to which a patient had achieved satisfactory social reintegration, but some studies have considered this aspect of recovery directly.

Thomsen (1974) interviewed the 50 patients in her study on average 30 months following their accidents, and found that their main problem was a lack of social contact: 'Most patients had lost contact with premorbid friends and they had very few possibilities of establishing new contacts, because they spent nearly all [their] time at home' (p. 182). Similarly, in the study by Levin *et al.* (1979a), 10 out of the 27 patients had been socially active young adults before sustaining a severe head injury, but when they were followed up on average 12 months afterwards had withdrawn to solitary activities (such as listening to music and watching television) and tended to avoid group situations. Thomsen (1984) subsequently followed up 40 of her patients between 10 and 15 years after their original injury, and she found that a loss of social contact remained the patients' most disabling handicap in their daily life.

Oddy *et al.* (1978b) interviewed the close relatives of 50 patients about the social activities of the latter during the month before they had sustained a severe closed head injury and during the two months preceding a follow-up assessment six months after the injury. Although 19 (or 38 per cent) of these patients showed some reduction in their leisure activities, this was attributed to the interruption in their normal routine rather than to brain injury, since a similar reduction was observed in a control group of 30 patients who had sustained traumatic limb fractures. Neither group showed any significant reduction in their overall amount of social contact. Nevertheless, the patients who had suffered very severe closed head injuries (as evidenced by a PTA lasting longer than seven days) did show a significant fall in the number of their close friends, in their amount of contact with close friends, and in the number of visits exchanged with their friends; in some patients the latter had led to social isolation. Moreover, single patients within this subgroup had tended to become more dependent upon their parents. Because the control patients had not become socially isolated either through physical disability or through absence from work, Oddy *et al.* concluded that the social problems of the patients with very severe head injuries were a reflection of personality changes such as restlessness, irritability, and impatience. Oddy and Humphrey (1980) followed up these patients at 12 and 24 months after their injury. Half of the head-injured patients continued to engage in fewer leisure activities than before their accidents, but this seemed to be the result of a lack of motivation rather than any appreciable physical disability. These patients reported fewer social excursions, and those with very severe head injuries continued to receive fewer social visits, although by the 24-month follow-up they no longer had fewer close friends than before their accidents and their family relationships also appeared to have returned to normal.

A similar investigation was carried out by Weddell *et al.* (1980) of 44 young adult patients who had been admitted to a rehabilitation centre following very severe head injury. Information concerning their social recovery was obtained from interviews carried out with close relatives roughly two years after their accidents. The findings were compared with the reports of relatives of 43 other patients with severe head injuries who were interviewed within a month of the relevant accidents and asked to describe the latter patients' social activities during the two months before their injuries. The patients with very severe head injuries were found to have fewer close friends, to make and receive fewer social visits, to date less frequently, and to have fewer interests and hobbies. Social contacts were curtailed especially in those patients who manifested post-traumatic personality changes or cognitive impairment. The number of acquaintances showed no difference between the two groups of patients, which indicated that the reduction in social contact was based on a change in the nature rather than in the number of personal relationships after very severe head injury, though six of the head-injured patients seemed to have no friends or acquaintances at all. Not surprisingly, the head-injured patients were regarded as being significantly more lonely than the comparison group, and nearly half of them had no friends whom they saw as often as once a week. Although only six of their relatives considered loneliness to be a major problem, Weddell *et al.* observed that evidence in the psychiatric field had demonstrated the necessity of close relationships for the maintenance of emotional stability.

An interesting suggestion in much of this research is that a persistent change in social behaviour following severe closed head injury is related to concomitant deficits in cognition and communication. In the study by Thomsen (1974), for instance, the proportion of patients who complained of loneliness was greater in those described as 'aphasics' (71 per cent) than in those described as 'nonaphasics' (52 per cent), although only one fifth of the former patients thought that problems involving language or speech might be the main reason for their loneliness. Oddy and Humphrey (1980) found that limited social contact among head-injured patients was related to poor performance on a test of associative learning and on the Logical Memory subtest of the Wechsler Memory Scale, while Weddell *et al.* (1980) found that it was related to a score on the Standard Progressive Matrices test that was equivalent to an IQ of less than 70. Hayden and Hart (1986) specifically argued that

> many of the personality changes reported by head injured patients or their relatives may be conceptualized as secondary to cognitive deficits which have a sweeping impact on typical patterns of behaviour. For example, the patient who is unable to follow or contribute to conversations because of information processing inefficiency may eventually give up the attempt, earning the label of 'socially withdrawn'. (p. 213)

Indeed, as these authors pointed out, any attempt to regain normal social functioning in the face of the severe and global cognitive deficits that may result from closed head injury would necessitate drastic changes in the patient's previous behaviour patterns and routines.

The Process of Recovery

Recovery Curves

The previous discussion has at various points alluded to the pattern of recovery at progressively increasing intervals after closed head injury. In principle this can be studied either by comparing different groups of patients tested at various intervals after their accidents or by testing the same patients on a number of occasions during the course of recovery. Both of these research strategies have inherent methodological weaknesses, some of which have already been mentioned. In the former case, unless the different patient groups are carefully matched with regard to the severity of their injuries, those patients with the more severe injuries will make a disproportionate contribution to the results obtained at later follow-up sessions because they were simply untestable at the earlier sessions (cf. Levin and Eisenberg, 1979a). In the latter case, repeated testing of the same patients tends to confound the effects of recovery *per se* with those of practice on a specific task and of familiarity with the general testing situation (Baddeley *et al.*, 1980; *see* Chapter 5, pp. 153–7). With both of these strategies, the interpretation of the results will depend on the specific choice of comparison or control group (Brooks *et al.*, 1984; *see* Chapter 4, pp. 118–9).

Conkey (1938) was the first investigator to express an interest in the pattern of recovery of psychological functions following closed head injury. On the basis of the results obtained with 25 head-injured cases, she noted that the recovery of psychological functions lagged behind that of physical signs and symptoms, that simple mental functions exhibited recovery earlier than more complex mental functions, and that the recovery of learning and memory lagged behind that of other mental functions. Her results also indicated that the greater part of the recovery had occurred within the first eight months or so following closed head injury. One problem with Conkey's study which was mentioned in Chapter 5 (p. 129) is that only four of her patients completed the entire programme of serial assessment over the first year following closed head injury, although she was able to show that these four patients had produced essentially the same pattern of results as the group as a whole. High attrition rates were also a problem in an otherwise potentially interesting longitudinal study of head-injured children reported by Black *et al.* (1971). As Brooks *et al.* (1984) noted, precautions need to be taken in research on the effects of brain damage to minimize patient drop-out and hence to achieve an optimum follow-up of the original clinical sample.

Nevertheless, subsequent research has confirmed that the pattern of recovery following closed head injury depends on the nature and complexity of the particular functions under examination. For instance, it has been noted already in this chapter that short-term memory tends to recover more rapidly and completely than long-term memory (e.g., Brooks, 1975) and that Verbal IQ tends to recover more rapidly and completely than Performance IQ (e.g., Mandleberg and Brooks, 1975). As extreme examples, the recovery of consciousness normally occurs within a matter of hours or days, while the restitution of higher mental functions can take many months (Carlsson *et al.*, 1968; Knill-Jones, 1975). In accordance with Conkey's conclusion, Black *et al.* (1971) found that in head-injured children most recovery of neurological deficits occurred within the first three months, though Jennett and Bond (1975) suggested that in severely injured patients neurological sequelae may continue to improve 'on a scale of years rather than months' (p. 482). Dikmen *et al.* (1983) identified different patterns of recovery amongst the component subtests of the Halstead-Reitan battery, and they agreed that 'deficits appear to be most consistent on the more complex and demanding neuropsychological tests' (p. 336). More speculatively, Eson *et al.* (1978) suggested that the underlying pattern of recovery from severe head injury reflected the sequence in which different functions were acquired during the course of normal human development.

It is in principle important to distinguish between case studies of individual patients and those which measure recovery of function in terms of the proportion of patients who have achieved a certain standard (e.g., Bricolo *et al.*, 1980, on eye opening; Guthkelch, 1980, on return to work) or in terms of the average test performance across a sample of patients. The pattern of recovery in individual patients may be quite different from the overall pattern of recovery across the clinical samples to which they belong. Indeed, Brooks and Aughton (1979a) found that only eight out of a group of 24 severely injured patients produced a monotonically increasing pattern of scores on the Progressive Matrices test across three successive sessions, whereas 12 patients showed a pattern that involved a decrement between two successive tests. In practice, however, such deviant patterns of scores may merely be tapping test-retest unreliability or else indicate idiosyncratic variations in practice effects or test sophistication.

In the vast majority of published reports the pattern of recovery in patients with closed head injury exemplifies the same characteristic form, regardless of the underlying research methodology. As in Conkey's (1938) original analysis, the most rapid improvement tends to occur during the first few months following the head injury, but the rate of improvement gradually slows and there is relatively little change in performance after the first year. Dikmen and Reitan (1976) found that the initial rate of improvement was greater in patients who showed a more pronounced initial impairment, though the latter continued to demonstrate greater residual deficits when retested 18 months later (*see also* Chadwick *et al.*, 1981a). Newcombe (1982) noted that head-injured patients and their relatives may need to be reassured that the characteristic slowing down of the recovery process is a normal phenomenon, but Jennett *et al.* (1981) emphasized that unrealistic expectations for further substantial recovery may impede the acceptance of disability and subsequent rehabilitative efforts.

When represented as a graph, the performance of head-injured patients in a series of testing sessions tends to follow a negatively accelerating curve which gradually approaches a limit or *asymptote* (Eson *et al.*, 1978; Newcombe, 1982). The initial point of this curve marks the beginning of significant recovery (which is typically later than the occurrence of the injury itself), the rate of recovery varies both among individual patients and among individual tasks, and the asymptote may or may not correspond to a normal functional level (Brooks *et al.*, 1984). In most instances such a shape is at least in part an artefact because there will be an upper limit upon performance: that is, a score of 100 if the measure of recovery is percentage correct performance and a score of zero if the relevant measure is response time. Dikmen *et al.* (1983) also noted that the performance of head-injured patients must have an upper limit that corresponds to that of normal control subjects. In other instances, there will be an upper limit on a patient's performance insofar as there are bounds to the sheer extent of clinical recovery. In any case it can be inferred that each successive increase in performance reduces the scope for any subsequent improvement, and this will generate a negatively accelerated recovery function which approaches some asymptotic level of performance.

However, many researchers feel that 'the study of such curves may throw light on natural or spontaneous recovery processes' (Newcombe *et al.*, 1975b, p. 132). In particular, Dikmen *et al.* (1983) considered that

> accurate and quantitative information about patterns of spontaneous improvement or recovery curves for higher-level brain functions . . . should yield insights regarding mechanisms of recovery, provide a framework against which the effectiveness of various treatments can be assessed, and allow formulation of rational treatment strategies. (p. 333)

The simplest theoretical model of functional recovery would assume that the level of performance on a specific test improved at a constant rate (k, say), which would predict that performance would be a linear function of the time elapsed since the head injury and would improve indefinitely without limit. However, as has just been noted, the level of performance in most situations will in practice be bounded by either a logical or an empirical upper limit. Under these circumstances, the rate of improvement will be a constant proportion of the increase in performance that has still to be attained. If y is the observed level of performance and α is the asymptotic level, then the rate of change in y is given by $k(\alpha - y)$. Solving this differential equation with respect to the elapsed time since the onset of recovery, t, yields the solution

$$y = \alpha - \beta \rho^t,$$

where $\alpha - \beta$ is the initial level of performance and ρ reflects the rate of recovery such that k equals the natural logarithm of $1/\rho$. The constant β is positive if y is a measure of accuracy or speed and negative if y is a measure of error rate or response time. In the latter version, the formula above was applied to the number of errors made by head-injured patients in reading aloud single words and in naming objects presented as line drawings by Newcombe *et al.* (1975a, 1975b; Hiorns and Newcombe, 1979), and it was applied to the response latencies produced by neurosurgical patients in carrying out a visual search task by Artiola i Fortuny and Hiorns (1979).

On this account the general form of recovery curves following closed head injury will be exponential in nature. Such curves are also loosely described as 'logarithmic' functions (e.g., Brooks *et al.*, 1984), insofar as the logarithm of the measure of performance is a linear function of the time elapsed since the onset of recovery (Carlsson *et al.*, 1968). It can in fact be formally proved that an exponential function of this type will describe any process in which some definite quantity changes in such a way that the change ratio depends only upon the duration of the time interval over which the change occurs and not upon the original value of that quantity. In the present case, the quantity in question is the amount of residual impairment relative to the asymptotic level of performance: in other words, $(\alpha - y)$ if one is measuring accuracy or speed, and $(y - \alpha)$ if one is measuring errors or latencies. Nevertheless, exponential functions of this general form can be used to describe a wide variety of processes in the natural and social sciences. Other examples include the growth of capital under continuously compound interest, the natural increase of a population, the decay of radioactive material, and the intensity of light being transmitted through a homogeneous absorbing medium (Ostrowski, 1968, pp. 280–1). Carlsson *et al.* (1968) showed that such a function yielded an excellent fit to fatality rates following severe head injury.

The fact that exponential functions are of such general applicability helps to illuminate both their strengths and their weaknesses. On the one hand, they offer a convenient notation in which to describe any physical system that is subject to constant processes of growth or decay, and to that extent provide a simple means of characterizing the 'natural history' of recovery from closed head injury (cf. Newcombe, 1982). On the other hand, recovery curves provide nothing more than a perspicuous survey of performance at various times following injury, and are quite uninformative with regard to the underlying mechanisms of recovery (Hiorns and Newcombe, 1979). In particular, they do not provide a reasoned basis for exploring possible *differences* among the recovery curves obtained from different tasks or different patients, or for distinguishing between the effects of recovery and those of practice. Moreover, while the basic assumption of an exponential relationship between performance and time since injury can be justified on a priori grounds, there is little in the way of any direct empirical evidence for such a relationship (Brooks *et al.*, 1984), since in most cases the data that are obtained would be equally compatible with the assumption that recovery proceeded in an essentially linear manner through several discrete stages of improvement (Hiorns and Newcombe, 1979).

Finally, some researchers have pointed out some possible exceptions to this general pattern of recovery. In analysing patients' performance on 12 subtests of the Halstead-Reitan battery, Dikmen *et al.* (1983) found that in nine cases performance was a linear function of time since injury between an initial assessment on average 16 days after injury, an initial follow-up assessment 12 months later, and a second follow-up assessment 18 months later. They concluded that these findings gave little support for the idea that the recovery of neuropsychological function following closed head injury slowed appreciably after the first year. Unfortunately, their conclusion rested upon only three observations per patient; it is nowadays generally recognized that adequate estimation of the parameters defining a recovery curve depends upon the collection of data across a sufficiently extended period of time to reflect the nonlinear pattern of performance (Hiorns and Newcombe, 1979; Newcombe *et al.*, 1975b). Nevertheless, it is also appreciated that improvement may continue beyond the first two years in the case of some patients and some functions (*see* Brooks *et al.*, 1984; Newcombe 1982).

In contrast to these different patterns of *improvement* following head injury, McKinlay *et al.* (1981) found that certain aspects of impairment tended to become more rather than less frequent over the course of time, at least according to the reports of patients' close relatives. This was particularly true of emotional difficulties and behavioural problems, such as reports of mood swings, bad temper, and social withdrawal, which showed large increases from three to 12 months after injury (*see also* McKinlay and Brooks, 1984). McKinlay *et al.* suggested two possible causal mechanisms that might underlie such reports. First, these changes might be a direct and immediate result of closed head injury but are only acknowledged at a later stage in the course of recovery. This might be because they are not observed or admitted by the patients' relatives, or else because they are considered unremarkable in the early stages of recovery. Second, changes of this nature might reflect adverse psychological reactions to disability (for instance, to restricted social activities or persistence of symptoms) which develop over the course of time. Regardless of their aetiology, the incidence of these symptoms shows no sign of any subsequent reduction, and reports of personality change and threats of violence continue to increase up to five years after severe closed head injury (Brooks *et al.*, 1986a; *see also* Black *et al.*, 1971).

Age and Recovery

It is often assumed that the long-term effects of brain damage tend to increase with the age of the individual to whom that damage has occurred, reflecting the relative resilience or plasticity of the young brain as opposed to the relative vulnerability of the elderly brain. According to Schneider (1979), Hans-Lukas Teuber attributed the principle that 'It is better to have your brain lesion early' to the work of Kennard (1938), though it is worth noting that the latter was concerned solely with the restitution of motor function following ablation of major areas of the cerebral cortex. It is true that experimental research with infrahuman species has demonstrated that identical lesions may have quite different consequences when sustained earlier rather than later in life. However, Schneider's own observations on lesions of the optic tract in the hamster showed that in detail the nature of these changes depends on the specific site of damage and the specific function that is under consideration.

Russell (1934) suggested that 'the most important single factor which influences the ultimate prognosis in a case of head injury is the age of the patient' (p. 139). This conclusion was based on observations obtained from an unselected sample of 200 patients admitted to hospital following head injury. When they were classified into successive age groups, the proportion of patients with postconcussional symptoms persisting more than two months after their discharge increased continuously from 46 per cent in the case of those aged 10–20 years to 100 per cent in the case of those of over 50 years of age, although 66 per cent of children aged up to ten years also suffered from such symptoms. More recent research has tended to find nonsignificant increases in the incidence of persistent postconcussional symptoms with advancing age (Rutherford *et al.*, 1977, 1979). In Russell's study, however, this increase was largely attributable to increases in the incidence of dizziness and loss of memory or mental ability rather than in the incidence of headaches, nervousness, or behavioural disturbances, and this pattern was confirmed in subsequent research (*see* Brenner *et al.*, 1944; Friedman *et al.*, 1945). Moreover, the increase in postconcussional symptoms among young children was largely attributable to increases in the incidence of disturbance of behaviour or personality. Dillon and Leopold (1961) and Black *et al.* (1969) confirmed that persistent postconcussional symptoms tend to be somatic in adults but predominantly behavioural in children. Finally, Russell (1934) demonstrated that in adult patients the duration of incapacity for previous work tended to vary directly with age; this also has been widely replicated in more recent work (*see* Humphrey and Oddy, 1980).

However, in evaluating the consequences of closed head injury, there are at least four considerations that militate against the possibility of making meaningful comparisons across different age groups of patients. First, as was pointed out in Chapter 1 (pp. 24–5), closed head injuries are much more common among young adults, so that unselected samples of head-injured patients may include relatively few individuals from the extremes of the age range. Kapur (1988, p. 108) noted that a paucity of elderly patients would explain why at least some studies (e.g., Brooks *et al.*, 1980; Lezak, 1979) had failed to find correlations between age and cognitive outcome following closed head injury. A second problem is that the sorts of accidents that give rise to closed head injury may be quite different in different age groups. As was also mentioned in Chapter 1 (pp. 32–8), domestic accidents and falls tend to be the major cause of head injuries among children and the elderly, whereas injuries to adults below the age of 65 are much more likely to be the result of traffic accidents, assaults, and occupational accidents. As a consequence, both the type of injury and the severity of the injury may well vary among these three different subgroups of patients (Kapur, 1988, p. 108).

A third difficulty is that staff working in accident and emergency departments may differentiate among the three groups in terms of the criteria for admission. For instance, a hospital might admit for observation any child with a history of head injury whatsoever (perhaps as a precautionary measure or because of difficulties in their clinical examination), whereas adult patients would be admitted only when a loss of consciousness had occurred. Jennett (1976c) noted that such a policy would give rise to a disproportionate number of less severely affected cases in samples of paediatric head injuries, and that this artefact would give the impression that young children could anticipate a more favourable outcome. Finally, it is possible that individuals in different age groups have different pathophysiological responses to closed head injury or else different levels of susceptibility to complications. Recent work on fatal head injury has tended to emphasize the similarities between the types of brain damage seen in children, adults of working age, and elderly patients (Adams *et al.*, 1989b; Graham *et al.*, 1989a). There are however some clear exceptions to this: in particular intracranial haematomas are more common among older patients, whereas hypoxic brain damage, elevated intracranial pressure, and especially generalized cerebral swelling are more common in children. It was mentioned earlier in this chapter that Carlsson *et al.* (1968) had demonstrated that the increased mortality following head injury in older patients could be attributed entirely to the occurrence of extracerebral complications such as pneumonia or cardiovascular problems. Johnston and Mellits (1980) argued that a lower incidence of complications might also explain any trend towards decreased mortality and morbidity in head-injured children, though there is little direct evidence on this.

It is quite clear that patients in different age groups who are admitted to hospital following closed head injury may well vary in the severity of their injuries, either because of the intrinsic nature of the injuries themselves or because of current hospital admissions policies. Recent studies of the role of age in recovery from closed head injury have usually attempted to handle this problem by including only those patients whose injuries exceed a particular level of severity. Unfortunately, this still may not be sufficient to ensure comparable degrees of brain damage. In a study of 40 children with traumatic or nontraumatic coma of at least 24 hours' duration, Johnston and Mellits (1980) found that the median coma duration was 14 days in those aged less than eight but 74 days in those aged eight years or more.

Head Injuries in Children

In neurophysical terms, most children who are admitted to hospital after closed head injury appear to make a good recovery (Gaidolfi and Vignolo, 1980; Klonoff *et al.*, 1977). However, such an assessment may well tend to obscure serious residual difficulties (Miner *et al.*, 1986). The somewhat limited amount of research literature suggests that head-injured children show persistent deficits of memory and cognition that are qualitatively similar to those shown by head-injured adults (*see* Levin *et al.*, 1982a, pp. 198–201; 1988a). In particular, they tend to be impaired in the acquisition of new information in long-term memory, and this is of obvious practical significance because it appears to be a major cause of academic difficulties that were not present before injury (Brink *et al.*, 1970; Fuld and Fisher, 1977; Klonoff *et al.*, 1977; Levin and Eisenberg, 1979a, 1979b; Richardson, 1963). Such an outcome seems to be especially likely in the case of severely injured children in whom the duration of coma is longer than two weeks (Heiskanen and Kaste, 1974) or in whom the duration of PTA is longer than three weeks (Chadwick *et al.*, 1981a). Indeed, precisely because brain damage tends to impair the learning of new information Rutter (1981) argued that its effects in young children might well be expected to be disproportionately severe, simply because they had more new learning still to do and less accumulated knowledge and fewer established skills on which to rely. As a result, even mild learning deficits may cumulatively lead to poor academic achievement in later years, or else they may only become evident in intellectually demanding tasks. More fundamentally, as Rutter pointed out, 'cognitive tasks may have a different meaning at different ages' (p. 1539).

Woo-Sam *et al.* (1970) compared two groups of children who had sustained head injuries leading to a period of coma lasting at least one week. Out of 25 children aged less than eight years at the time of injury, 22 (or 88 per cent) were assessed as being of below normal intelligence; however, out of 21 children aged more than ten years at the time of injury, only ten (or 48 per cent) were assessed as being of below normal intelligence. This was not because of differences in the severity of the resulting injuries, since the older children tended if anything to have suffered longer periods of coma, nor was there any evidence that it was attributable to differences in socio-economic status, premorbid intellectual functioning, or the amount of practice between the two age groups. Woo-Sam *et al.* interpreted the results to mean that intellectual prognosis after head injury was likely to be poorer for younger children than for older children. Unfortunately, a wide variety of different psychometric instruments were used to assess intelligence in individual patients, and it is conceivable that some of the variations in test adminstration might explain these differences in IQ estimates.

Bruce *et al.* (1978) studied the effects of severe head injury in 53 children between the ages of four months and 17 years. These patients were selected on the basis of the criteria that had been used in the international collaborative study of head injuries in Scotland, the Netherlands, and the United States which was mentioned towards the beginning of this chapter (p. 227): in other words, a period of unconsciousness lasting longer than six hours, defined as an inability to obey commands, to utter recognizable words, or to open the eyes. All of the patients were assessed six months after injury on the Glasgow Outcome Scale. The results showed that 48 (or 91 per cent) of the sample had made a good recovery or had only moderate disability, and indeed all but one of those over five years of age in this group had returned to school. Only one of their patients had been left in a vegetative state following the injury and only three patients had died. One of these deaths was associated with uncontrollable hypertension, but the other two deaths did not seem to be the direct result of head injury.

Despite their careful efforts to make their sample as comparable as possible with those in the international collaborative study, Bruce *et al.* noted that they had obtained markedly lower levels of both mortality and morbidity. They cited previous studies of severe head injury in children which had also produced better outcomes than research with adult series, and identified certain distinctive features of their own sample that might explain this trend. First, the incidence of mass lesions was rather less than that found in the international study. Fewer of their patients had shown evidence of intracranial haematoma, and despite the fact the 49 of them had undergone computerized tomography (CT) immediately after their admission to hospital, none of the latter patients had shown any signs of haemorrhagic contusions. Bruce *et al.* noted that the latter finding was consistent with earlier *post mortem* studies of head injuries in children, in which cerebral contusions proved to be relatively rare. Nevertheless, 18 of these patients had shown signs of diffuse cerebral swelling (namely, compressed ventricles and absent basal cisterns on CT scans), and this had been identified in previous research as the most common clinical sign in children dying after head injury (*see* Chapter 2, p. 61).

These considerations led Bruce *et al.* to suggest that the symptomatology and pathophysiology of head injury were different in children and adults, and in particular that children had a lower threshold for acute neurophysiological dysfunction. From this it would follow that 'a coma score that in an adult would be associated with severe parenchymal injury and a poor prognosis for recovery may be associated with less cerebral injury and, therefore, a better prognosis for recovery in the child' (p. 685). However, these researchers noted that this would not explain why the level of outcome in their series was also markedly better than that obtained in previous studies of the effects of severe head injury in children. They commented that their investigation was the first such study in which CT had been routinely used in the early assessment of head-injured patients. This had permitted the prompt diagnosis of intracranial mass lesions, thus enabling rapid surgical intervention when necessary, as well as the effective control of intracranial hypertension (which had been recorded in 22 of the 27 patients in whom intracranial pressure had been monitored).

Levin and Eisenberg (1979a) administered a neuropsychological battery to 22 children between six and 12 years of age and 42 adolescents between 13 and 18 years of age, and in each case compared the results with data from normal individuals of the same ages. Memory deficits tended to be more common among the children, but other types of impairment were rather more frequent among the adolescents; however, in no case was the relationship between age and impairment statistically significant. Levin and Eisenberg (1979b) found a nonsignificant trend for children to be more impaired than adolescents, but they also made a specific observation that the incidence of post-traumatic aphasia appeared to be somewhat lower in children and in adolescents than in adults. They took this to be consistent with Hécaen's (1976) notion that the child's brain has greater potential for functional reorganization among the regions that subserve language. The latter idea is also supported by the results of the study by Chadwick *et al.* (1981c) which were described in Chapter 5 (pp. 160–1).

Levin *et al.* (1982b) suggested that the supposed greater neural plasticity of the young brain might well facilitate the reorganization of cognitive function following focal lesions, but that it would confer no particular advantage in recovery from the sort of diffuse insult that was typically produced by severe closed head injury. They compared 30 head-injured children (aged between two and 12 years at the time of injury) with 30 head-injured adolescents (aged between 13 and 19 years) in terms of verbal recall using the selective reminding procedure, continuous visual recognition memory for familiar objects, and intellectual functioning according to the age-appropriate Wechsler intelligence scale. In each age group, half of the patients had sustained severe head injuries (defined by a Glasgow Coma Sale score on admission of 8 or less), while half had sustained minor head injuries (defined by a Glasgow Coma Scale score on admission of more than 8). At a follow-up assessment several months or years after their accidents, the severely injured patients in both age groups performed worse on all three tests than those with minor injuries, but there was no suggestion of any greater residual impairment among the adolescents. Indeed, when compared with age-matched normal controls, the children were somewhat more likely to show persistent memory impairments. Moreover, of the severely injured children, five had a Verbal IQ of less than 80 and six had a Performance IQ of less than 80, whereas none of the adolescents showed any subnormal intellectual functioning in this sense. Although the two age groups had been matched in terms of their Glasgow Coma Scale scores, Levin *et al.* suggested that their adolescent patients might if anything be expected to have suffered more severe injuries than the children in their study because of their more frequent involvement in high-speed vehicular accidents. They concluded that their findings 'provide no evidence that the young brain confers an advantage with respect to the development and restitution of higher functions after traumatic brain injury' (p. 672).

Mechanisms of Recovery

The discussion so far has described recovery following closed head injury as if it were a unitary process, and this is certainly implicit in the exponential model of the relationship between objective performance and the time since the injury. Nevertheless, it is nowadays generally agreed that there are two qualitatively different types of mechanism underlying the process of recovery from brain damage (Bond, 1986; Cronholm, 1972). First, there are a number of mechanisms of primary recovery that operate at a neuronal level from the instant that the injury has occurred. Their effects are manifested in the neurological outcome and especially in the recovery of motor function (Bond, 1979). The available evidence suggests that in these terms recovery is complete or else reaches a plateau within six months of a closed head injury (e.g., Livingston and Livingston, 1985). Second, the possibility of improvement beyond this 6-month period depends upon the patient's adaptation to residual deficits and the development of compensatory strategies (Humphrey and Oddy, 1980; Jennett and Bond, 1975). These in turn demand the patient's awareness of the nature and extent of his or her disability, and hence they begin with the restitution of full consciousness at the end of the period of PTA (*see* Bond, 1979; Bond and Brooks, 1976). The literature that was reviewed earlier in this chapter suggests that the processes of spontaneous recovery of higher cognitive functions and the establishment of changes in personality and in social behaviour also occur predominantly within the first six months following a closed head injury (Bond, 1979), but the key to rehabilitative endeavours is that in principle such processes may persist for much longer.

Until relatively recently, the effects of brain damage were discussed solely in terms of the direct morphological changes to nerve cells, and it was widely assumed that cells within the central nervous system lacked any capacity for regeneration. On this assumption recovery must consist in a process of relearning, involving the development of other neural pathways. This can take the form either of vicarious functioning of undamaged neural tissue, in which some region of the brain takes on a function for which it previously had no responsibility; or of behavioural substitution, in which undamaged systems retain their original function but are also deployed in the service of novel goals (*see* Rutter, 1981). However, the possibility of recovery at a purely physiological level is indicated by the findings of magnetic resonance imaging (MRI) in head-injured patients. As mentioned in Chapter 2 (pp. 46, 54), MRI can indicate lesions of the grey and white matter of the brain in greater quantity and of larger volume than are visualized by means of CT scans. These lesions generally resolve within 1 to 3 months: moreover, they do not in themselves appear to demand any changes in the clinical management of head-injured patients, although they may be related to the persistence and nature of cognitive sequelae (Levin *et al.*, 1987a).

There are a number of short-term processes that promote the recovery of neuronal function in the immediate period after a closed head injury, including the replenishment of neurotransmitters and the restoration of cell membrane potential, in addition to the reversal of complications such as vascular constriction and brain swelling (Rutter, 1981; Teasdale and Mendelow, 1984). However, it is now quite clear that lesions of the brain have longer-term implications of both a positive and a negative sort. In an authoritative review, Schoenfeld and Hamilton (1977) argued that these secondary changes may be more significant in terms of their effects upon behaviour than the primary damage itself. In particular, it now appears that there is considerable potential for structural reorganization within the brain as the result of regenerative growth and sprouting that involves both damaged and intact neurones (*see also* Eccles, 1987). There is also evidence that damage to the central nervous system can lead to heightened sensitivity of deafferented tissue. There is however very little support for the classical notion of 'diaschisis', which was assumed to constitute a transient and reversible form of shock that affected neurones remote from the site of damage when they were deprived of afferent input (von Monakow, 1914, pp. 26–34). Pavlov and other Soviet psychologists speculated that this inhibitory process served to protect the intact areas of the brain, concussion being seen as a prime example (*see* Luria *et al.*, 1969, p. 370). Nevertheless, Schoenfeld and Hamilton considered that diaschisis lacked an adequate operational definition, and experimental tests of the notion have proved unsuccessful (e.g., West *et al.*, 1976).

The possibility of adaptation and compensation obviously depends upon the nature of the patients' residual deficits, but also upon the quality of the interactions between the patients and the individuals who are responsible for their continuing care and rehabilitation. The latter are themselves vulnerable to emotional changes that may in turn influence the patients' recovery (Bond, 1986; McKinlay and Brooks, 1984). At this level recovery following closed head injury is both a psychosocial process and a neurophysiological one. The coping strategies, successful or otherwise, that patients and their families adopt in such circumstances will depend on their cognitive, emotional, and motivational resources and on the amount and quality of the support that they receive (Barth *et al.*, 1983; Newcombe, 1982).

Rehabilitation

Traditional approaches to the treatment of head-injured patients tended to emphasize the need for conservative management. Symonds (1962) quoted the Victorian surgeon John Hilton thus:

> The brain after concussion is at first unequal to its ordinary duties .... It recovers itself slowly; it then soon becomes fatigued from use; and if claims are made upon it too soon after the injury — that is before the structural and physiological integrity is re-acquired — the patient is very likely to suffer. Cerebral exercise or mental occupation should always be short of fatigue. (p. 4)

Experiences during the Second World War brought about a marked change in clinical attitudes in favour of more active forms of rehabilitation such as occupational therapy, physiotherapy, and intellectual and recreational pursuits (Lewis, 1942; Symonds, 1942; *see also* Relander *et al.*, 1972). Nevertheless, rehabilitative efforts were focused almost exclusively upon the remediation of physical deficits with the primary aim of facilitating the patient's return to gainful employment; indeed, it was often assumed that very little could be done to promote the restoration of cognitive and behavioural functioning (*see* Bigler, 1987; Bond, 1975). Weddell *et al.* (1980) speculated that such an emphasis might have been reinforced by head-injured patients themselves and by their relatives since physical deficits were more easily recognized and accepted. For similar reasons, resources tended to be aimed towards severely disabled patients, despite the fact that those with moderate disability were more numerous and more likely to benefit from early active rehabilitation (Aitken *et al.*, 1982).

During the 1970s, however, a number of factors encouraged a growing awareness of the need for a deeper understanding of the broader aspects of recovery from closed head injury. First, it became apparent that even occupational resettlement depended upon residual cognitive and behavioural deficits as well as upon physical recovery. Second, residual deficits of this nature were seen to be of even greater significance in determining general social recovery, and hence to constitute a fundamental obstacle to rehabilitation. Third, clinical neuropsychologists began to take a more active professional interest in questions of treatment and rehabilitation as opposed to observation and assessment (*see* Brooks, 1979; Oddy and Humphrey, 1980). As a result, in recent years there has been a trend towards the view that the effective rehabilitation of head-injured patients demands an interdisciplinary approach that integrates traditional forms of treatment with cognitive retraining and behaviour modification, as well as counselling for both the patients and their relatives (*see* e.g., Bond, 1979; Cohen and Titonis, 1985; Eames and Wood, 1989; Evans, 1981; Livingston, 1986; Malkmus, 1983; Najenson *et al.*, 1978).

Questions of effectiveness and efficiency in the context of rehabilitation can only be answered by careful evaluative trials of different techniques, which need explicit descriptions of the relevant procedures such that they can be replicated in different centres as well as sensitive and reliable measures of the outcome (*see* Levin and Eisenberg, 1979b; Newcombe, 1982). In essence, such research would differentiate between genuine effects of treatment and improvements that could merely be attributed to spontaneous recovery or to familiarity with a particular testing procedure, although the latter may still form the basis of a useful training programme. For instance, Miller (1980) showed substantial learning with severely injured patients on a single version of the Minnesota Spatial Relations Test and good transfer to alternative versions of the test. His control group of neurologically normal subjects showed much less improvement, so that the performance of the head-injured group gradually approached that of the controls over the course of the experiment. However, when subgroups of subjects were matched in terms of their initial levels of performance, the head-injured patients showed a slower rate of improvement, which indicated that they might still be suffering from an impairment of learning. Miller suggested that his results were comparable to those obtained from subjects with severe mental subnormality, and that they vindicated the use of work on training in subnormality as a starting point for examining the problem of training in severe head injury. Obrzut and Hynd (1987) made a similar suggestion with regard to outcome and treatment in children with acquired brain injury compared to those with developmental learning disabilities.

Nevertheless, most researchers consider that it is vital to separate the effects of practice on a particular task in the rehabilitation setting from generalized improvement when patients have returned to the community, and this requires comparison with other head-injured patients who have not received the training programme under evaluation. For ethical reasons, as Aitken *et al.* (1982) pointed out, the latter should still receive routine or standard treatment. Indeed, it may turn out to be the dedication and commitment of the rehabilitation team that promotes recovery rather than any particular therapeutic technique, and they themselves might regard it as unethical to deviate from their established methods (Baddeley *et al.*, 1980; Newcombe, 1982). However, this points to a more fundamental goal of research: to identify the specific causal mechanisms underlying recovery both with and without rehabilitative intervention (Parsons and Prigatano, 1978). The latter is inherently a less tractable problem because many of the available findings are purely correlational in nature. For instance, Brooks *et al.* (1987) found a positive association between the incidence of emotional and behavioural deficits in head-injured patients and problems in occupational resettlement; they also identified a positive association between the latter problems and the input of social work services. They concluded that emotional and behavioural deficits caused difficulties in returning to work and that social work services were provided in response to such difficulties. Nevertheless, this conclusion imposes a particular interpretation on the findings, which are equally compatible with causal mechanisms operating in the reverse direction: in other words, persistent difficulties in occupational resettlement might give rise to emotional and behavioural deficits, and the availability of social work services might serve as a disincentive to patients to return to work.

Field (1976) stated that 'there is an almost total lack of objective data on the value of rehabilitation in recovery from head injury–either rehabilitation programmes in general or the various elements that go to make up those programmes' (p. 66), and the situation unfortunately seems barely to have changed in the intervening interval. Given the amount of resources being committed to such programmes (which so far as the UK is concerned is admittedly wholly inadequate) and the personal and economic benefits that would accrue from the development of successful programmes, this paucity of evaluative research is quite outrageous. Three studies have sought to examine the effectiveness of the more traditional forms of rehabilitation, but in each case the outcome has been far from reassuring.

First, Relander *et al.* (1972) compared matched groups of head-injured patients who were allocated at random to receive 'routine' or 'active' treatment:

> Patients allocated to routine treatment were treated by the registrar or house officer in charge of that particular ward. They were usually allowed to get up when they felt like it, but no special effort was made to get them up. They were given information about their injury if and when they asked for it. No arrangements were made for them to see the same doctor at follow-up clinics.
>
> Patients allocated to active treatment were managed by the doctor who assessed them initially. They were seen daily, the nature of their injury was explained to them, they were encouraged to get up as early as possible, and physiotherapy was started. This was supervised by the same physiotherapist for all actively treated patients, and she also saw the patients twice a week in the outpatient department until the end of treatment. The patients were encouraged to attend follow-up clinics, where they were seen by the same doctor who had treated them in hospital. (p. 778)

As Field (1976) wryly commented, even the 'active' treatment in this study seems to have been little more than an expected standard of medical care. In the event there was no significant difference between the two groups in terms of the duration of bed rest or the length of stay in hospital. The amount of time each patient was off work was significantly less following 'active' treatment, which Relander *et al.* felt to be a worthwhile outcome. In a subsequent study information and encouragement from the medical staff seemed to be important factors for younger patients, whereas physiotherapy was more important for older patients and those who had fears about their condition. Nevertheless, when some of the patients in the original study were followed up a year after head injury, there was no difference between those who had had active treatment and those who had had routine treatment in terms of the incidence of either postconcussional symptoms or residual disability. Similar results were obtained by Cope and Hall (1982) in an evaluation of the benefits of early as opposed to late rehabilitation (that is, commencing within 35 days of head injury or later). This study found a substantial difference between early and late admissions to the rehabilitation programme in terms of the duration of their subsequent hospitalization, but it is unclear whether this reflected the benefits of early intervention or the deleterious effects of delayed rehabilitation.

A second example concerns speech therapy. It has been suggested that subclinical disturbances of language function may have a disproportionate impact upon the benefits to be gained from other forms of therapy and upon subsequent occupational resettlement (Evans *et al.*, 1975). David *et al.* (1979) carried out a preliminary evaluation of speech therapy in the case of 13 stroke patients. Seven received conventional individual treatment from a speech therapist, whereas six received an equal amount of attention from an untrained volunteer. The former group adventitiously demonstrated slightly better communicative performance at their initial assessment and throughout the subsequent treatment, and most recovery in both groups took place during the first month of treatment. Nevertheless, despite a fairly intensive programme (40 hours of treatment over 12 weeks), the group which received speech therapy did not show a greater amount of improvement than the control group; indeed, if anything, there was a slight tendency in the opposite direction. There appears to be no equivalent study in the case of patients with closed head injury. Moreover, it has been suggested that the wide variety of persistent communicative deficits seen in head-injured patients are different from those which most speech therapists are trained to deal with, and should be seen as demanding adjustment and compensation rather than restoration (Milton and Wertz, 1986).

Finally, the recent study by Brooks *et al.* (1987) investigated the relationship between occupational resettlement and whether or not patients had had access to a variety of services, including occupational therapy, physiotherapy, speech therapy, clinical psychology, psychiatry, social work, nursing, and a Government-sponsored rehabilitation service that was aimed specifically at vocational rehabilitation. In no case was there a significant positive association between whether a patient had received a particular service according to the report of a relative and whether or not the patient was working seven years after head injury. One major reason for this result is that in spite of persistent difficulties in cognition, communication, and occupational resettlement few of the patients had had any access to formal rehabilitation at all. Indeed, many criticisms have been expressed of the inadequate provision in the UK of facilities for the progressive care and rehabilitation of the permanently disabled survivors of closed head injury.

In this context, one might also consider the role of pharmacological treatment in head-injured patients. There is a paucity of well-controlled studies of the medical treatment of post-traumatic psychiatric conditions, and the use of psychoactive medication is mainly justified by its efficacy in treating behavioural disorders with other aetiologies (*see* Gualtieri, 1988; McGuire and Sylvester, 1987). An interesting account of the risks and benefits of the pharmacological treatment of head-injured patients has recently been given by Eames (1989). This might be especially suitable in dealing with post-traumatic memory impairment, since a number of different systems of neurochemical transmission have been implicated in memory function and drugs that modulate the efficiency of these systems might thus be expected to influence memory performance (*see* Richardson, 1989a). In particular, the neuropeptide vasopressin and its synthetic analogues appear to enhance the encoding and retrieval of information in long-term episodic memory as well as ease of access to semantic memory. However, double-blind trials involving head-injured patients with persistent memory dysfunction have failed to find any significant improvement as a result of administering vasopressin or its analogues desmopressin or desglycinamide vasopressin (Jenkins *et al.*, 1981; Koch-Henriksen and Nielsen, 1981). The magnitude of any improvement found with other clinical groups has in any case been too small to be of any practical significance (Wolkowitz *et al.*, 1985).

The cholinergic system is certainly known to play an important role in long-term memory, and there is some evidence that cholinergic agonists facilitate learning and remembering in both normal volunteers and clinical patients. Walton (1982) suggested that techniques aimed at increasing the amount of centrally available acetylcholine could promote the restoration of memory and cognitive functioning in head-injured individuals. On the basis of his clinical experience with just two patients, Walton concluded that orally administered lecithin (the normal dietary source of choline) combined with the intramuscular administration of physostigmine (which is also known as eserine and which inhibits the metabolism of acetylcholine) would improve cognitive function and might also alleviate post-traumatic behavioural disorders. Indeed, in a double-blind study involving a single head-injured patient with persistent memory impairment, Goldberg *et al.* (1982a, 1982b) found that oral physostigmine salicylate and lecithin led to a significant improvement in performance on the Wechsler Memory Scale (the Memory Quotient increasing from 102.5 to 115) and in the free recall of a list of words using the selective reminding procedure, though not in performance on a visual retention test or the Progressive Matrices test.

Nevertheless, the effects of cholinergic agonists in research studies with other clinical groups have once again been generally disappointing (*see* Bartus *et al.*, 1985; Kopelman, 1986; Wolkowitz *et al.*, 1985). The rationale for using lecithin as a direct source of choline is in any case relatively weak, as only about 1 per cent of tissue choline is utilized for acetylcholine and consequently nearly all the material administered will find its way into other metabolic pathways (McGeer, 1984). A recent double-blind trial of chronic oral physostigmine did find a statistically significant increase in memory performance among patients with Alzheimer's disease (Thal *et al.*, 1989), which suggests that this might be a more useful treatment. Paradoxically, however, there are findings from animal studies which suggest that both the initial disturbance of consciousness and the persistent neurological deficits that result from head injury are mediated by increased activation of cholinergic pathways and hence can be treated by *anti*cholinergic drugs such as scopolamine (Hayes *et al.*, 1989).

In general it remains the case that considerable work still needs to be done on the scientific evaluation of programmes of clinical treatment and rehabilitation following closed head injury. As Newcombe (1982) concluded from her own assessment of the situation: 'In the absence of definitive knowledge of the efficacy of rehabilitation techniques, each case becomes a diagnostic and therapeutic experiment, requiring a balanced sequence of test-treat-test, checked with matched controls' (pp. 124–5).

Counselling and Psychotherapy

Treatment that goes beyond conventional forms of rehabilitation would seem to be most apposite in dealing with persistent postconcussional symptoms. As Long and Novack (1986) noted, how these symptoms should be treated does not depend critically upon whether or not they define a clinical syndrome. Moreover, whether or not one accepts that any such syndrome is entirely an iatrogenic disease (i.e., one resulting from an unsupportive attitude on the part of the patient's doctor: *see* Chapter 6, p. 196), it is obvious that the clinician's attitude may be of major importance in determining whether the patient is able to resolve any psychic conflict that results from the trauma of a closed head injury. Russell (1934) emphasized the importance of 'simple reassurance' in ensuring the disappearance of postconcussional symptoms, though Lewis (1942) argued that 'direct psychological treatment' would sometimes be called for (p. 613) and Symonds (1942) went so far as to suggest that psychotherapy 'has a place in the treatment of every case of this kind' (p. 605). In a similar manner Björkesten (1971) argued that the postconcussional syndrome could be reduced by active mobilization, by appropriate psychotherapy and by good encouragement regarding the eventual prognosis, while Martin (1974) suggested that 'adequate initial treatment of the syndrome, sympathy, recognition of its reality and reassurance that it is only temporary will usually prevent the appearance of a neurosis' (p. 117; *see also* Wrightson and Gronwall, 1981). Conversely, the genesis of postconcussional symptoms and other psychosocial problems in patients with closed head injury tends to be attributed to the lack of provision for counselling and follow-up services (e.g., Jennett, 1975b; McMillan and Glucksman, 1987).

An early attempt to evaluate such ideas was carried out by Hjern and Nylander (1964) using a consecutive series of 305 children hospitalized following head injury over the course of a year. The mothers of children admitted during the first six months were systematically advised before the patient's discharge that concussion was a trivial complaint which did not give rise to permanent after-effects and that the best way to encourage the disappearance of any transient symptoms was gradually to train the patient to become fully active both physically and psychically. In contrast, the mothers of those admitted during the second six months were merely informed that the children had suffered concussion and were advised to contact the hospital in the event of any problems arising after their discharge. The proportion of children showing residual psychiatric symptoms according to the results of enquiries six months after the injury increased significantly between the two groups from 6 per cent to 17 per cent. However, the first group had also been investigated more intensively both during the initial period of hospitalization and by means of a 1-month follow-up examination. Moreover, the main findings were apparently based on postal enquiries, and direct clinical examination was carried out only when 'symptoms worthy of note' had been reported by the children's parents (p. 9). A similar study was performed by Minderhoud *et al.* (1980), who compared 352 patients with cerebral concussion who received no systematic treatment during the period of their hospitalization and 180 patients who received a strict programme of treatment that involved information, explanation and encouragement. With the exception of those of over 60 years of age, the latter patients reported fewer postconcussional symptoms both three weeks and six months after their head injuries, and in particular were less likely to complain of irritability, loss of memory, and loss of concentration. These findings were taken to support the hypothesis that postconcussional sequelae start from an organic basic but that the persistence of symptoms following minor head injury is caused by psychogenic and especially by iatrogenic factors.

As was mentioned in the previous chapter (pp. 200–1), Gronwall and Wrightson (1974) hypothesized that persistent postconcussional symptoms represented a neurotic reaction to a subtle yet transient impairment of information-processing capacity in the absence of adequate information and support from medical staff. They concluded that the effective management of patients with closed head injury depended not merely upon a supportive attitude on the part of their physicians, but also upon the monitoring and assessment of cognitive functioning throughout the period of recovery in order to ensure that the intellectual demands involved in returning to work did not exceed a patient's available information-processing capacity. During the course of a single year, Gronwall and Wrightson monitored 80 head-injured patients in this manner. Five patients were identified as being 'at risk' for the development of a postconcussional syndrome on the basis of the delayed recovery of performance on the paced auditory serial addition task (PASAT). They were 'guided to eventual complete recovery' (p. 608) by means of a formal rehabilitation programme aimed at gradually building up tolerance to fatigue and at developing the abilities to work at speed, to tolerate noise, and to ignore distraction (*see also* Gronwall, 1977). This was a somewhat ambitious project that involved a full-time research fellow, two part-time occupational therapists and two part-time physiotherapists; however, Gronwall and Wrightson considered that the expenditure represented by these resources was not excessive.

Just as Gronwall and Wrightson (1974) used the PASAT to monitor the recovery of cognitive functioning in adult patients returning to gainful employment, Levin and Eisenberg (1979a) observed that in the recovery of children following closed head injury 'the degree of improvement over time in verbal learning and memory using the selective reminding test provides an indication of the patient's readiness to cope with the mnemonic demands of schoolwork' (p. 401). More recently Malkmus (1983) and Long and Novack (1986) advocated a similar approach to rehabilitation, based upon matching the information-processing demands of environmental tasks to the patient's cognitive capabilities at each stage of recovery after closed head injury.

Nowadays more intensive rehabilitation programmes tend to incorporate psychotherapeutic interventions that are specifically intended to develop in head-injured patients 'increased awareness and acceptance of the injury and residual deficits' and 'an understanding of their particular emotional and motivational disturbances and their personal reactions to the injury' (Prigatano *et al.*, 1984, p. 507; *see also* Prigatano *et al.*, 1986, Chaps. 5 and 6). Nevertheless, Hayden and Hart (1986) considered that full-blown psychodynamically orientated psychotherapy was typically not appropriate for dealing with head-injured patients because they often lacked the necessary level of abstraction and needed much more structure than was provided by psychodynamic methods. Similarly, McGuire and Sylvester (1987) suggested that when applied to head-injured children or adolescents traditional individual psychotherapy was often impeded by post-traumatic cognitive impairment and 'a premorbid, externally oriented personality lacking in introspective tendencies' (p. 592), as well as by inconsistent expectations and possibly outright conflict between a child's family and professional staff with whom the child had frequent contact.

Cognitive Retraining

Cognitive deficits are of course ubiquitous in head-injured patients, and it was thus hardly surprising that they became a major focus of attention when researchers and professional workers came to reconsider the goals of rehabilitation following closed head injury. This was also encouraged by concomitant theoretical developments in the field of cognitive psychology during the 1970s. Cognitive retraining tackles the direct remediation of deficits in higher intellectual functions by providing practice on tasks which exercise the defective skills or which encourage the development of new cognitive strategies (Hayden and Hart, 1986). As Cicerone and Tupper (1986) explained, the treatment of a word-finding impairment might proceed through repetitive vocabulary-link exercises, the use of visual imagery as an aid to word retrieval, or the development of circumlocutory strategies. To take a somewhat different example, head-injured patients might be given systematic training on Gronwall and Wrightson's (1974) PASAT in an attempt to enhance their central processing capacity (*see* Newcombe, 1982).

In everyday life, cognitive dysfunction leads to a failure to respond adequately or appropriately to the demands of one's immediate environment. In an institutional setting, the remediation of cognitive dysfunction can also be encouraged by increasing the amount of structure that is afforded by that external environment, both social and physical. This goal can be achieved by eliminating (or, at least, reducing) sources of ambiguity and by ensuring that the environment contains prompts which elicit appropriate forms of behaviour. For instance, Hayden and Hart (1986) recommended that professional staff should use verbal cues that elicit particular cognitive or behavioural strategies (or 'scripts') designed to cope with problematic situations. Such an approach obviously requires the collaboration of all of the staff concerned (Malkmus, 1983). However, it also suffers from the limitation that explicit structure is unlikely to be encountered in daily life, and so techniques of this sort will be of little practical benefit unless patients can also be trained to generate their own internal cues.

Generally speaking, cognitive remediation in brain-damaged patients is based upon the notion of behavioural substitution which was described earlier in this chapter (pp. 262–3); that is, the assumption that undamaged systems within the brain can be deployed towards different goals (Rutter, 1981). Cicerone and Tupper (1986) observed that this is an essentially subversive approach to rehabilitation because it implicitly contradicts the concept of 'deficit testing' in neuropsychological assessment: the latter assumes a uniform level of competence within the intact individual that constitutes a single benchmark against which to evaluate intellectual impairment in brain-damaged patients (*see* e.g., Lezak, 1984). Cognitive remediation instead assumes that the potential for recovery and retraining in brain-damaged patients varies from one cognitive function to another, and that the same behavioural goal can be achieved by deploying different functional systems or by taking different routes through the same system. The scope for rehabilitation therefore depends more upon the complexity of the tasks confronting the patient and upon his or her executive control of alternative strategies than upon any single overall measure of attainment.

Cognitive retraining methods are often considered to be useful ways of encouraging the rehabilitation of head-injured patients, though controlled studies demonstrating their clinical efficacy have mostly been carried out with stroke patients in whom brain damage may well be more circumscribed (Hayden and Hart, 1986). Prigatano *et al.* (1984) evaluated the benefits of a neuropsychological rehabilitation programme that included intensive cognitive retraining of selected residual deficits and psychotherapeutic intervention in addition to traditional rehabilitation (*see also* Prigatano *et al.*, 1986, chaps 6 and 7). An experimental group of 18 patients with closed head injury was compared with 17 matched control patients (who only received traditional rehabilitation) in terms of their IQs on the Wechsler Adult Intelligence Scale before and after a 6-month period. The two groups were very similar in terms of their baseline scores, which were clearly impaired in the case of Performance IQ but not in the case of Verbal IQ. After cognitive retraining there was a significant difference between the groups in terms of their mean Performance IQs that was mainly attributable to the Block Design subtest. Unfortunately, the magnitude of this difference was less than four points when corrected for the patients' baseline scores. Moreover, many of the control patients had specifically declined to participate in the intensive neuropsychological rehabilitation programme; consequently, these findings might simply have resulted from subject selection artefacts (Schacter and Glisky, 1986).

Memory Retraining and Remediation

Much of the work on cognitive remediation following closed head injury has been concerned specifically with memory impairment. Apart from being the most apparent form of residual dysfunction, this has an obvious impact on academic attainment in children and young people and on learning capacity in general, and it tends to constrain the effectiveness of other forms of rehabilitation (such as social skills training) that depend upon adequate mnemonic and cognitive functioning (McGuire and Sylvester, 1987). Harris (1984) classified methods for improving memory into four broad categories: physical treatments (i.e., drugs); external devices; repetitive practice; and mnemonic strategies. The use of drugs seems to be of little practical value in alleviating memory disorders (*see above*, pp. 268–9), but Harris and Sunderland (1981) found that the three remaining categories were widely used in British rehabilitation units.

External memory aids include devices for storing information (such as notepads and computer files) and devices for cueing action (such as alarm cooking timers and shopping lists). Harris (1978) found that such devices were widely used in everyday life and warranted further investigation, and there are a few published case studies that involve neurological patients. However, there is still very little formal discussion of their role in the rehabilitation of memory following closed head injury (cf. Newcombe, 1982). Under this heading Schacter and Glisky (1986) also mentioned structured environments that reduce or eliminate the need for remembering, such as a kitchen in which the contents of cupboards are labelled.

Repetitive practice involves the continual administration of memory games (such as Kim's game) or conventional laboratory tasks. Harris and Sunderland (1981) commented that its widespread use 'is apparently based on the assumption that memory responds like a "mental muscle", and that exercising it on one task will strengthen it for use on other tasks' (p. 208). Schacter and Glisky (1986) reported that they had met similar ideas in informal discussions with professional rehabilitation workers in North America. Harris and Sunderland argued that repetitive practice might be rewarding for head-injured patients and that it might conceivably promote neural regeneration, but they acknowledged that there was little evidence that it was of any practical benefit for either normal or impaired memory. In the study mentioned above, Prigatano *et al.* (1984; 1986, chap.7) found that cognitive retraining in head-injured patients led to a statistically significant improvement in terms of their Memory Quotients according to the Wechsler Memory Scale, though not in terms of their performance on any of the constituent subtests. Quite apart from the problem of possible subject selection artefacts, Schacter and Glisky (1986) pointed out that the improvement in question corresponded to a net increase of one item per patient on each subtest as the result of roughly 625 hours of training. They concluded that repetitive drill or practice did not produce general improvements in memory function.

From a psychological point of view, the most interesting category of rehabilitative intervention is training in the use of particular mnemonic strategies. Instructions to use imagery mnemonics in particular are well known to produce substantial improvements in laboratory experiments with normal subjects, and during the 1970s there were a great many attempts to adapt these techniques for use with neurological patients (*see* Richardson *et al.*, 1987). There is some evidence that imagery mnemonics might help to alleviate memory impairment following severe head injury, but patients appear to have considerable difficulty in transferring such strategies to learning situations in everyday life (Crosson and Buenning, 1984; Crovitz *et al.*, 1979; Glasgow *et al.*, 1977). In common with other patients with acquired memory disorders, they do not seem to be able to continue to use these strategies in the absence of explicit instructions or prompting, or to generalize their use to learning tasks and situations other than the ones used for training; instead they revert to the use of external memory aids (Richardson *et al.*, 1987; Schacter and Glisky, 1986). There has been little or no research on the use of verbal mnemonics and other devices in the case of head-injured patients, but similar considerations are likely to apply. Cicerone and Tupper (1986) argued that the ability to maintain and transfer cognitive strategies depended upon higher executive function and the patient's awareness and knowledge of how and when such strategies might be employed (*see also* Richardson *et al.*, 1987). Even if the latter 'metacognitive' skills were imparted to patients with closed head injury, deficits of higher executive function of the sort discussed in Chapter 5 (pp. 132–46) would still constrain the efficacy of mnemonic training.

Of course, one reason for these disappointing results might be that patients with closed head injury are not a heterogeneous population, but exhibit a wide variety of different memory disorders. It follows that no one form of rehabilitative intervention will prove helpful in all or even most cases. Wilson (1984) stressed the need for flexibility and ingenuity in dealing with memory impairment and offered a flow diagram as a starting point in selecting particular treatment strategies (Figure 7.1). This has the further implication that single-case experimental designs will be more useful than group studies in assessing the effectiveness of rehabilitation for brain-damaged patients (Wilson, 1987b). A quite separate argument is that a retraining perspective is overly restrictive as a basis for helping such patients; state-of-the-art accounts of 'cognitive rehabilitation' use this expression to describe 'any intervention strategy or technique which intends to enable clients or patients and their families to live with, manage, bypass, reduce or come to terms with cognitive deficits precipated by injury to the brain' (Wilson, 1989, p. 117).

However, Schacter and Glisky (1986) suggested instead that research on normal human memory motivated an interest in the retention of information relating to particular domains of knowledge. To be more specific, information about pragmatically important conceptual domains tends to be represented in modular knowledge structures (*see* Richardson, 1989b). Rather than seeking to improve memory function in a global fashion, it follows that the goal of rehabilitation should be that of facilitating the acquisition and retention of knowledge within domains of practical significance to patients. As an example of domain-specific knowledge Schacter and Glisky chose terminology relating to the operations and commands used in interacting with a microcomputer. They were however concerned to deny that there was anything intrinsically significant about this particular knowledge domain or that the use of a computer had any inherent therapeutic properties.

A number of previous researchers had claimed that microcomputers had an important role to play in cognitive rehabilitation (e.g., Newcombe, 1982). Kerner and Acker (1985) tested 12 patients with closed head injury on a battery of memory tests at least three months after their accidents, and found highly significant gains in performance as the result of a memory retraining programme that was delivered by a microcomputer in 12 sessions over the course of 30 days. Two control groups of subjects who used the microcomputer to produce creative graphics for a similar amount of time or who had no exposure to the microcomputer at all exhibited no significant improvement over this period. The patients in the experimental group also seemed to have more positive feelings about themselves as well as enhanced motivation for academic and vocational pursuits, and some continued to use the computer voluntarily beyond the end of the study. The contents of the programme were not described in detail, but they seem to have included repetitive practice on a memory-span task and also training in the use of mental imagery and simple stories as mediating devices in verbal learning tasks (cf. Gianutsos and Grynbaum, 1983). However, Schacter and Glisky argued that there was no evidence that computerized programmes differed from cognitive retraining presented by other means in terms of their effects, or that such programmes had any generalized effect upon memory function.

Schacter and Glisky also remarked that previous attempts to promote the use of

Figure 7.1   Deciding on a treatment strategy for a memory impaired patient

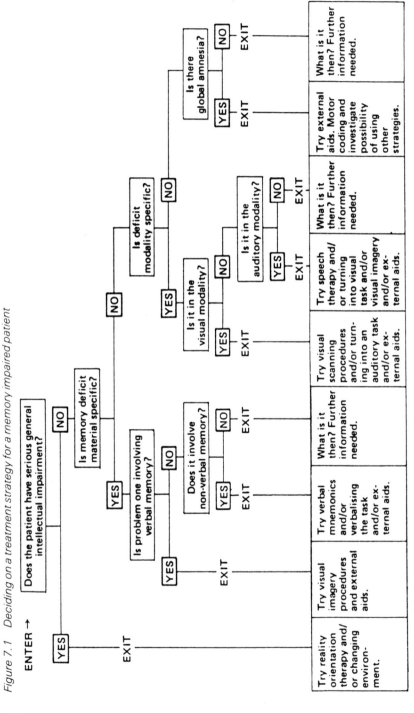

Source: Wilson, B. (1984) 'Memory therapy in practice', in Wilson, B. A. and Moffat, N. (Eds), *Clinical Management of Memory Problems*, London, Croom Helm, pp. 89–111. Reprinted by permission.

computers as external memory aids for memory-impaired patients had been bedevilled by the patients' inability to learn even the simplest commands and would therefore require novel modes of stimulus presentation. To this end, they showed that patients with memory impairment (in several cases as a result of closed head injury) could acquire a reasonably large vocabulary of terms relating to the use of computers, provided that items were tested by the 'method of vanishing cues', a technique based upon the presentation of successively fewer letter fragments on successive trials (*see* Glisky *et al.*, 1986b). These patients learned much more slowly than a control group of unimpaired subjects, but their retention over a 6-week interval was remarkably good. Schacter and Glisky then showed that such patients could learn to use the relevant terms to write simple programs and perform disk operations on a microcomputer (*see* Glisky *et al.*, 1986a). As these authors noted, this would then enable memory-impaired patients to use a microcomputer as an external aid or prosthetic device in learning about other complex domains of knowledge. Schacter and Glisky added that their methodology was especially applicable to the task of acquiring or indeed reacquiring the body of knowledge needed to perform a particular job, and was therefore of potential benefit in occupational resettlement.

Behaviour Modification

Newcombe *et al.* (1980) observed that personality changes and behavioural disorders often constituted serious barriers to effective rehabilitation in head-injured patients; this seemed to be associated with the patients' impaired ability to monitor their own behaviour as a result of damage to the frontal lobes (cf. Deaton, 1987; Luria, 1963). They suggested that behaviour therapy was likely to be the most useful technique in treating these severe behavioural disorders, although at the time it was only just beginning to be systematically exploited in the treatment of brain-damaged patients. Nowadays, rehabilitation of patients with severe head injuries typically involves a combination of cognitive remediation and behavioural techniques (Brooks, 1984).

Behaviour therapy is the process of modifying undesirable behaviour by means of operant conditioning, in which the probability of a specific response being repeatedly emitted in the context of a particular stimulus is affected by the consequences of the individual's behaviour. This can be used to increase the likelihood of desirable behaviour through reward or positive reinforcement, to reduce the likelihood of undesirable behaviour through punishment or negative reinforcement, and also to shape existing forms of behaviour into more complex or appropriate ones (Deaton, 1987). An operant analysis is most often applied to social behaviour, but it is also applicable to cognitive behaviour such as remembering (Moffat, 1984). An institution in the UK with considerable experience of the use of such methods in dealing with post-traumatic behaviour disorders is the Kemsley Unit at St Andrews Hospital in Northampton, which was set up in 1979 to provide a full range of rehabilitative therapies combined with behaviour modification techniques (*see* Eames and Wood, 1985a, 1985b; Wood and Eames, 1981). Positive reinforcement takes the form of rewards, privileges, attention, and praise as well as tokens which might later be exchanged for these rewards. Negative reinforcement usually takes the form of strict avoidance of such rewards (or 'time out from positive reinforcement'), often with some form of social isolation.

Wood and Eames (1981) described their initial experience in the use of behaviour therapy to manage behaviour disorders following severe head injury. Operant conditioning appeared to take much longer in the case of head-injured patients and to require schedules of reinforcement that were virtually continuous; these circumstances were difficult to arrange given the normal pressures on staff in a ward setting. Such patients were also vulnerable to reduced motivation, which meant that they tended to produce less spontaneous behaviour and were less responsive to reinforcers. They nevertheless exhibited the acquisition of positively reinforced responses and the loss or extinction of negatively reinforced ones within a specific context and to build up units of behaviour into coherent activities (such as those involved in getting up in the morning), though they tended not to develop learning sets that generalized to new situations. Finally, some behavioural disturbances, such as those produced by epileptic discharges, were less tractable and required pharmacological treatment, though Deaton (1987) noted that such medications might interfere with learning ability.

Eames and Wood (1985a) carried out an evaluation of behaviour therapy in the case of 24 severely damaged patients of whom 12 had suffered closed head injury. Since the major impact of the patients' behaviour disorders had been to make them unacceptable in conventional settings devoted either to rehabilitation or to continuing care, the effect of therapy was defined in terms of a scale of possible placements from self-care in patients' own homes to institutionalization in a psychiatric, psycho-geriatric, or mental handicap hospital. The patients' carers also completed rating scales that were concerned with changes in behaviour and 'activities of daily living'. Three-quarters of the patients demonstrated an improvement in the overall outcome, and more than half were discharged to their own homes. This was broadly maintained at a follow-up assessment between six months and three years later. A similar impression was given by the assessment of activities of daily living, which in ten patients approached normal achievement in five out of the seven areas examined at the follow-up session.

Eames and Wood considered that a high proportion of severely damaged individuals 'could achieve dramatic and lasting improvements in behaviour and (thanks to consequent accessibility to rehabilitative interventions) in personal and social independence' (p. 618). They also emphasized that these improvements had been achieved in spite of long delays between brain injury and the beginning of rehabilitation; indeed, the average interval between the injury and admission to the rehabilitation unit was 45 months. Eames and Wood interpreted their findings as being inconsistent with the notion that any improvement in the outcome was to be expected during the first two or three years following closed head injury. They concluded 'that, even years after injury, persistent and comprehensive rehabilitation can achieve changes significant enough to make worthwhile improvements in the quality of life' (p. 618).

Finally, Eames and Wood (1985b) noted that problems in monitoring and controlling behaviour should be tackled by means of behaviour therapy with groups of patients together, not least because many of these problems were in the area of social behaviour. Deaton (1987) claimed that interventions of this nature provided peer support, feedback, and social modelling, and might therefore be particularly appropriate for head-injured children and adolescents who might be seeking acceptance from their peer group. Deaton argued that behaviour modification could serve to increase adaptive skills such as eating or socializing that were often important to the development of a patient's self-esteem and independence. She also suggested that a carefully structured environment might circumvent problems in behaviour modification that resulted from cognitive deficits, memory impairment, and poor self-monitoring skills.

Support for Families

Livingston *et al.* (1985a) noted that the relatives of patients with severe head injury themselves showed a significant level of psychiatric morbidity (*see* Chapter 6, pp. 210–8). The occurrence of such problems varied with the level of the patients' subjective complaints but not with the severity of the injury, which entailed that it could not be predicted in individual families at the time of the patients' initial hospitalization. Livingston *et al.* concluded that 'these findings suggest the need for comprehensive rehabilitation of head-injury patients and their relatives' (p. 876). It has also been suggested that good family relationships tend to facilitate successful rehabilitation (Oddy and Humphrey, 1980); while Jennett (1975b) considered that 'prophylactic and on-going psychosocial counselling of the patient and the family' might influence the outcome of closed head injury more significantly than physical rehabilitation (p. 270). Quine *et al.* (1988) even suggested that relatives could be recruited as lay-therapists in the task of rehabilitating head-injured patients, although they did acknowledge that this burden would tend to fall upon female relatives who had other family responsibilities.

Bond (1979) recommended that while head-injured patients were still in coma their relatives should receive individual counselling with regard to the likely course of recovery to prevent them from developing unrealistic expectations. Complaints from relatives concerning a lack of information from medical staff about the patient's condition and prognosis seem to be fairly common (e.g., Oddy *et al.*, 1978a), but it is really unclear to what extent such complaints are justified. Thomsen (1974) found that they came exclusively from working-class families, which she interpreted as evidence for a genuine difficulty in doctor-patient communication. However, others regard such complaints as expressions of anger towards professional staff, perhaps arising out of unresolved denial during earlier stages of recovery (e.g., Levin *et al.*, 1982a, p. 209). Gans (1983) made the important point that rehabilitation specialists might mistakenly accept such criticisms at face value as a challenge to their professional competence, rather than as manifestations of family members' unconscious need to share their pain and struggle with their overwhelming negative feelings.

Once head-injured patients demonstrate relative independence in basic functions of self-care, they tend to be discharged to their homes, even if they exhibit severe physical or mental deficits (Livingston *et al.*, 1985a; Timming *et al.*, 1982). Jennett (1975b) suggested that some families might well insist on taking patients home out of desperation at the lack of any adequate rehabilitation facilities within an institutional setting, though Newcombe (1982) suggested that an early return to a well-known environment did tend to promote recovery. Continuing support for relatives is clearly important at this juncture, but it is generally agreed that this should go well beyond general advice and include more constructive and dynamic forms of treatment such as family therapy, group therapy and psychotherapy (*see* e.g., Aitken *et al.*, 1982; Bond, 1979; Lewin *et al.*, 1979; McGuire and Sylvester, 1987; Rosenbaum *et al.*, 1978). Hayden and Hart (1986) argued that models of grief and bereavement provided a useful perspective from which to view the difficulties encountered by the families of patients following severe closed head injury: namely, as resulting from the inevitable disruption of the normal grieving process by the uncertainty concerning the precise nature of the loss and the challenge of maintaining a relationship with the 'lost' individual. Finally, and especially in the absence of adequate rehabilitation facilities, families of head-injured patients must rely on voluntary self-help and support groups such as those organized in the UK by Headway, the National Head Injuries Association, and in the US by the National Head Injury Foundation. Similar structures and mechanisms at an institutional level are of equal value in providing support for rehabilitation personnel themselves (*see* Gans, 1983).

Concluding Summary

Most deaths attributable to closed head injury occur within the first few days as the result of primary brain damage. Mortality rates are higher in older victims as the result of extracranial complications, but the picture is unclear in the case of children. A relatively small number of severely injured patients may survive for up to several years in a vegetative state for which any effective rehabilitation has yet to be discovered. In other cases, the quality of survival can be judged in terms of the neurophysical outcome, occupational resettlement, or social outcome; the Glasgow Outcome Scale provides a convenient way of categorizing patients in terms of their social dependence or independence.

Recovery of function can be measured in terms of subjective complaints or in terms of objective performance, but in either case the most obvious long-term deficits among patients with severe head injury are in the areas of memory, cognition, and communication. These have obvious implications for these patients' ability to cope with situations at work, at school, or in public life more generally which demand skilled and efficient learning, thinking, and social skills. Substantial restitution of these functions usually takes place during the first six months, but the rate of improvement gradually slows, and there may be relatively little change after the first year. In contrast, after a minor head injury, performance usually returns to broadly normal levels during the first month or so.

Quantitative data can often be fitted well by a simple exponential function that describes many other processes of natural and social change. Brooks *et al.* (1984) suggested that as a general rule the more severe the injury, the more likely it is that complex functions will be affected, the more slowly such functions will recover, the lower will be the asymptotic level that they will eventually recover to, and the more likely it is that the pattern of recovery will exemplify an exponential function. However, there are some exceptions to this general pattern of recovery; personality changes and behavioural problems in particular continue to increase during the five years following severe closed head injury, at least according to the reports of patients' relatives. There is a good deal of evidence that the effects of closed head injury are rather more pronounced in older patients than in young adults, confirming that the elderly brain is more vulnerable to brain damage. However, there is no unambiguous evidence that children are any less susceptible to functional impairment after closed head injury than adults by virtue of the supposed plasticity of the young brain. The mechanisms underlying recovery of function are still poorly understood but involve both neural regeneration and behavioural adaptation.

Effective rehabilitation following closed head injury depends upon an interdisciplinary approach combining occupational therapy, physiotherapy, medical management, counselling, psychotherapy, cognitive retraining, and behaviour modification. Unfortunately, evaluative research concerned with identifying the effective causal constituents of different rehabilitation techniques is as yet poorly developed. Counselling is an important means of dealing with postconcussional symptoms, especially when it is informed by continuing neuropsychological assessment; however, persistent cognitive deficits may militate against the use of psychoanalytically-based methods. Cognitive retraining is usually based upon the use of repetitive practice or alternative strategies, but neither technique seems to be of much value in everyday life and patients may rely more on external aids or structured environments. Nevertheless, some success has been reported in the use of micro-computers with head-injured patients and in the use of partial cueing techniques to teach particular domains of knowledge. Formal programmes of behaviour therapy can lead to substantial and persistent improvements in patients' daily activities which may well be a prerequisite for attempting any other forms of rehabilitative intervention. Finally, it is now widely recognized that patients' families should be involved in such intervention not simply because they can promote successful rehabilitation, but because family members may themselves exhibit a significant degree of psychiatric morbidity. Individual counselling needs to begin even during the period of coma, while continuing support for the relatives and carers (including family therapy and psychotherapy) needs to be available after the patients are discharged to their homes.

Suggestions for Further Reading

Epidemiology

Although now somewhat dated, J. H. Field's report for the UK Department of Health and Social Security is an essential source for anyone interested in the epidemiology of closed head injuries:

Field, J. H. (1976) *Epidemiology of Head Injuries in England and Wales*, London, Her Majesty's Stationery Office.

This summarized an extensive amount of material and reviewed the various lines of research being carried out in the UK during the mid-1970s. More important, perhaps, it also provides a careful discussion of the range of methodological and statistical problems that are involved in using some of the principal sources of information on the incidence of head injuries. The following paper provides a more up-to-date account of the same issues, with specific attention to studies carried out in the United States during the 1970s and early 1980s:

Frankowski, R. F. (1986) 'Descriptive epidemiologic studies of head injury in the United States: 1974–1984', in Peterson, L. G. and, O'Shanick, G. J. (Eds), *Psychiatric Aspects of Trauma* (*Advances in Psychosomatic Medicine*, Vol. 16), Basel, Karger, pp. 153–72.

Management of Closed Head Injury

The authoritative work on all matters concerning the clinical management of head-injured patients is that by Jennett and Teasdale (1981). A second edition is due to be published shortly:

Jennett, B. and Teasdale, G. (1990) *Management of Head Injuries*, 2nd ed., Philadelphia, PA, Davis.

The following paper gives an exceptionally clear summary of the structural neuro-pathology of closed head injury:

Adams, J. H. (1988) 'The autopsy in fatal non-missile head injuries', in Berry, C. L. (Ed.) *Neuropathology* (*Current Topics in Pathology*, Vol. 76), Berlin, Springer-Verlag, pp. 1–22.

Another useful textbook and one which contains an extensive discussion of the nature, diagnosis and treatment of intracranial haematoma is:

Bakay, L. and Glasauer, F. E. (1980) *Head Injury*, Boston, MA, Little, Brown and Company

The authoritative text on post-traumatic epilepsy is still undoubtedly:

Jennett, B. (1975) *Epilepsy After Non-missile Head Injuries*, 2nd ed., London, Heinemann.

Psychological Assessment

There are several useful references on the psychological assessment of head-injured patients:

Bond, M. R. (1986) 'Neurobehavioural sequelae of closed head injury', in Grant, I. and Adams, K. M. (Eds) *Neuropsychological Assessment of Neuropsychiatric Disorders*, New York, Oxford University Press, pp. 347–73.

Kapur, N. (1988) *Memory Disorders in Clinical Practice*, London, Butterworths, Chap. 1.

Levin, H. S. (1981) 'Aphasia in closed head injury', in Sarno, M. T. (Ed.) *Acquired Aphasia*, New York, Academic Press, pp. 427–63.

Prigatano, G. P., Pepping, M. and Klonoff, P. (1986) 'Cognitive, personality, and psychosocial factors in the neuropsychological assessment of brain-injured patients', in Uzzell, B. P. and Gross, Y. (Eds), *Clinical Neuropsychology of Intervention*, Boston, MA, Martinus Nijhoff, pp. 135–66.

Minor Head Injury

Two interesting collections of papers have recently appeared specifically concerned with the nature, management and sequelae of minor head injury:

Hoff, J., Anderson, T. and Cole, T. (Eds) (1989) *Mild to Moderate Head Injury*, Boston, MA, Blackwell.

Levin, H. S., Eisenberg, H. M. and Benton, A. L. (Eds) (1989) *Mild Head Injury*, New York, Oxford University Press.

Outcome, Recovery and Rehabilitation

The following collection provides an analysis of the methodological issues involved in studying the outcome of head injury:

Levin, H. S., Grafman, J. and Eisenberg, H. M. (1987) *Neurobehavioral Recovery from Head Injury*, New York, Oxford University Press.

There are several good accounts of aspects of recovery and rehabilitation following closed head injury:

Hayden, M. E. and Hart, T. (1986) 'Rehabilitation of cognitive and behavioral dysfunction in head injury', in Peterson, L. G. and O'Shanick, G. J. (Eds) *Psychiatric Aspects of Trauma* (*Advances in Psychosomatic Medicine*, Vol. 16), Basel, Karger, pp. 194–229.

Rosenthal, M., Griffith, E. R., Bond, M. R. and Miller, J. D. (Eds) (1983) *Rehabilitation of the Head Injured Adult*, Philadelphia, PA, Davis.

Wood, R. L. and Eames, P. (Eds) (1989) *Models of Brain Injury Rehabilitation*, London, Chapman and Hall.

Ylvisaker, M. (Ed.) (1985) *Head Injury Rehabilitation: Children and Adolescents*, San Diego, CA, College-Hill Press (London, Taylor and Francis).

Two papers provide a particular focus upon the issues involved in dealing with persistent deficits of communication skills and memory, respectively:

Milton, S. B. and Wertz, R. T. (1986) Management of persisting communication deficits in patients with traumatic brain injury. In Uzzell, B. P. and Gross, Y. (Eds), *Clinical Neuropsychology of Intervention*, Boston, MA, Martinus Nijhoff, pp. 225–56.

Schacter, D. L. and Glisky, E. L. (1986) 'Memory remediation: Restoration, alleviation, and the acquisition of domain-specific knowledge', in Uzzell, B. P. and Gross, Y. (Eds) *Clinical Neuropsychology of Intervention*, Boston, MA, Martinus Nijhoff, pp. 257–82.

Support for Relatives

A thoughtful account of the impact of severe head injury on the families and relatives of patients is contained in:

Brooks, N. (1984) 'Head injury and the family', in Brooks, N. (Ed.), *Closed Head Injury: Psychological, Social, and Family Consequences*, Oxford, Oxford University Press, pp. 123–47.

Headway publications can be obtained from the National Head Injuries Association, 200 Mansfield Road, Nottingham NG1 3HX, UK. The address of the National Head Injury Foundation, Inc., is 333 Turnpike Road, Southborough, Massachusetts 01772, USA.

Bibliography

ADAMS, J. H. (1988) 'The autopsy in fatal non-missile head injuries', in BERRY, C. L. (Ed.) *Neuropathology (Current Topics in Pathology*, Vol. 76), Berlin, Springer–Verlag, pp. 1–22.

ADAMS, J. H., DOYLE, D., FORD, I., GENNARELLI, T. A., GRAHAM, D. I. and McLELLAN, D. R. (1989a) 'Diffuse axonal injury in head injury: Definition, diagnosis and grading', *Histopathology*, **15**, pp. 49–59.

ADAMS, J. H., DOYLE, D., FORD, I., GRAHAM, D. I., McGEE, M. and McLELLAN, D. R. (1989b) 'Brain damage in fatal non-missile head injury in relation to age and type of injury', *Scottish Medical Journal*, **34**, pp. 399–401.

ADAMS, J. H., DOYLE, D., GRAHAM, D. I., LAWRENCE, A. E. and McLELLAN, D. R. (1984) 'Diffuse axonal injury in head injuries caused by a fall', *Lancet*, **2**, pp. 1420–2.

(1986a) 'Deep intracerebral (basal ganglia) haematomas in fatal non-missile head injury in man', *Journal of Neurology, Neurosurgery, and Psychiatry*, **49**, pp. 1039–43.

(1986b) 'Gliding contusions in nonmissile head injury in humans', *Archives of Pathology and Laboratory Medicine*, **110**, pp. 485–8.

ADAMS, J. H., DOYLE, D., GRAHAM, D. I., LAWRENCE, A. E., McLELLAN, D. R., GENNARELLI, T. A., PASTUSKO, M. and SAKAMOTO, T. (1985) 'The contusion index: A reappraisal in human and experimental non-missile head injury', *Neuropathology and Applied Neurobiology*, **11**, pp. 299–308.

ADAMS, H. and GRAHAM, D. I. (1972) 'The pathology of blunt head injuries', in CRITCHLEY, M., O'LEARY, J. L. and JENNETT, B. (Eds) *Scientific Foundations of Neurology*, London, Heinemann, pp. 478–91.

(1976) 'The relationship between ventricular fluid pressure and the neuropathology of raised intracranial pressure', *Neuropathology and Applied Neurobiology*, **2**, pp. 323–32.

ADAMS, J. H., GRAHAM, D. I. and GENNARELLI, T. A. (1982a) 'Neuropathology of acceleration-induced head injury in the subhuman primate', in GROSSMAN, R. G. and GILDENBERG, P. L. (Eds) *Head Injury: Basic and Clinical Aspects*, New York, Raven Press, pp. 141–50.

(1983) 'Head injury in man and experimental animals: Neuropathology', *Acta Neurochirurgica*, Suppl. 32, pp. 15–30.

ADAMS, J. H., GRAHAM, D. I., MURRAY, L. S. and SCOTT, G. (1982b) 'Diffuse axonal injury due to nonmissile head injury in humans: An analysis of 45 cases', *Annals of Neurology*, **12**, pp. 557–63.

ADAMS, J. H., GRAHAM, D. I., SCOTT, G., PARKER, L. S. and DOYLE, D. (1980a) 'Brain damage in fatal non-missile head injury', *Journal of Clinical Pathology*, **33**, pp. 1132–45.

ADAMS, J. H., MITCHELL, D. E., GRAHAM, D. I. and DOYLE, D. (1977) 'Diffuse brain damage of immediate impact type: Its relationship to "primary brain-stem damage" in head injury', *Brain*, **100**, pp. 489–502.

ADAMS, J. H., SCOTT, G., PARKER, L. S., GRAHAM, D. I. and DOYLE, D. (1980b) 'The contusion index: A quantitative approach to cerebral contusions in head injury', *Neuropathology and Applied Neurobiology*, **6**, pp. 319–24.

ADAMS, R. D. (1969) 'Comments on the morbid anatomy of concussion and the protracted traumatic deficits of cerebral function', in WALKER, A. E., CAVENESS, W. F. and CRITCHLEY, M. (Eds) *The Late Effects of Head Injury*, Springfield, IL, Thomas, pp. 524–6.

ADLER, A. (1945) 'Mental symptoms following head injury: A statistical analysis of two hundred cases', *Archives of Neurology and Psychiatry*, **53**, pp. 34–43.

AITKEN, C., BADDELEY, A., BOND, M. R, BROCKLEHURST, J. C., BROOKS, D. N., HEWER, R. L., JENNETT, B., LONDON, P., MEADE, T., NEWCOMBE, F., SHAW, D. A., SMITH, M. and JAMES, D. R. (1982) 'Research aspects of rehabilitation after acute brain damage in adults', *Lancet*, **2**, pp. 1034–6.

AKBAROVA, N. A. (1972) ['Aspects of memory dysfunction in patients with closed cranio-cerebral trauma of mild and moderate severity'] (in Russian), *Zhurnal Nevropatologii i Psikhiatrii*, **72**, pp. 1641–6.

ALAJOUANINE, T., CASTAIGNE, P., LHERMITTE, F., ESCOUROLLE, R. and DE RIBAUCOURT, B. (1957) 'Étude de 43 cas d'aphasie post-traumatique: Confrontation anatomo-clinique et aspects évolutifs', *Encéphale*, **46**, pp. 1–45.

ALBERT, M. L., SILVERBERG, R., RECHES, A. and BERMAN, M. (1976) 'Cerebral dominance for consciousness', *Archives of Neurology*, **33**, pp. 453–4.

ALEXANDRE, A., COLOMBO, F., NERTEMPI, P. and BENEDETTI, A. (1983) 'Cognitive outcome and early indices of severity of head injury', *Journal of Neurosurgery*, **59**, pp. 751–61.

ALEXANDRE, A., COLOMBO, F., RUBINI, L. and BENEDETTI, A. (1980) 'Evaluation of sleep EEG alterations during post-traumatic coma in order to predict cognitive defects', in GROTE, W., BROCK, M., CLAR, H.-E., KLINGER, M. and NAU, H.-E. (Eds) *Surgery of Cervical Myelopathy. Infantile Hydrocephalus: Long-Term Results (Advances in Neurosurgery*, Vol. 8), Berlin, Springer–Verlag, pp. 374–80.

ALEXANDRE, A., NERTEMPI, P., FARINELLO, C. and RUBINI, L. (1979) 'Recognition memory alterations after severe head injury: Preliminary results in a series of 50 patients', *Journal of the Neurosurgical Sciences*, **23**, pp. 201–6.

ALLEN, I. V., SCOTT, R. and TANNER, J. A. (1982) 'Experimental high-velocity missile head injury', *Injury*, **14**, pp. 183–93.

AMERICAN PSYCHIATRIC ASSOCIATION (1980) *Diagnostic and Statistical Manual of Mental Disorders*, 3rd ed., Washington, DC, American Psychiatric Association.

ANDERSON, D. W. and KALSBEEK, W. D. (1980) 'The National Head and Spinal Cord Injury Survey: Assessment of some uncertainties affecting the findings', *Journal of Neurosurgery*, **53**, pp. 532–4.

ANDERSON, D. W., KALSBEEK, W. D. and HARTWELL, T. D. (1980) 'The National Head and Spinal Cord Injury Survey: Design and methodology', *Journal of Neurosurgery*, **53**, pp. S11–S18.

ANNEGERS, J. F., GRABOW, J. D., KURLAND, L. T. and LAWS, E. R., Jr. (1980) 'The incidence, causes, and secular trends of head trauma in Olmsted County, Minnesota, 1935–1974', *Neurology*, **30**, pp. 912–9.

ANONYMOUS (1961) 'The best yardstick we have', *Lancet*, **2**, pp. 1445–6.

ARSENI, C., CONSTANTINOVICI, A., ILIESCU, D., DOBROTÁ, I. and GAGEA, A. (1970) 'Considerations on post-traumatic aphasia in peace time', *Psychiatria Neurologia Neurochirurgia*, **73**, pp. 105–12.

ARTIOLA I FORTUNY, L., BRIGGS, M., NEWCOMBE, F., RATCLIFF, G. and THOMAS, C. (1980) 'Measuring the duration of post-traumatic amnesia', *Journal of Neurology, Neurosurgery, and Psychiatry*, **43**, pp. 377–9.

ARTIOLA I FORTUNY, L. and HIORNS, R. W. (1979) 'Recovery curves in a visual search task', *International Rehabilitation Medicine*, **1**, pp. 177–81.

ASHTON, S. J., PEDDER, J. B. and MACKAY, G. M. (1977) 'Pedestrian injuries and the car exterior'. Paper presented at the Society of Automotive Engineers' International Automotive Engineering Congress and Exposition, Detroit, MI.

ATKINSON, R. C. and SHIFFRIN, R. M. (1968) 'Human memory: A proposed system and its control processes', in SPENCE, K. W. and SPENCE, J. T. (Eds) *The Psychology of Learning and Motivation: Advances in Research and Theory*, New York, Academic Press, pp. 89–195.

BABCOCK, H. (1930) 'An experiment in the measurement of mental deterioration', *Archives of Psychology*, Whole No. 117.

BADDELEY, A. D. (1976) *The Psychology of Memory*, New York, Basic Books.

(1986) *Working Memory*, Oxford, Oxford University Press.

(1988) 'Imagery and working memory', in DENIS, M., ENGELKAMP, J. and RICHARDSON, J. T. E. (Eds) *Cognitive and Neuropsychological Approaches to Mental Imagery*, Dordrecht, Martinus Nijhoff, pp. 169–80.

BADDELEY, A. D. and HITCH, G. J. (1974) 'Working Memory', in BOWER, G. H. (Ed.) *The Psychology of Learning and Motivation: Advances in Research and Theory*, Vol. 8, New York, Academic Press, pp. 47–90.

BADDELEY, A., MEADE, T. and NEWCOMBE, F. (1980) 'Design problems in research on rehabilitation after brain damage', *International Rehabilitation Medicine*, **2**, pp. 138–42.

BADDELEY, A. D. and PATTERSON, K. (1971) 'The relation between long-term and short-term memory', *British Medical Bulletin*, **27**, pp. 237–42.

BADDELEY, A. and WILSON, B. (1985) 'Phonological coding and short-term memory in patients without speech', *Journal of Memory and Language*, **24**, pp. 490–502.

BAKAY, L. and GLASAUER, F. E. (1980) *Head Injury*, Boston, MA, Little, Brown and Company.

BARBER, H. M. (1973) 'Horse-play: Survey of accidents with horses', *British Medical Journal*, **3**, pp. 532–4.

BARIN, J. J., HANCHETT, J. M., JACOB, W. L. and SCOTT, M. B. (1985) 'Counseling the head injured patient', in YLVISAKER, M. (Ed.) *Head Injury Rehabilitation: Children and Adolescents*, San Diego, CA, College–Hill Press (London, Taylor and Francis), pp. 361–79.

BARONA, A., REYNOLDS, C. R. and CHASTAIN, R. (1984) 'A demographically based index of premorbid intelligence for the WAIS–R', *Journal of Consulting and Clinical Psychology*, **52**, pp. 885–7.

BARTH, J. T., ALVES, W. M., RYAN, T. V., MACCIOCCHI, S. N., RIMEL, R. W., JANE, J. A. and NELSON, W. E. (1989) 'Mild head injury in sports: Neuropsychological sequelae and recovery of function', in LEVIN, H. S., EISENBERG, H. M. and BENTON, A. L. (Eds) *Mild Head Injury*, New York, Oxford University Press, pp. 257–75.

BARTH, J. T., MACCIOCCHI, S. N., GIORDANI, B., RIMEL, R., JANE, J. A. and BOLL, T. J. (1983) 'Neuropsychological sequelae of minor head injury', *Neurosurgery*, **13**, pp. 529–33.

BARTUS, R. T., DEAN, R. L., PONTECORVO, M. J. and FLICKER, C. (1985) 'The cholinergic hypothesis: A historical overview, current perspective, and future directions', *Annals of the New York Academy of Sciences*, **444**, pp. 332–58.

BECKER, B. (1975) 'Intellectual changes after closed head injury', *Journal of Clinical Psychology*, **31**, pp. 307–9.

BECKER, D. P. (1979) 'Comments', *Neurosurgery*, **4**, p. 289.

BEHRMAN, S. (1977) 'Migraine as a sequela of blunt head injury', *Injury*, **9**, pp. 74–6.

BENNETT-LEVY, J. M. (1984) 'Long-term effects of severe closed head injury on memory: Evidence from a consecutive series of young adults', *Acta Neurologica Scandinavica*, **70**, pp. 285–98.

BENNETT-LEVY, J. and POWELL, G. E. (1980) 'The Subjective Memory Questionnaire (SMQ): An investigation into the self-reporting of "real life" memory skills', *British Journal of Social and Clinical Psychology*, **19**, pp. 177–88.

BENSON, D. F., GARDNER, H. and MEADOWS, J. C. (1976) 'Reduplicative paramnesia', *Neurology*, **26**, pp. 147–51.

BENSON, D. F. and GESCHWIND, N. (1967) 'Shrinking retrograde amnesia', *Journal of Neurology, Neurosurgery, and Psychiatry*, **30**, pp. 539–44.

BENTON, A. L. (1967) 'Problems of test construction in the field of aphasia', *Cortex*, **3**, pp. 32–58.

(1968) 'Differential behavioral effects in frontal lobe disease', *Neuropsychologia*, **6**, pp. 53–60.

(1969) 'Development of a multilingual aphasia battery: Progress and problems', *Journal of the Neurological Sciences*, **9**, pp. 39–48.

BENTON, A. L., VAN ALLEN, M. W. and FOGEL, M. L. (1964) 'Temporal orientation in cerebral disease', *Journal of Nervous and Mental Disease*, **139**, pp. 110–9.

BIGLER, E. D. (1987) 'Acquired cerebral trauma: Behavioral, neuropsychiatric, psychoeducational assessment and cognitive retraining issues', *Journal of Learning Disabilities*, **20**, pp. 579–80.

BINDER, L. M. (1986) 'Persisting symptoms after mild head injury: A review of the postconcussive syndrome', *Journal of Clinical and Experimental Neuropsychology*, **8**, pp. 323–46.

BJÖRKESTEN, G. AF (1971) 'Summary', in *Head Injuries: Proceedings of an International Symposium*, Edinburgh, Churchill Livingstone, pp. 341–2.

BLACK, F. W. (1973) 'Cognitive and memory performance in subjects with brain damage secondary to penetrating missile wounds and closed head injury', *Journal of Clinical Psychology*, **29**, pp. 441–2.

BLACK, P., BLUMER, D., WELLNER, A. M. and WALKER, A. E. (1971) 'The head-injured child: Time-course of recovery, with implications for rehabilitation', in *Head Injuries: Proceedings of an International Symposium*, Edinburgh, Churchill Livingstone, pp. 131–7.

BLACK, P., JEFFRIES, J. J., BLUMER, D., WELLNER, A. and WALKER, A. E. (1969) 'The post-traumatic syndrome in children: Characteristics and incidence', in WALKER, A. E., CAVENESS, W. F. and CRITCHLEY, M. (Eds) *The Late Effects of Head Injury*, Springfield, IL, Thomas, pp. 142–9.

BLOMERT, D. M. and SISLER, G. C. (1974) 'The measurement of retrograde post-traumatic amnesia', *Canadian Psychiatric Association Journal*, **19**, pp. 185–92.

BOLLER, F. C., ALBERT, M. L., LeMAY, M. and KERTESZ, A. (1972) 'Enlargement of the Sylvian aqueduct: A sequel of head injuries', *Journal of Neurology, Neurosurgery, and Psychiatry*, **35**, pp. 463–7.

BOND, M. R. (1975) 'Assessment of the psychosocial outcome after severe head injury', in *Outcome of Severe Damage to the Central Nervous System*, Ciba Foundation Symposium No. 34 (new series), Amsterdam, Elsevier/Excerpta Medica/North-Holland, pp. 141–57.

(1976) 'Assessment of the psychosocial outcome of severe head injury', *Acta Neurochirurgica*, **34**, pp. 57–70.

(1979) 'The stages of recovery from severe head injury with special reference to late outcome', *International Rehabilitation Medicine*, **1**, pp. 155–9.

(1986) 'Neurobehavioral sequelae of closed head injury', in GRANT, I. and ADAMS, K. M. (Eds) *Neuropsychological Assessment of Neuropsychiatric Disorders*, New York, Oxford University Press, pp. 347–73.

BOND, M. R. and BROOKS, D. N. (1976) 'Understanding the process of recovery as a basis for the investigation of rehabilitation for the brain injured', *Scandinavian Journal of Rehabilitation Medicine*, **8**, pp. 127–33.

BOWERS, S. A. and MARSHALL, L. F. (1980) 'Outcome in 200 consecutive cases of severe head injury treated in San Diego County: A prospective analysis', *Neurosurgery*, **6**, pp. 237–42.

BRAAKMAN, R., AVEZAAT, C. J. J., MAAS, A. I. R., ROEL, M. and SCHOUTEN, H. J. A. (1977) 'Inter observer agreement in the assessment of the motor response of the Glasgow "coma" scale', *Clinical Neurology and Neurosurgery*, **80**, pp. 100–6.

BRENNER, C., FRIEDMAN, A. P., MERRITT, H. H. and DENNY-BROWN, D. E. (1944) 'Post-traumatic headache', *Journal of Neurosurgery*, **1**, pp. 379–91.

BRICOLO, A., TURAZZI, S. and FERIOTTI, G. (1980) 'Prolonged post-traumatic unconsciousness: Therapeutic assets and liabilities', *Journal of Neurosurgery*, **52**, pp. 625–34.

BRIERLEY, J. B. (1976) 'Cerebral hypoxia', in BLACKWOOD, W. and CORSELLIS, J. A. N. (Eds) *Greenfield's Neuropathology*, 3rd ed., London, Edward Arnold, pp. 43–85.

BRINK, J. D., GARRETT, A. L., HALE, W. R., WOO-SAM, J. and NICKEL, V. L. (1970) 'Recovery of motor and intellectual function in children sustaining severe head injuries', *Developmental Medicine and Child Neurology*, **12**, pp. 565–71.

BROADBENT, D. E. (1958) *Perception and Communication*, Oxford, Pergamon.

    (1971) *Decision and Stress*, London, Academic Press.

BROCK, S. (1960) 'General considerations in injuries of the brain and spinal cord and their coverings', in BROCK, S. (Ed.) *Injuries of the Brain and Spinal Cord and Their Coverings*, 4th ed., London, Cassell, pp. 1–22.

BROOKS, D. N. (1972) 'Memory and head injury', *Journal of Nervous and Mental Disease*, **155**, pp. 350–5.

    (1974a) 'Recognition memory after head injury: A signal detection analysis', *Cortex*, **11**, pp. 224–30.

    (1974b) 'Recognition memory, and head injury', *Journal of Neurology, Neurosurgery, and Psychiatry*, **37**, pp. 794–801.

    (1975) 'Long and short term memory in head injured patients', *Cortex*, **11**, pp. 329–40.

    (1976) 'Wechsler Memory Scale performance and its relationship to brain damage after severe closed head injury', *Journal of Neurology, Neurosurgery, and Psychiatry*, **39**, pp. 593–601.

    (1979) 'Psychological deficits after severe blunt head injury: Their significance and rehabilitation', in OBORNE, D. J., GRUNEBERG, M. M. and EISER, J. R. (Eds) *Research in Psychology and Medicine: Vol. II. Social Aspects: Attitudes, Communication, Care and Training*, London, Academic Press, pp. 469–76.

    (1984) 'Cognitive deficits after head injury', in BROOKS, N. (Ed.) *Closed Head Injury: Psychological, Social, and Family Consequences*, Oxford, Oxford University Press, pp. 44–73.

BROOKS, D. N. and AUGHTON, M. E. (1979a) 'Cognitive recovery during the first year after severe blunt head injury', *International Rehabilitation Medicine*, **1**, pp. 166–72.

    (1979b) 'Psychological consequences of blunt head injury', *International Rehabilitation Medicine*, **1**, pp. 160–5.

BROOKS, D. N., AUGHTON, M. E., BOND, M. R., JONES, P. and RIZVI, S. (1980) 'Cognitive sequelae in relationship to early indices of severity of brain damage after severe blunt head injury', *Journal of Neurology, Neurosurgery, and Psychiatry*, **43**, pp. 529–34.

BROOKS, N., CAMPSIE, L., SYMINGTON, C., BEATTIE, A. and MCKINLAY, W. (1986a) 'The five year outcome of severe blunt head injury: A relative's view', *Journal of Neurology, Neurosurgery, and Psychiatry*. **49**, pp. 764–70.

BROOKS, D. N., DEELMAN, B. G., VAN ZOMEREN, A. H., VAN DONGEN, H., VAN HARSKAMP, F. and AUGHTON, M. E. (1984) 'Problems in measuring cognitive recovery after acute brain injury', *Journal of Clinical Neuropsychology*, **6**, pp. 71–85.

BROOKS, D. N., HOSIE, J., BOND, M. R., JENNETT, B. and AUGHTON, M. (1986b) 'Cognitive sequelae of severe head injury in relation to the Glasgow Outcome Scale', *Journal of Neurology, Neurosurgery, and Psychiatry*, **49**, pp. 549–53.

BROOKS, D. N. and MCKINLAY, W. (1983) 'Personality and behavioural change after severe blunt head injury: A relative's view', *Journal of Neurology, Neurosurgery, and Psychiatry*, **46**, pp. 336–44.

BROOKS, N., MCKINLAY, W., SYMINGTON, C., BEATTIE, A. and CAMPSIE, L. (1987) 'Return to work within the first seven years of severe head injury', *Brain Injury*, **1**, pp. 5–19.

BROUWER, W. H. and VAN WOLFFELAAR, P. C. (1985) 'Sustained attention and sustained effort after closed head injury: Detection and 0.10 Hz heart rate variability in a low event rate vigilance task', *Cortex*, **21**, pp. 111–9.

BROWN, G., CHADWICK, O., SHAFFER, D., RUTTER, M. and TRAUB, M. (1981) 'A prospective study of children with head injuries in adulthood: III. Psychiatric sequelae', *Psychological Medicine*, **11**, pp. 63–78.

BRUCE, D. A., ALAVI, A., BILANIUK, L., DOLINSKAS, C., OBRIST, W. and UZZELL, B. (1981) 'Diffuse cerebral swelling following head injuries in children: The syndrome of "malignant brain edema" ', *Journal of Neurosurgery*, **54**, pp. 170–8.

BRUCE, D. A., SCHUT, L., BRUNO, L. A., WOOD, J. H. and SUTTON, L. N. (1978) 'Outcome following severe head injuries in children', *Journal of Neurosurgery*, **48**, pp. 679–88.

BRUCKNER, F. E. and RANDLE, A. P. H. (1972) 'Return to work after severe head injuries', *Rheumatology and Physical Medicine*, **11**, pp. 344–8.

BRYDEN, J. (1989) 'How many head-injured? The epidemiology of post head injury disability', in WOOD, R. L. and EAMES, P. (Eds) *Models of Brain Injury Rehabilitation*, London, Chapman and Hall, pp. 17–27.

BURKINSHAW, J. (1960) 'Head injuries in children', *Archives of Diseases in Childhood*, **35**, pp. 205–14.

BUSCHKE, H. (1973) 'Selective reminding for analysis of memory and learning', *Journal of Verbal Learning and Verbal Behavior*, **12**, pp. 543–50.

BUSCHKE, H. and FULD, P. (1974) 'Evaluating storage, retention, and retrieval in disordered memory and learning', *Neurology*, **24**, pp. 1019–25.

CAFFEY, J. (1972) 'On the theory and practice of shaking infants: Its potential residual effects of permanent brain damage and mental retardation', *American Journal of Diseases of Children*, **124**, pp. 161–9.

    (1974) 'The whiplash shaken infant syndrome: Manual shaking by the extremities with whiplash-induced intracranial and intraocular bleedings, linked with residual permanent brain damage and mental retardation', *Pediatrics*, **54**, pp. 396–403.

CAINE, E. D., EBERT, M. H. and WEINGARTNER, H. (1977) 'An outline for the analysis of dementia: The memory disorder of Huntingtons disease', *Neurology*, **27**, pp. 1087–92.

CANAVAN, A. G. M., DUNN, G. and MCMILLAN, T. M. (1986) 'Principal components of the WAIS-R', *British Journal of Clinical Psychology*, **25**, pp. 81–5.

CARLSSON, C.-A., VON ESSEN, C. and LÖFGREN, J. (1968) 'Factors affecting the clinical course of patients with severe head injuries', *Journal of Neurosurgery*, **29**, pp. 242–51.

CASEY, R., LUDWIG, S. and MCCORMICK, M. C. (1986) 'Morbidity following minor head trauma in children', *Pediatrics*, **78**, pp. 497–502.

CATTELL, R. B. (1963) 'Theory of fluid and crystallized intelligence: A critical experiment', *Journal of Educational Psychology*, **54**, pp. 1–22.

    (1965) 'Higher order factor structures and reticular-vs-hierarchical formulae for their interpretation', in BANKS, C. and BROADHURST, P. L. (Eds) *Studies in Psychology Presented to Cyril Burt*, London, University of London Press, pp. 223–66.

CAVENESS, W. F. (1979) 'Incidence of craniocerebral trauma in the United States in 1976 with trend from 1970 to 1975', *Advances in Neurology*, **22**, pp. 1–3.

CHADWICK, O. (1985) 'Psychological sequelae of head injury in children', *Developmental Medicine and Child Neurology*, **27**, pp. 72–5.

CHADWICK, O., RUTTER, M., BROWN, G., SHAFFER, D. and TRAUB, M. (1981a) 'A prospective study of children with head injuries: II. Cognitive sequelae', *Psychological Medicine*, **11**, pp. 49–61.

CHADWICK, O., RUTTER, M., SHAFFER, D. and SHROUT, P. E. (1981b) 'A prospective study of children with head injuries: IV. Specific cognitive deficits', *Journal of Clinical Neuropsychology*, **3**, pp. 101–20.

CHADWICK, O., RUTTER, M., THOMPSON, J. and SHAFFER, D. (1981c) 'Intellectual performance and reading skills after localized head injury in childhood', *Journal of Child Psychology and Psychiatry*, **22**, pp. 117–39.

CHAMPION, H. R., SACCO, W. J., COPES, W. S., GANN, D. S., GENNARELLI, T. A. and FLANAGAN, M. E. (1989) 'A revision of the Trauma Score', *Journal of Trauma*, **29**, pp. 623–9.

CICERONE, K. D. and TUPPER, D. E. (1986) 'Cognitive assessment in the neuropsychological treatment of head-injured adults', in UZZELL, B. P. and GROSS, Y. (Eds) *Clinical Neuropsychology of Intervention*, Boston, MA, Martinus Nijhoff, pp. 59–83.

CLIFTON, G. L., GROSSMAN, R. G., MAKELA, M. E., MINER, M. E., HANDEL, S. and SADHU, V. (1980) 'Neurological course and correlated computerized tomography findings after severe closed head injury', *Journal of Neurosurgery*, **52**, pp. 611–24.

COHEN, S. B. and TITONIS, J. (1985) 'Head injury rehabilitation: Management issues', in YLVISAKER, M. (Ed.) *Head Injury Rehabilitation: Children and Adolescents*, London, Taylor and Francis, pp. 429–43.

COLE, E. M. (1945) 'Intellectual impairment in head injury', in *Trauma of the Central Nervous System (Research Publications of the Association for Research in Nervous and Mental Disease*, Vol. 24), Baltimore, MD, Williams and Wilkins, pp. 473–9.

CONKEY, R. C. (1938) 'Psychological changes associated with head injuries', *Archives of Psychology*, **33**, Whole No. 232.

COOK, J. B. (1969) 'The effects of minor head injuries sustained in sport and the post-concussional syndrome', in WALKER, A. E., CAVENESS, W. F. and CRITCHLEY, M. (Eds) *The Late Effects of Head Injury*, Springfield, IL, Thomas, pp. 408–13.

(1972) 'The post-concussional syndrome and factors influencing recovery after minor head injury admitted to hospital', *Scandinavian Journal of Rehabilitation Medicine*, **4**, pp. 27–30.

COOPER, K., TABADDOR, K., HAUSER, W., SHULMAN, K., FEINER, C. and FACTOR, P. (1983) 'The epidemiology of head injury in the Bronx', *Neuroepidemiology*, **2**, pp. 70–88.

COOPER, P. R. (1982a) 'Epidemiology of head injury', in COOPER, P. R. (Ed.) *Head Injury*, Baltimore, MD, Williams and Wilkins, pp. 1–14.

(1982b) 'Post-traumatic intracranial mass lesions', in COOPER, P. R. (Ed.) *Head Injury*, Baltimore, MD, Williams and Wilkins, pp. 185–232.

COPE, D. N. (1987) 'Combined head and spinal cord injury', in MINER, M. E. and WAGNER, K. A. (Eds) *Neurotrauma: Treatment, Rehabilitation, and Related Issues, No. 2*, Boston, MA, Butterworths, pp. 99–102.

COPE, D. N. and HALL, K. (1982) 'Head injury rehabilitation: Benefit of early intervention', *Archives of Physical Medicine and Rehabilitation*, **63**, pp. 433–7.

CORKIN, S., COHEN, N. J., SULLIVAN, E. V., CLEGG, R. A., ROSEN, T. J. and ACKERMAN, R. H. (1985) 'Analyses of global memory impairments of different etiologies', *Annals of the New York Academy of Sciences*, **444**, pp. 10–40.

CORRIGAN, J. D., ARNETT, J. A., HOUCK, L. J. and JACKSON, R. D. (1985) 'Reality orientation for brain injured patients: group treatment and monitoring of recovery', *Archives of Physical Medicine and Rehabilitation*, **66**, pp. 626–30.

CORRIGAN, J. D. and HINKELDEY, N. S. (1987) 'Comparison of intelligence and memory in patients with diffuse and focal injury', *Psychological Reports*, **60**, pp. 899–906.

COURVILLE, C. B. (1942) 'Coup–contrecoup mechanism of craniocerebral injuries: Some observations', *Archives of Surgery*, **45**, pp. 19–43.

CROMPTON, M. R. (1971) 'Hypothalmic lesions following closed head injury', *Brain*, **94**, pp. 165–72.

CRONHOLM, B. (1972) 'Evaluation of mental disturbances after head injury', *Scandinavian Journal of Rehabilitation Medicine*, **4**, pp. 35–8.

CROSSON, B. and BUENNING, W. (1984) 'An individualized memory retraining program after closed-head injury: A single-case study', *Journal of Clinical Neuropsychology*, **6**, pp. 287–301.

CROVITZ, H. F., HARVEY, M. T. and HORN, R. W. (1979) 'Problems in the acquisition of imagery mnemonics: Three brain-damaged cases', *Cortex*, **15**, pp. 225–34.

CROVITZ, H. F., HORN, R. W. and DANIEL, W. F. (1983) 'Inter-relationships among retrograde amnesia, post-traumatic amnesia, and time since head injury: A retrospective study', *Cortex*, **19**, pp. 407–12.

CULLUM, C. M. and BIGLER, E. D. (1985) 'Late effects of haematoma on brain morphology and memory in closed head injury', *International Journal of Neuroscience*, **28**, pp. 279–83.

CYR, J. J. and BROOKER, B. H. (1984) 'Use of appropriate formulas for selecting WAIS–R short forms', *Journal of Consulting and Clinical Psychology*, **52**, pp. 903–5.

DAHLSTROM, W. G., WELSH, G. S. and DAHLSTROM, L. E. (1972) *An MMPI Handbook. Vol. 1: Clinical Interpretation*, Minneapolis, MN, University of Minnesota Press.

DAILEY, C. A. (1956) 'Psychologic findings five years after head injury', *Journal of Clinical Psychology*, **12**, pp. 349–52.

DANIEL, M. S. (1987) 'Memory and depression following brain injury', *Dissertation Abstracts International*, **47B**, p. 3514.

DAVID, R. M., ENDERBY, P. and BAINTON, D. (1979) 'Progress report on an evaluation of speech therapy for aphasia', *British Journal of Disorders of Communication*, **14**, pp. 85–8.

DAVIDOFF, G., MORRIS, J., ROTH, E. and BLEIBERG, J. (1985) 'Closed head injury in spinal cord injured patients: Retrospective study of loss of consciousness and post-traumatic amnesia', *Archives of Physical Medicine and Rehabilitation*, **66**, pp. 41–3.

DAVIDOFF, G., ROTH, E., MORRIS, J. and BLEIBERG, J. (1987) 'Evaluation of closed head injury and cognitive deficits in patients with traumatic spinal cord injury', in MINER, M. E. and WAGNER, K. A. (Eds) *Neurotrauma: Treatment, Rehabilitation, and Related Issues, No. 2*, Boston, MA, Butterworths, pp. 127–35.

DAVIDOFF, G., ROTH, E., MORRIS, J., BLEIBERG, J. and MEYER, P. R., Jr. (1986) 'Assessment of closed head injury in trauma-related spinal cord injury', *Paraplegia*, **24**, pp. 97–104.

DEATON, A. V. (1987) 'Behavioral change strategies for children and adolescents with severe brain injury', *Journal of Learning Disabilities*, **20**, pp. 581–9.

DE MORSIER, G. (1972) 'Les hallucinations survenant après les traumatismes cranio-cérébraux: La schizophrénie traumatique', *Annales médico-psychologiques*, **130**, pp. 183–94.

(1973) 'Sur 23 cas d'aphasie traumatique', *Psychiatria Clinica*, **6**, pp. 226–39.

DENCKER, S. J. (1958) 'A follow-up study of 128 closed head injuries in twins using co-twins as controls', *Acta Psychiatrica et Neurologica Scandinavica*, **33**, Suppl. 123.

(1960) 'Closed head injury in twins: Neurologic, psychometric, and psychiatric follow-up study of consecutive cases, using co-twins as controls', *Archives of General Psychiatry*, **2**, pp. 569–75.

DENCKER, S. J. and LÖFVING, B. (1958) 'A psychometric study of identical twins discordant for closed head injury', *Acta Psychiatrica et Neurologica Scandinavica*, **33**, Supp. 122.

DENNY-BROWN, D. (1945a) 'Disability arising from closed head injury, *Journal of the American Medical Association*, **127**, pp. 429–36.

(1945b) 'Intellectual deterioration resulting from head injury', in *Trauma of the Central Nervous System* (*Research Publications of the Association for Research in Nervous and Mental Disease*, Vol. 24), Baltimore, MD, Williams and Wilkins, pp. 467–72.

DENNY-BROWN, D. E. and RUSSELL, W. R. (1941) 'Experimental cerebral concussion', *Brain*, **64**, pp. 93–164.

DE RENZI, E. and VIGNOLO, L. A. (1962) 'The Token Test: A sensitive test to detect receptive disturbances in aphasics', *Brain*, **85**, pp. 665–78.

DIKMEN, S. and REITAN, R. M. (1976) 'Psychological deficits and recovery of functions after head injury', *Transactions of the American Neurological Association*, **101**, pp. 72–7.

(1977) 'Emotional sequelae of head injury', *Annals of Neurology*, **2**, pp. 492–4.

DIKMEN, S., REITAN, R. M. and TEMKIN, N. R. (1983) 'Neuropsychological recovery in head injury', *Archives of Neurology*, **40**, pp. 333–8.

DILLON, H. and LEOPOLD, R. L. (1961) 'Children and the post-concussion syndrome', *Journal of the American Medical Association*, **175**, pp. 86–92.

DIXON, K. C. (1962) 'The amnesia of cerebral concussion', *Lancet*, **2**, pp. 1359–60.

DRACHMAN, D. A. and ARBIT, J. (1966) 'Memory and the hippocampal complex: II', *Archives of Neurology*, **15**, pp. 52–61.

DRESSER, A. C., MEIROWSKY, A. M., WEISS, G. H., MCNEEL, M. L., SIMON, G. A. and CAVENESS, W. F. (1973) 'Gainful employment following head injury', *Archives of Neurology*, **29**, pp. 111–6.

DUHAIME, A. -C., GENNARELLI, T. A., THIBAULT, L. E., BRUCE, D. A., MARGULIES, S. S. and WISER, R. (1987) 'The shaken baby syndrome: A clinical, pathological, and biomechanical study', *Journal of Neurosurgery*, **66**, pp. 409–15.

DUNN, J. and BROOKS, D. N. (1974) 'Memory and post traumatic amnesia', *IRCS (Research on Neurology and Neurosurgery; Psychiatry and Clinical Psychology; Psychology)*, **2**, p. 1497.

DYE, O. A., MILBY, J. B. and SAXON, S. A. (1979) 'Effects of early neurological problems following head trauma on subsequent neuropsychological performance', *Acta Neurologica Scandinavica*, **59**, pp. 10–4.

EAMES, P. (1989) 'Risk–benefit considerations in drug treatment', in WOOD, R. L. and EAMES, P. (Eds) *Models of Brain Injury Rehabilitation*, London, Chapman and Hall, pp. 164–79.

EAMES, P. and WOOD, R. (1985a) 'Rehabilitation after severe brain injury: A follow-up study of a behaviour modification approach', *Journal of Neurology, Neurosurgery, and Psychiatry*, **48**, pp. 613–9.

(1985b) 'Rehabilitation after severe brain injury: A special-unit approach to behaviour disorders', *International Rehabilitation Medicine*, **7**, pp. 130–3.

(1989) 'The structure and content of a head injury rehabilitation service', in WOOD, R. L. and EAMES, P. (Eds) *Models of Brain Injury Rehabilitation*, London, Chapman and Hall, pp. 31–47.

ECCLES, J. C. (1987) 'Regeneration of the mammalian brain following lesions', in MINER, M. E. and WAGNER, K. A. (Eds) *Neurotrauma: Treatment, Rehabilitation, and Related Issues, No. 2*, Boston, MA, Butterworths, pp. 55–64.

EDEN, K. and TURNER, J. W. A. (1941) 'Loss of consciousness in different types of head injury', *Proceedings of the Royal Society of Medicine*, **34**, pp. 685–91.

EDITORIAL (1973) 'The psychiatric sequelae of head injury', *Medical Journal of Australia*, **2**, pp. 873–4.

(1986) 'Psychosocial outcome of head injury', *Lancet*, **1**, pp. 1361–2.

EDNA, T. -H. and CAPPELEN, J. (1987) 'Late post-concussional symptoms in traumatic head injury: An analysis of frequency and risk factors', *Acta Neurochirurgica*, **86**, pp. 12–7.

EISENBERG, H. M. and WEINER, R. L. (1987) 'Input variables: How information from the acute injury can be used to characterize groups of patients for studies of outcome', in LEVIN, H. S., GRAFMAN, J. and EISENBERG, H. M. (Eds) *Neurobehavioral Recovery from Head Injury*, New York, Oxford University Press, pp. 13–29.

ELIA, J. (1974) 'Cranial injuries and the post-concussion syndrome', *Medical Trial Techniques Quarterly*, **21**, pp. 127–61.

ENGLISH, T. C. (1904) 'The after-effects of head injuries: Lecture II', *Lancet*, **1**, pp. 559–63.

ESON, M. E., YEN, J. K. and BOURKE, R. S. (1978) 'Assessment of recovery from serious head injury', *Journal of Neurology, Neurosurgery, and Psychiatry*, **41**, pp. 1036–42.

EVANS, C. D. (Ed.) (1981) *Rehabilitation after Severe Head Injury*, Edinburgh, Churchill Livingstone.

EVANS, C. (1989) 'Long-term follow-up', in WOOD, R. L. and EAMES, P. (Eds) *Models of Brain Injury Rehabilitation*, London, Chapman and Hall, pp. 183–204.

EVANS, C. D., BULL, C. P. I., DEVONPORT, M. J., HALL, P. M., JONES, J., MIDDLETON, F. R. I., RUSSELL, G., STICHBURY, J. C. and WHITEHEAD, B. (1975) 'Rehabilitation of the brain-damaged survivor', *Injury*, **8**, pp. 80–97.

EVANS, R. W. (1987) 'Postconcussive syndrome: An overview', *Texas Medicine*, **83**, pp. 49–53.

EYSENCK, H. J. and EYSENCK, S. B. G. (1975) *Eysenck Personality Questionnaire*, London, Hodder and Stoughton.

EYSENCK, M. W. (1979) 'Anxiety, learning, and memory: A reconceptualization', *Journal of Research in Personality*, **13**, pp. 365–85.

(1982) *Attention and Arousal: Cognition and Performance*, Berlin, Springer–Verlag.

FAHY, T. J., IRVING, M. H. and MILLAC, P. (1967) 'Severe head injuries: A six-year follow-up', *Lancet*, **2**, pp. 475–9.

FERGUSON, G. A. and TAKANE, Y. (1989) *Statistical Analysis in Psychology and Education*, 6th ed., New York, McGraw–Hill.

FIELD, J. H. (1976) *Epidemiology of Head Injuries in England and Wales*, London, Her Majesty's Stationery Office.

FISHER, C. M. (1966) 'Concussion amnesia', *Neurology*, **16**, pp. 826–30.

FLYNN, J. R. (1984) 'The mean IQ of Americans: Massive gains 1932 to 1978', *Psychological Bulletin*, **95**, pp. 29–51.

FODOR, I. E. (1972) 'Impairment of memory functions after acute head injury', *Journal of Neurology, Neurosurgery, and Psychiatry*, **35**, pp. 818–24.

FOSTER, J. B., LEIGUARDA, R. and TILLEY, P. J. B. (1976) 'Brain damage in National Hunt jockeys', *Lancet*, **1**, pp. 981–83.

FRANKOWSKI, R. F. (1986) 'Descriptive epidemiologic studies of head injury in the United States: 1974–1984', in PETERSON, L. G. and O'SHANICK, G. J. (Eds) *Psychiatric Aspects of Trauma* (*Advances in Psychosomatic Medicine*, Vol. 16), Basel, Karger, pp. 153–72.

FRAZEE, J. G. (1986) 'Head trauma', *Emergency Medicine Clinics of North America*, **4**, pp. 859–74.

FRIEDMAN, A. P., BRENNER, C. and DENNY-BROWN, D. (1945) 'Post-traumatic vertigo and dizziness', *Journal of Neurosurgery*, **2**, pp. 36–46.

FULD, P. A. and FISHER, P. (1977) 'Recovery of intellectual ability after closed head-injury', *Developmental Medicine and Child Neurology*, **19**, pp. 495–502.

GAIDOLFI, E. and VIGNOLO, L. A. (1980) 'Closed head injuries of school-age children: Neuropsychological sequelae in early adulthood', *Italian Journal of Neurological Sciences*, **2**, pp. 65–73.

GALBRAITH, S., MURRAY, W. R., PATEL, A. R. and KNILL-JONES, R. (1976a) 'The relationship between alcohol and head injury and its effect on the conscious level', *British Journal of Surgery*, **63**, pp. 128–30.

GALBRAITH, S., TEASDALE, G. and BLAIKLOCK, C. (1976b) 'Computerised tomography of acute traumatic intracranial haematoma: Reliability of neurosurgeons' interpretations', *British Medical Joaurnal*, **2**, pp. 1371–3.

GANDY, S. E., SNOW, R. B., ZIMMERMAN, R. D. and DECK, M. D. F. (1984) 'Cranial nuclear magnetic resonance imaging in head trauma', *Annals of Neurology*, **16**, pp. 254–7.

GANS, J. S. (1983) 'Hate in the rehabilitation setting', *Archives of Physical Medicine and Rehabilitation*, **64**, pp. 176–9.

GENNARELLI, T. A. (1983) 'Head injury in man and experimental animals: Clinical aspects', *Acta Neurochirurgica*, Suppl. 32, pp. 1–13.

GENNARELLI, T. A., CHAMPION, H. R., SACCO, W. J., COPES, W. S. and ALVES, W. M. (1989) 'Mortality of patients with head injury and extracranial injury treated in trauma centers', *Journal of Trauma*, **29**, pp. 1193–202.

GENNARELLI, T. A., SPIELMAN, G. M., LANGFITT, T. W., GILDENBERG, P. L., HARRINGTON, T., JANE, J. A., MARSHALL, L. F., MILLER, J. D. and PITTS, L. H. (1982) 'Influence of the type of intracranial-lesion on outcome from severe head injury: A multicenter study using a new classification system', *Journal of Neurosurgery*, **56**, pp. 26–32.

GENNARELLI, T. A., THIBAULT, L. E., ADAMS, J. H., GRAHAM, D. I., THOMPSON, C. J. and MARCINCIN, R. P. (1982) 'Diffuse axonal injury and traumatic coma in the primate', *Annals of Neurology*, **12**, pp. 564–74.

GENTILINI, M., NICHELLI, P. and SCHOENHUBER, R. (1989) 'Assessment of attention in mild head injury', in LEVIN, H. S., EISENBERG, H. M. and BENTON, A. L. (Eds) *Mild Head Injury*, New York, Oxford University Press, pp. 163–75.

GENTILINI, M., NICHELLI, P., SCHOENHUBER, R., BORTOLOTTI, P., TONELLI, L., FALASCA, A. and MERLI, G. A. (1985) 'Neuropsychological evaluation of mild head injury', *Journal of Neurology, Neurosurgery, and Psychiatry*, **48**, pp. 137–40.

GERBOTH, R. (1950) 'A study of the two forms of the Wechsler–Bellevue Intelligence Scale', *Journal of Consulting Psychology*, **14**, pp. 365–70.

GESCHWIND, N. (1971) 'Aphasia', *New England Journal of Medicine*, **284**, pp. 654–6.

GIANUTSOS, R. and GRYNBAUM, B. B. (1983) 'Helping brain-injured people to contend with hidden cognitive deficits', *International Rehabilitation Medicine*, **5**, pp. 37–40.

GILCHRIST, E. and WILKINSON, M. (1979) 'Some factors determining prognosis in young people with severe head injuries', *Archives of Neurology*, **36**, pp. 355–9.

GLANZER, M. and CUNITZ, A. R. (1966) 'Two storage mechanisms in free recall', *Journal of Verbal Learning and Verbal Behavior*, **5**, pp. 351–60.

GLASGOW, R. E., ZEISS, R. A., BARRERA, M., Jr. and LEWINSOHN, P. M. (1977) 'Case studies on remediating memory deficits in brain-damaged individuals', *Journal of Clinical Psychology*, **33**, pp. 1049–54.

GLISKY, E. L., SCHACTER, D. L. and TULVING, E. (1986a) 'Computer learning by memory-impaired patients: Acquisition and retention of complex knowledge', *Neuropsychologia*, **24**, pp. 313–28.

(1986b) 'Learning and retention of computer-related vocabulary in memory-impaired patients: Method of vanishing cues', *Journal of Clinical and Experimental Neuropsychology*, **8**, pp. 292–312.

GOLDBERG, D. (1978) *Manual of the General Health Questionnaire*, Windsor, Berks., NFER Publishing.

GOLDBERG, E., ANTIN, S. P., BILDER, R. M., Jr., GERSTMAN, L. J., HUGHES, J. E. O. and MATTIS, S. (1981) 'Retrograde amnesia: Possible role of mesencephalic reticular activation in long-term memory', *Science*, **213**, pp. 1392–4.

GOLDBERG, E., GERSTMAN, L. J., MATTIS, S., HUGHES, J. E. O., BILDER, R. M., Jr. and SIRIO, C. A. (1982a) 'Effects of cholinergic treatment on post-traumatic anterograde amnesia', *Archives of Neurology*, **39**, p. 581.

GOLDBERG, E., GERSTMAN, L. J., MATTIS, S., HUGHES, J. E. O., SIRIO, C. A. and BILDER, R. M., Jr. (1982b) 'Selective effects of cholinergic treatment on verbal memory in post-traumatic amnesia', *Journal of Clinical Neuropsychology*, **4**, pp. 219–34.

GOLDSMITH, W. (1972) 'Biomechanics of head injury', in FUNG, Y. C., PERRONE, N. and ANLIKER, M. (Eds) *Biomechanics: Its Foundations and Objectives*, Englewood Cliffs, NJ, Prentice–Hall, pp. 585–634.

GOLDSTEIN, K. (1936) 'The problem of the meaning of words based upon observation of aphasic patients', *Journal of Psychology*, **2**, pp. 301–16.

(1942) *After-effects of Brain Injuries in War: Their Evaluation and Treatment. The Application of Psychologic Methods in the Clinic*, London, Heinemann.

(1943) 'Brain concussion: Evaluation of the after-effects by special tests', *Diseases of the Nervous System*, **4**, pp. 325–34.

(1952) 'The effect of brain damage on the personality', *Psychiatry*, **15**, pp. 245–60.

GOODGLASS, H. and KAPLAN, E. (1972) *The Assessment of Aphasia and Related Disorders*, New York, Lea and Febiger.

GOSCH, H. H., GOODING, E. and SCHNEIDER, R. C. (1970) 'The lexan calvarium for the study of cerebral responses to acute trauma', *Journal of Trauma*, **10**, pp. 370–6.

GRAF, P. and SCHACTER, D. L. (1985) 'Implicit and explicit memory for new associations in normal and amnesic subjects', *Journal of Experimental Psychology: Learning, Memory and Cognition*, **2**, pp. 501–18.

GRAHAM, D. I. (1985) 'The pathology of brain ischaemia and possibilities for therapeutic intervention', *British Journal of Anaesthesia*, **57**, pp. 3–17.

GRAHAM, D. I., ADAMS, J. H. and GENNARELLI, T. A. (1988a) 'Mechanisms of non-penetrating head injury', in BOND, R. F. (ed.), *Perspectives in Shock Research (Progress in Clinical and Biological Research*, Vol. 264), New York, Alan R. Liss, pp. 159–68.

GRAHAM, D. I., FORD, I., ADAMS, J. H., DOYLE, D., LAWRENCE, A. E., McLELLAN, D. R. and NG, H. K. (1989a) 'Fatal head injury in children', *Journal of Clinical Pathology*, **42**, pp. 18–22.

GRAHAM, D. I., FORD, I., ADAMS, J. H., DOYLE, D., TEASDALE, G. M., LAWRENCE, A. E. and McLELLAN, D. R. (1989b) 'Ischaemic brain damage is still common in fatal non-missile head injury', *Journal of Neurology, Neurosurgery, and Psychiatry*, **52**, pp. 346–50.

GRAHAM, D. I., LAWRENCE, A. E., ADAMS, J. H., DOYLE, D. and McLELLAN, D. R. (1987) 'Brain damage in non-missile head injury secondary to high intracranial pressure', *Neuropathology and Applied Neurobiology*, **13**, pp. 209–17.

(1988b) 'Brain damage in fatal non-missile head injury without high intracranial pressure', *Journal of Clinical Pathology*, **41**, pp. 34–7.

GRAHAM, D. I., McLELLAN, D., ADAMS, J. H., DOYLE, D., KERR, A. and MURRAY, L. S. (1983) 'The neuropathology of the vegetative state and severe disability after non-missile head injury', *Acta Neurochirurgica*, Suppl. 32, pp. 65–7.

GRATTAN, E. and HOBBS, J. A. (1978) *Injuries to Occupants of Heavy Goods Vehicles* (TRRL Laboratory Report 854), Crowthorne, Berks., Transport and Road Research Laboratory.

(1980) *Permanent Disability in Road Traffic Accident Casualties* (TRRL Laboratory Report 924), Crowthorne, Berks., Transport and Road Research Laboratory.

GRATTAN, E., HOBBS, J. A. and KEIGAN, M. E. (1976) 'Anatomical sites and severities of injury in unprotected road users'. Paper presented to the 3rd International Conference of the International Research Committee on the Biokinetics of Impacts, Amsterdam, 7–8 September.

GRAVES, E. J. (1989) 'Detailed diagnoses and procedures, National Hospital Discharge Survey, 1987' (*Vital and Health Statistics*, Series 13, No. 100), DHHS Pub. No. (PHS) 89–1761, Hyattsville, MD, Public Health Service.

GROHER, M. (1977) 'Language and memory disorders following closed head trauma', *Journal of Speech and Hearing Research*, **20**, pp. 212–23.

GRONWALL, D. M. A. (1976) 'Performance changes during recovery from closed head injury', *Proceedings of the Australian Association of Neurologists*, **13**, pp. 143–7.

(1977) 'Paced auditory serial-addition task: A measure of recovery from concussion', *Perceptual and Motor Skills*, **44**, pp. 367–73.

GRONWALL, D. M. A. and SAMPSON, H. (1974) *The Psychological Effects of Concussion*, Auckland, Auckland University Press/Oxford University Press.

GRONWALL, D. and WRIGHTSON, P. (1974) 'Delayed recovery of intellectual function after minor head injury', *Lancet*, **2**, pp. 605–9.

(1975) 'Cumulative effect of concussion', *Lancet*, **2**, pp. 995–7.

(1980) 'Duration of post-traumatic amnesia after mild head injury', *Journal of Clinical Neuropsychology*, **2**, pp. 51–60.

(1981) 'Memory and information processing capacity after closed head injury', *Journal of Neurology, Neurosurgery, and Psychiatry*, **44**, pp. 889–95.

GRUNEBERG, R. (1970) 'The concept of accident neurosis', *Injury*, **1**, pp. 209–12.

GUALTIERI, C. T. (1988) 'Pharmacotherapy and the neurobehavioural sequelae of traumatic brain injury', *Brain Injury*, **2**, pp. 101–29.

GURDJIAN, E. S. (1971) 'Mechanisms of impact injury of the head', in *Head Injuries: Proceedings of an International Symposium*, Edinburgh, Churchill Livingstone, pp. 17–22.

GURDJIAN, E. S. and GURDJIAN, E. S. (1975) 'Re-evaluation of the biomechanics of blunt impact injury of the head', *Surgery, Gynecology, and Obstetrics*, **140**, pp. 845–50.

(1978) 'Acute head injuries', *Surgery, Gynecology, and Obstetrics*, **146**, pp. 805–20.

GUTHKELCH, A. N. (1980) 'Post-traumatic amnesia, post-concussional symptoms and accident neurosis', *European Neurology*, **19**, pp. 91–102.

HAAS, D. C. and ROSS, G. S. (1986) 'Transient global amnesia triggered by mild head trauma', *Brain*, **109**, pp. 251–57.

HAAS, J. F., COPE, D. N. and HALL, K. (1987) 'Premorbid prevalence of poor academic performance in severe head injury', *Journal of Neurology, Neurosurgery and Psychiatry*, **50**, pp. 52–6.

HAGEN, C., MALKMUS, D. and DURHAM, P. (1979) 'Levels of cognitive functioning', in *Rehabilitation of the Head Injured Adult: Comprehensive Physical Management*, Downey, CA, Professional Staff Association of Rancho Los Amigos Hospital, pp. 87–8.

HALL, K. M., COPE, D. N. and WILMOT, C. B. (1987) 'Occult head injury in spinal cord injury: Relationship to premorbid history and learning self-care', in MINER, M. E. and WAGNER, K. A. (Eds) *Neurotrauma: Treatment, Rehabilitation, and Related Issues, No. 2*, Boston, MA, Butterworths, pp. 113–25.

HALPERN, H., DARLEY, F. L. and BROWN, J. R. (1973) 'Differential language and neurologic characteristics in cerebral involvement', *Journal of Speech and Hearing Disorders*, **38**, pp. 162–73.

HALSTEAD, W. C. (1947) *Brain and Intelligence: A Quantitative Study of the Frontal Lobes*, Chicago, University of Chicago Press.

HAN, J. S., KAUFMAN, B., ALFRIDI, R. J., YEUNG, H. N., BENSON, J. E., HAAGA, J. R., EL YOUSEF, S. J., CLAMPITT, M. E., BONSTELLE, C. T. and HUSS, R. (1984) 'Head trauma evaluated by magnetic resonance and computed tomography: A comparison', *Radiology*, **150**, pp. 71–7.

HANLEY, I. G., MCGUIRE, R. J. and BOYD, W. D. (1981) 'Reality orientation and dementia: A controlled trial of two approaches', *British Journal of Psychiatry*, **138**, pp. 10–4.

HANNAY, H. J. and JAMES, C. M. (1981) 'Simulation of a memory deficit on the Continuous Recognition Memory Test', *Perceptual and Motor Skills*, **53**, pp. 51–8.

HANNAY, H. J. and LEVIN, H. S. (1985) 'Selective reminding test: An examination of the equivalence of four forms', *Journal of Clinical and Experimental Neuropsychology*, **7**, pp. 251–63.

HANNAY, H. J., LEVIN, H. S. and GROSSMAN, R. G. (1979) 'Impaired recognition memory after head injury', *Cortex*, **15**, pp. 269–83.

HANNAY, H. J., LEVIN, H. S. and KAY, M. (1982) 'Tachistoscopic visual perception after closed head injury', *Journal of Clinical Neuropsychology*, **4**, pp. 117–129.

HARDMAN, J. M. (1979) 'The pathology of traumatic brain injuries', *Advances in Neurology*, **22**, pp. 15–50.

HARRIS, J. E. (1978) 'External memory aids', in GRUNEBERG, M. M., MORRIS, P. E. and SYKES, R. N. (Eds) *Practical Aspects of Memory*, London, Academic Press, pp. 172–9.
(1984) 'Methods of improving memory', in WILSON, B. A. and MOFFAT, N. (Eds) *Clinical Management of Memory Problems*, London, Croom Helm, pp. 46–62.

HARRIS, J. E. and SUNDERLAND, A. (1981) 'A brief survey of the management of memory disorders in rehabilitation units in Britain', *International Rehabilitation Medicine*, **3**, pp. 206–9.

HAWTHORNE, V. M. (1978) 'Epidemiology of head injuries', *Scottish Medical Journal*, **23**, p. 92.

HAYDEN, M. E. and HART, T. (1986) 'Rehabilitation of cognitive and behavioral dysfunction in head injury', in PETERSON, L. G. and O'SHANICK, G. J. (Eds) *Psychiatric Aspects of Trauma* (*Advances in Psychosomatic Medicine*, Vol. 16), Basel, Karger, pp. 194–229.

HAYES, R. L., LYETH, B. G. and JENKINS, L. W. (1989) 'Neurochemical mechanisms of mild and moderate head injury: Implications for treatment', in LEVIN, H. S., EISENBERG, H. M. and BENTON, A. L. (Eds) *Mild Head Injury*, New York, Oxford University Press, pp. 54–79.

HÉCAEN, H. (1976) 'Acquired aphasia in children and the ontogenesis of hemispheric functional specialization', *Brain and Language*, **3**, pp. 114–34.

HEIDEN, J. S., SMALL, R., CATON, W., WEISS, M. and KURZE, T. (1983) 'Severe head injury: Clinical assessment and outcome', *Physical Therapy*, **63**, pp. 1946–51.

HEILMAN, K. M., SAFRAN, A. and GESCHWIND, N. (1971) 'Closed head trauma and aphasia', *Journal of Neurology, Neurosurgery, and Psychiatry*, **34**, pp. 265–9.

HEISKANEN, O. and KASTE, M. (1974) 'Late prognosis of severe brain injury in children', *Developmental Medicine and Child Neurology*, **16**, pp. 11–4.

HEISKANEN, O. and SIPPONEN, P. (1970) 'Prognosis of severe brain injury', *Acta Neurologica Scandinavica*, **46**, pp. 343–8.

HENDRICK, E. B., HARWOOD-HASH, D. C. F. and HUDSON, A. R. (1964) 'Head injuries in children: A survey of 4465 consecutive cases at the Hospital for Sick Children, Toronto, Canada', *Clinical Neurosurgery*, **11**, pp. 46–65.

HENRY, S. (1979) 'Physicians from two continents review management of brain-injured patients', *Canadian Medical Association Journal*, **121**, pp. 1535–7.

HICK, W. E. (1952) 'On the rate of gain of information', *Quarterly Journal of Experimental Psychology*, **4**, pp. 11–26.

HIGASHI, K., SAKATA, Y., HATANO, M., ABIKO, S., IHARA, K., KATAYAMA, S., WAKUTA, Y., OKAMURA, T., UEDA, H., ZENKE, M. and AOKI, H. (1977) 'Epidemiological studies on patients with a persistent vegetative state', *Journal of Neurology, Neurosurgery, and Psychiatry*, **40**, pp. 876–85.

HILL, J. F. (1979) 'Blunt injury with particular reference to recent terrorist bombing incidents', *Annals of the Royal College of Surgeons of England*, **61**, pp. 4–11.

HILLBOM, E. (1960) 'After-effects of brain-injuries: Research on the symptoms causing invalidism of persons in Finland having sustained brain-injuries during the wars of 1939–1940 and 1941–1944', *Acta Psychiatrica et Neurologica Scandinavica*, **35**, Suppl. 142.

HIORNS, R. W. and NEWCOMBE, F. (1979) 'Recovery curves: Uses and limitations', *International Rehabilitation Medicine*, **1**, pp. 173–6.

HIRSCH, A. E. and OMMAYA, A. K. (1972) 'Head injury caused by underwater explosion of a firecracker: Case report', *Journal of Neurosurgery*, **37**, pp. 95–9.

HJERN, B. and NYLANDER, I. (1964) 'Acute head injuries in children: Traumatology, therapy and prognosis', *Acta Pediatrica*, Suppl. 152.

HOBBS, C. A. (1978) *The Effectiveness of Seat Belts in Reducing Injuries to Car Occupants* (TRRL Laboratory Report No. 811), Crowthorne, Berks., Transport and Road Research Laboratory.

   (1981) *Car Occupant Injury Patterns and Mechanisms* (TRRL Scientific Report No. 648), Crowthorne, Berks., Transport and Road Research Laboratory.

HODGES, W. F. and SPIELBERGER, C. D. (1969) 'Digit-span: An indicant of trait or state anxiety?' *Journal of Consulting and Clinical Psychology*, **33**, pp. 430–4.

HOLBOURN, A. H. S. (1943) 'Mechanics of head injuries', *Lancet*, **2**, pp. 438–41.

   (1945) 'The mechanics of brain injuries', *British Medical Bulletin*, **3**, pp. 147–9.

HOOPER, R. S., MCGREGOR, J. M. and NATHAN, P. W. (1945) 'Explosive rage following head injury', *Journal of Mental Science*, **91**, pp. 458–71.

HOROWITZ, I., COSTEFF, H., SADAN, N., ABRAHAM, E., GEYER, S. and NAJENSON, T. (1983) 'Childhood head injuries in Israel: Epidemiology and outcome', *International Rehabilitation Medicine*, **5**, pp. 32–6.

HPAY, H. (1971) 'Psycho-social effects of severe head injury', in *Head Injuries: Proceedings of an International Symposium*, Edinburgh, Churchill Livingstone, pp. 110–9.

HUMPHREY, M. and ODDY, M. (1978) 'The social costs of head injuries', *New Society*, **45**, pp. 452–4.

(1980) 'Return to work after head injury: A review of post-war studies', *Injury*, **12**, pp. 107–14.

INGLIS, J. (1959) 'A paired–associate learning test for use with elderly psychiatric patients', *Journal of Mental Science*, **105**, pp. 440–3.

JACOBSON, S. A. (1969) 'Mechanisms of the sequelae of minor craniocervical trauma', in WALKER, A. E., CAVENESS, W. F. and CRITCHLEY, M. (Eds) *The Late Effects of Head Injury*, Springfield, IL, Thomas, pp. 35–45.

JAGGER, J., LEVINE, J., JANE, J. and RIMEL, R. (1984) 'Epidemiologic features of head injury in a predominantly rural population', *Journal of Trauma*, **24**, pp. 40–4.

JAMIESON, K. G. (1971a) *A First Notebook of Head Injury*, 2nd ed., London, Butterworths.

(1971b) 'Prevention of head injury', in *Head Injuries: Proceedings of an International Symposium*, Edinburgh, Churchill Livingstone, pp. 12–15.

JAMIESON, K. G. and YELLAND, J. D. N. (1968) 'Extradural hematoma: Report of 167 cases', *Journal of Neurosurgery*, **29**, pp. 13–23.

(1972) 'Traumatic intracerebral hematoma: Report of 63 surgically treated cases', *Journal of Neurosurgery*, **37**, pp. 528–32.

JANE, J. A., RIMEL, R. W., POBERESKIN, L. H., TYSON, G. W., STEWARD, O. and GENNARELLI, T. A. (1982) 'Outcome and pathology of head injury', in GROSSMAN, R. G. and GILDENBERG, P. L. (Eds) *Head Injury: Basic and Clinical Aspects*, New York, Raven Press, pp. 229–37.

JANE, J. A., STEWARD, O. and GENNARELLI, T. (1985) 'Axonal degeneration induced by experimental noninvasive minor head injury', *Journal of Neurosurgery*, **62**, 96–100.

JENKINS, A., TEASDALE, G., HADLEY, M. D. M., MACPHERSON, P. and ROWAN, J. O. (1986) 'Brain lesions detected by magnetic resonance imaging in mild and severe head injuries', *Lancet*, **2**, pp. 445–6.

JENKINS, J. S., MATHER, H. M., COUGHLAN, A. K. and JENKINS, D. G. (1981) 'Desmopressin and desglycinamide vasopressin in post-traumatic amnesia', *Lancet*, **1**, p. 39.

JENNETT, B. (1969) 'Early traumatic epilepsy: Definition and identity', *Lancet*, **1**, pp. 1023–5.

(1972) 'Head injuries in children', *Developmental Medicine and Child Neurology*, **14**, pp. 137–47.

(1973) 'Epilepsy after non-missile head injuries', *Scottish Medical Journal*, **18**, pp. 8–13.

(1974) 'Early traumatic epilepsy: Incidence and significance after nonmissile injuries', *Archives of Neurology*, **30**, pp. 394–8.

(1975a) 'Epilepsy and acute traumatic intracranial haematoma', *Journal of Neurology, Neurosurgery, and Psychiatry*, **38**, pp. 378–81.

(1975b) 'Who cares for head injuries?' *British Medical Journal*, **3**, pp. 267–70.

(1976a) 'Assessment of the severity of head injury', *Journal of Neurology, Neurosurgery, and Psychiatry*, **39**, pp. 647–55.

(1976b) 'Predicting outcome after head injury', *Proceedings of the Royal Society of Medicine*, **69**, pp. 140–1.

(1976c) 'Prognosis of severe head injury', in MCLAURIN, R. L. (Ed.) *Head Injuries: Proceedings of the Second Chicago Symposium on Neural Trauma*, New York, Grune and Stratton, pp. 45–7.

(1976d) 'Resource allocation for the severely brain damaged', *Archives of Neurology*, **33**, pp. 595–7.

(1979) 'Defining brain damage after head injury', *Journal of the Royal College of Physicians of London*, **13**, pp. 197–200.

(1983) 'Scale and scope of the problem', in ROSENTHAL, M., GRIFFITH, E. R., BOND, M. R., and MILLER, J. D. (Eds) *Rehabilitation of the Head Injured Adult*, Philadelphia, PA, Davis, pp. 3–8.

(1984) 'The measurement of outcome', in BROOKS, N. (Ed.) *Closed Head Injury: Psychological, Social, and Family Consequences*, Oxford, Oxford University Press, pp. 37–43.

JENNETT, B. and BOND, M. (1975) 'Assessment of outcome after severe brain damage', *Lancet*, **1**, pp. 480–4.

JENNETT, B. and CARLIN, J. (1978) 'Preventable mortality and morbidity after head injury', *Injury*, **10**, pp. 31–39.

JENNETT, B. and GALBRAITH, S. (1983) *An Introduction to Neurosurgery*, 4th ed., London, Heinemann.

JENNETT, W. B. and LEWIN, W. (1960) 'Traumatic epilepsy after closed head injuries', *Journal of Neurology, Neurosurgery, and Psychiatry*, **23**, pp. 295–301.

JENNETT, B. and MACMILLAN, R. (1981) 'Epidemiology of head injury', *British Medical Journal*, **282**, pp. 101–4.

JENNETT, B., MILLER, J. D. and BRAAKMAN, R. (1974) 'Epilepsy after nonmissile depressed skull fracture', *Journal of Neurosurgery*, **41**, pp. 208–16.

JENNETT, B., MURRAY, A., CARLIN, J., MCKEAN, M., MACMILLAN, R. and STRANG, I. (1979a) 'Head injuries in three Scottish neurosurgical units: Scottish Head Injury Management Study', *British Medical Journal*, **2**, pp. 955–8.

JENNETT, B., MURRAY, A., MACMILLAN, R., MACFARLANE, J., BENTLEY, C., STRANG, I. and HAWTHORNE, V. (1977a) 'Head injuries in Scottish hospitals: Scottish Head Injury Management Study', *Lancet*, **2**, pp. 696–8.

JENNETT, B. and PLUM, F. (1972) 'Persistent vegetative state after brain damage: A syndrome in search of a name', *Lancet*, **1**, pp. 734–7.

JENNETT, B., SNOEK, J., BOND, M. R. and BROOKS, N. (1981) 'Disability after severe head injury: Observations on the use of the Glasgow Outcome Scale', *Journal of Neurology, Neurosurgery, and Psychiatry*, **44**, pp. 285–93.

JENNETT, B. and TEASDALE, G. (1977) 'Aspects of coma after severe head injury', *Lancet*, **1**, pp. 878–81.

(1981) *Management of Head Injuries*, Philadelphia, PA, Davis.

JENNETT, B., TEASDALE, G., BRAAKMAN, R., MINDERHOUD, J., HEIDEN, J. and KURZE, T. (1979b) 'Prognosis of patients with severe head injury', *Neurosurgery*, **4**, pp. 283–9.

JENNETT, B., TEASDALE, G., BRAAKMAN, R., MINDERHOUD, J. and KNILL-JONES, R. (1976) 'Predicting outcome in individual patients after severe head injury', *Lancet*, **1**, pp. 1031–4.

JENNETT, B., TEASDALE, G., GALBRAITH, S., PICKARD, J., GRANT, H., BRAAKMAN, R., AVEZAAT, C., MAAS, A., MINDERHOUD, J., VECHT, C. J., HEIDEN, J., SMALL, R., CATON, W. and KURZE, T. (1977b) 'Severe head injuries in three countries', *Journal of Neurology, Neurosurgery, and Psychiatry*, **40**, pp. 291–8.

JENNETT, B., TEASDALE, G. M. and KNILL-JONES, R. P. (1975a) 'Predicting outcome after head injury', *Journal of the Royal College of Physicians of London*, **9**, pp. 231–7.

JENNETT, B., TEASDALE, G. and KNILL-JONES, R. (1975b) 'Prognosis after severe head injury', in *Outcome of Severe Damage to the Central Nervous System*, Ciba Foundation Symposium No. 34 (new series), Amsterdam, Elsevier/Excerpta Medica/North–Holland, pp. 309–24.

JENNETT, B., TEATHER, D. and BENNIE, S. (1973) 'Epilepsy after head injury: Residual risk after varying fit-free intervals since injury', *Lancet*, **2**, pp. 652–3.

JOHNSTON, R. B. and MELLITS, E. D. (1980) 'Pediatric coma: Prognosis and outcome', *Developmental Medicine and Child Neurology*, **22**, pp. 3–12.

JOINT COMMITTEE ON INJURY SCALING (1976) *The Abbreviated Injury Scale*, Morton Grove, IL, American Association for Automotive Medicine.

JONES, J. G. (Ed.) (1989) *Depth of Anaesthesia* (*Baillière's Clinical Anaesthesiology*, Vol. 3, No. 3), London, Baillière Tindall.

JONES-GOTMAN, M. and MILNER, B. (1977) 'Design fluency: The invention of nonsense drawings after focal cortical lesions', *Neuropsychologia*, **15**, pp. 653–74.

KALISKY, Z., GOLDMAN, A. M., MORRISON, D. P. and VON LAUFEN, A. (1987) 'Comparison of results with CT scanning and magnetic resonance imaging of brain-injured patients undergoing rehabilitation', in MINER, M. E. and WAGNER, K. A. (Eds) *Neurotrauma: Treatment, Rehabilitation, and Related Issues, No. 2*, Boston, MA, Butterworths, pp. 89–97.

KALSBEEK, W. D., MCLAURIN, R. L., HARRIS, B. S. H., III and MILLER, J. D. (1980) 'The National Head and Spinal Cord Injury Survey: Major findings', *Journal of Neurosurgery*, **53**, pp. S19–31.

KAPUR, N. (1988) *Memory Disorders in Clinical Practice*, London, Butterworths.

KAPUR, N. and PEARSON, D. (1983) 'Memory symptoms and memory performance of neurological patients', *British Journal of Psychology*, **74**, pp. 409–15.

KAY, D. W. K., KERR, T. A. and LASSMAN, L. P. (1971) 'Brain trauma and the post-concussional syndrome', *Lancet*, **2**, pp. 1052–5.

KEAR-COLWELL, J. J. and HELLER, M. (1980) 'The Wechsler Memory Scale and closed head injury', *Journal of Clinical Psychology*, **36**, pp. 782–7.

KELLY, R. (1975) 'The post-traumatic syndrome: An iatrogenic disease', *Forensic Science*, **6**, pp. 17–24.

KENNARD, M. A. (1938) 'Reorganization of motor function in the cerebral cortex of monkeys deprived of motor and premotor areas in infancy', *Journal of Neurophysiology*, **1**, pp. 477–96.

KERNER, M. J. and ACKER, M. (1985) 'Computer delivery of memory retraining with head injured patients', *Cognitive Rehabilitation*, **3**, 6, pp. 26–31.

KERR, T. A., KAY, D. W. K. and LASSMAN, L. P. (1971) 'Characteristics of patients, type of accident, and mortality in a consecutive series of head injuries admitted to a neurosurgical unit', *British Journal of Preventive and Social Medicine*, **25**, pp. 179–85.

KIMURA, D. (1963) 'Right temporal lobe damage', *Archives of Neurology*, **8**, pp. 264–71.

KLAUBER, M., BARRETT-CONNOR, E., MARSHALL, L. and BOWERS, S. (1978) 'The epidemiology of head injury: A prospective study of an entire community — San Diego County, California', *American Journal of Epidemiology*, **113**, pp. 500–9.

KLENSCH, H. (1973) 'Die diagnostische Valenz der Reaktionszeitmessung bei verschiedenen zerebralen Erkrankungen', *Fortschritte der Neurologie, Psychiatrie, und ihrer Grenzgebiete*, **41**, pp. 575–81.

KLINE, N. A. (1979) 'Reversal of post-traumatic amnesia with lithium', *Psychosomatics*, **20**, pp. 363–4.

KLONOFF, H. (1971) 'Head injuries in children: Predisposing factors, accident conditions, accident proneness, and sequelae', *American Journal of Public Health*, **61**, pp. 2405–17.

KLONOFF, H. and LOW, M. (1974) 'Disordered brain function in young children and early adolescents: Neuropsychological and electroencephalographic correlates', in REITAN, R. M. and DAVISON, L. A. (Eds) *Clinical Neuropsychology: Current Status and Applications*, Washington, DC, Winston, pp. 121–78.

KLONOFF, H., LOW, M. D. and CLARK, C. (1977) 'Head injuries in children: A prospective five year follow-up', *Journal of Neurology, Neurosurgery, and Psychiatry*, **40**, pp. 1211–9.

KLONOFF, H. and PARIS, R. (1974) 'Immediate, short-term and residual effects of acute head injuries in children: Neuropsychological and neurological correlates', in REITAN, R. M. and DAVISON, L. A. (Eds) *Clinical Neuropsychology: Current Status and Applications*, Washington, DC, Winston, pp. 179–210.

KLONOFF, H. and THOMPSON, G. B. (1969) 'Epidemiology of head injuries in adults: A pilot study', *Canadian Medical Association Journal*, **100**, pp. 235–41.

KLØVE, H. and CLEELAND, C. S. (1972) 'The relationship of neuropsychological impairment to other indices of severity of head injury', *Scandinavian Journal of Rehabilitation Medicine*, **4**, pp. 55–60.

KNILL-JONES, R. (1975) 'Recovery curves', in *Outcome of Severe Damage to the Nervous System*, Ciba Foundation Symposium 34 (new series), Amsterdam, Elsevier/Excerpta Medica/North-Holland, pp. 330–1.

KOCH-HENRIKSEN, N. and NIELSEN, H. (1981) 'Vasopressin in post-traumatic amnesia', *Lancet*, **1**, pp. 38–9.

KOLLEVOLD, T. (1976) 'Immediate and early cerebral seizures after head injuries: Part I', *Journal of the Oslo City Hospitals*, **26**, pp. 99–114.

(1978) 'Immediate and early cerebral seizures after head injuries: Part III', *Journal of the Oslo City Hospitals*, **28**, pp. 77–86.

(1979) 'Immediate and early cerebral seizures after head injuries: Part IV', *Journal of the Oslo City Hospitals*, **29**, pp. 35–47.

KOPANIKY, D. R. and WAGNER, K. A. (1987) 'Incidence of combined head and spinal cord injury and potential for errors in diagnosis', in MINER, M. E. and WAGNER, K. A. (Eds) *Neurotrauma: Treatment, Rehabilitation, and Related Issues, No. 2*, Boston, MA, Butterworths, pp. 103–12.

KOPELMAN, M. D. (1986) 'The cholinergic neurotransmitter system in human memory and dementia: A review', *Quarterly Journal of Experimental Psychology*, **38A**, pp. 535–73.

KOZOL, H. L. (1945) 'Pretraumatic personality and psychiatric sequelae of head injury: I. Categorical pretraumatic personality status correlated with general psychiatric reaction to head injury based on analysis of two hundred cases', *Archives of Neurology and Psychiatry*, **53**, pp. 358–64.

(1946) 'Pretraumatic personality and psychiatric sequelae of head injury: II. Correlation of multiple, specific factors in the pretraumatic personality and psychiatric reaction to head injury, based on analysis of one hundred and one cases', *Archives of Neurology and Psychiatry*, **56**, pp. 245–75.

KRAUS, J. F. (1978) 'Epidemiologic features of head and spinal cord injury', *Advances in Neurology*, **19**, pp. 261–78.

(1980) 'Injury to the head and spinal cord: The epidemiological relevance of the medical literature published from 1960 to 1978', *Journal of Neurosurgery*, **53**, pp. S3–10.

KRAUS, J. F., BLACK, M. A., HESSOL, N., LEY, P., ROKAW, W., SULLIVAN, C., BOWERS, S., KNOWLTON, S. and MARSHALL, L. (1984) 'The incidence of acute brain injury and serious impairment in a defined population', *American Journal of Epidemiology*, **119**, 186–201.

LAMPERT, P. W. and HARDMAN, J. M. (1984) 'Morphological changes in brains of boxers', *Journal of the American Medical Association*, **251**, pp. 2676–9.

LANDESMAN, S. and COOPER, P. R. (1982) 'Infectious complications of head injury', in COOPER, P. R. (Ed.) *Head Injury*, Baltimore, MD, Williams and Wilkins, pp. 343–62.

LANDY, P. J. (1968) 'The post-traumatic syndrome in closed head injuries accident neurosis', *Proceedings of the Australian Association of Neurologists*, **5**, pp. 463–6.

LANGFITT, T. W. and GENNARELLI, T. A. (1982) 'A holistic view of head injury including a new clinical classification', in GROSSMAN, R. G. and GILDENBERG, P. L. (Eds) *Head Injury: Basic and Clinical Aspects*, New York, Raven Press, pp. 1–14.

LARRABEE, G. J. (1987) 'Further cautions in interpretation of comparisons between the WAIS–R and the Wechsler Memory Scale', *Journal of Clinical and Experimental Neuropsychology*, **9**, pp. 456–60.

LEE, K. F., WAGNER, L. K. and KOPANIKY, D. R. (1987) 'Protective effect of facial fractures on closed head injuries', in MINER, M. E. and WAGNER, K. A. (Eds) *Neurotrauma: Treatment, Rehabilitation, and Related Issues, No. 2*, Boston, MA, Butterworths, pp. 15–29.

LEVENTHAL, B. L. and MIDELFORT, H. B. (1986) 'The physical abuse of children: A hurt greater than pain', in PETERSON, L. G. and O'SHANICK, G. J. (Eds) *Psychiatric Aspects of Trauma (Advances in Psychosomatic Medicine, Vol. 16)*, Basel, Karger, pp. 48–83.

LEVIN, H. S. (1981) 'Aphasia in closed head injury', in SARNO, M. T. (Ed.) *Acquired Aphasia*, New York, Academic Press, pp. 427–63.

LEVIN, H. S., AMPARO, E., EISENBERG, H. M., WILLIAMS, D. H., HIGH, W. M., Jr., MCARDLE, C. B. and WEINER, R. L. (1987a) 'Magnetic resonance imaging and computerized tomography in relation to the neurobehavioral sequelae of mild and moderate head injuries', *Journal of Neurosurgery*, **66**, pp. 706–13.

LEVIN, H. S., BENTON, A. L. and GROSSMAN, R. G. (1982a) *Neurobehavioral Consequences of Closed Head Injury*, New York, Oxford University Press.

LEVIN, H. S. and EISENBERG, H. M. (1979a) 'Neuropsychological impairment after closed head injury in children and adolescents', *Journal of Pediatric Psychology*, **4**, pp. 389–402.

(1979b) 'Neuropsychological outcome of closed head injury in children and adolescents', *Child's Brain*, **5**, pp. 281–92.

(1986) 'The relative durations of coma and post-traumatic amnesia after severe nonmissile head injury: Findings from the pilot phase of the National Traumatic Coma Data Bank', in MINER, M. E. and WAGNER, K. A. (Eds) *Neurotrauma: Treatment, Rehabilitation, and Related Issues, No. 1*, Boston, MA, Butterworths, pp. 89–97.

LEVIN, H. S., EISENBERG, H. M., WIGG, N. R. and KOBAYASHI, K. (1982b) 'Memory and intellectual ability after head injury in children and adolescents', *Neurosurgery*, **11**, pp. 668–73.

LEVIN, H. S., GARY, H. E., Jr. and EISENBERG, H. M. (1989) 'Duration of impaired consciousness in relation to side of lesion after severe head injury', *Lancet*, **1**, pp. 1001–3.

LEVIN, H. S., GARY, H. E., Jr., HIGH, W. M., Jr., MATTIS, S., RUFF, R. M., EISENBERG, H. M., MARSHALL, L. F. and TABADDOR, K. (1987b) 'Minor head injury and the post-concussional syndrome: Methodological issues in outcome studies', in LEVIN, H. S., GRAFMAN, J. and EISENBERG, H. M. (Eds) *Neurobehavioral Recovery from Head Injury*, New York, Oxford University Press, pp. 262–75.

LEVIN, H. S. and GOLDSTEIN, F. C. (1986) 'Organization of verbal memory after severe closed-head injury', *Journal of Clinical and Experimental Neuropsychology*, **8**, pp. 643–56.

LEVIN, H. S. and GROSSMAN, R. G. (1978) 'Behavioral sequelae of closed head injury: A quantitative study', *Archives of Neurology*, **35**, pp. 720–7.

LEVIN, H. S., GROSSMAN, R. G. and KELLY, P. J. (1976a) 'Aphasic disorder in patients with closed head injury', *Journal of Neurology, Neurosurgery, and Psychiatry*, **39**, pp. 1062–70.

(1976b) 'Short-term recognition memory in relation to severity of head injury', *Cortex*, **12**, pp. 175–82.

(1977a) 'Assessment of long-term memory in brain-damaged patients', *Journal of Consulting and Clinical Psychology*, **45**, pp. 684–8.

(1977b) 'Impairment of facial recognition after closed head injuries of varying severity', *Cortex*, **13**, pp. 119–30.

LEVIN, H. S., GROSSMAN, R. G., ROSE, J. E. and TEASDALE, G. (1979a) 'Long-term neuropsychological outcome of closed head injury', *Journal of Neurosurgery*, **50**, pp. 412–22.

LEVIN, H. S., GROSSMAN, R. G., SARWAR, M. and MEYERS, C. A. (1981a) 'Linguistic recovery after closed head injury', *Brain and Language*, **12**, pp. 360–74.

LEVIN, H. S., HANDEL, S. F., GOLDMAN, A. M., EISENBERG, H. M. and GUINTO, F. C., Jr. (1985a) 'Magnetic resonance imaging after "diffuse" nonmissile head injury: A neurobehavioral study', *Archives of Neurology*, **42**, pp. 963–8.

LEVIN, H. S., HIGH, W. M., Jr., EWING-COBBS, L., FLETCHER, J. M., EISENBERG, H. M., MINER, M. E. and GOLDSTEIN, F. C. (1988a) 'Memory functioning during the first year after closed head injury in children and adolescents', *Neurosurgery*, **22**, pp. 1043–52.

LEVIN, H. S., HIGH, W. M., MEYERS, C. A., VON LAUFEN, A., HAYDEN, M. E. and EISENBERG, H. M. (1985b) 'Impairment of remote memory after closed head injury', *Journal of Neurology, Neurosurgery, and Psychiatry*, **48**, pp. 556–63.

LEVIN, H. S., KALISKY, Z., HANDEL, S. F., GOLDMAN, A. M., EISENBERG, H. M., MORRISON, D. and VON LAUFEN, A. (1985c) 'Magnetic resonance imaging in relation to the sequelae and rehabilitation of diffuse closed head injury: Preliminary findings', *Seminars in Neurology*, **5**, pp. 221–32.

LEVIN, H. S., MATTIS, S., RUFF, R. M., EISENBERG, H. M., MARSHALL, L. F., TABADDOR, K., HIGH, W. M., Jr. and FRANKOWSKI, R. F. (1987c) 'Neurobehavioral outcome following minor head injury: A three-center study', *Journal of Neurosurgery*, **66**, pp. 234–43.

LEVIN, H. S., MEYERS, C. A., GROSSMAN, R. G. and SARWAR, M. (1981b) 'Ventricular enlargement after closed head injury', *Archives of Neurology*, **38**, pp. 623–9.

LEVIN, H. S., O'DONNELL, V. M. and GROSSMAN, R. G. (1979b) 'The Galveston Orientation and Amnesia Test: A practical scale to assess cognition after head injury', *Journal of Nervous and Mental Disease*, **167**, pp. 675–84.

LEVIN, H. S., PAPANICOLAOU, A. and EISENBERG, H. M. (1984) 'Observations on amnesia after nonmissile head injury', in SQUIRE, L. R. and BUTTERS, N. (Eds) *Neuropsychology of Memory*, New York, Guilford Press, pp. 247–57.

LEVIN, H. S. and PETERS, B. H. (1976) 'Neuropsychological testing following head injuries: Prosopagnosia without visual field defect', *Diseases of the Nervous System*, **37**, pp. 68–71.

LEVIN, H. S., WILLIAMS, D., CROFFORD, M. J., HIGH, W. M., Jr., EISENBERG, H. M., AMPARO, E. G., GUINTO, F. C., Jr., KALISKY, Z., HANDEL, S. F. and GOODMAN, A. M. (1988b) 'Relationship of depth of brain lesions to consciousness and outcome after closed head injury', *Journal of Neurosurgery*, **69**, pp. 861–6.

LEVY, D. E., BATES, D., CARONNA, J. J., CARTLIDGE, N. E. F., KNILL-JONES, R. P., LAPINSKI, R. H., SINGER, B. H., SHAW, D. A. and PLUM, F. (1981) 'Prognosis in nontraumatic coma', *Annals of Internal Medicine*, **94**, pp. 293–301.

LEVY, P. (1968) 'Short-form tests: A methodological review', *Psychological Bulletin*, **69**, pp. 410–6.

LEWIN, W. (1970) 'Rehabilitation needs of the brain-damaged patient', *Proceedings of the Royal Society of Medicine*, **63**, pp. 8–12.

LEWIN, W., MARSHALL, T. F. DE C. and ROBERTS, A. H. (1979) 'Long-term outcome after severe head injury', *British Medical Journal*, **2**, pp. 1533–8.

LEWIS, A. (1942) 'Discussion on differential diagnosis and treatment of post-contusional states', *Proceedings of the Royal Society of Medicine*, **35**, pp. 607–14.

LEZAK, M. D. (1978) 'Living with the characterologically altered brain injured patient', *Journal of Clinical Psychiatry*, **39**, pp. 592–8.

　　(1979) 'Recovery of memory and learning functions following traumatic brain injury', *Cortex*, **15**, pp. 63–72.

　　(1982) 'The problem of assessing executive functions', *International Journal of Psychology*, **17**, pp. 281–97.

　　(1984) 'An individualized approach to neuropsychological assessment', in LOGUE, P. E. and SCHEAR, J. M. (Eds) *Clinical Neuropsychology: A Multidisciplinary Approach*, Springfield, IL, Thomas, pp. 29–49.

(1987) 'Making neuropsychological assessment relevant to head injury', in LEVIN, H. S., GRAFMAN, J. and EISENBERG, H. M. (Eds) *Neurobehavioral Recovery from Head Injury*, New York, Oxford University Press, pp. 116–28.

LIDVALL, H. F., LINDEROTH, B. and NORLIN, B. (1974) 'Causes of the post-concussional syndrome', *Acta Neurologica Scandinavica*, **50**, Suppl. 56.

LIEBERT, R. M. and MORRIS, L. W. (1967) 'Cognitive and emotional components of test anxiety: A distinction and some initial data', *Psychological Reports*, **20**, pp. 975–8.

LINDENBERG, R. and FREYTAG, E. (1960) 'The mechanism of cerebral contusions', *Archives of Pathology and Laboratory Medicine*, **69**, pp. 440–69.

(1969) 'Morphology of brain lesions from blunt trauma in early infancy', *Archives of Pathology*, **87**, pp. 298–305.

LINDSAY, K. W., MCLATCHIE, G. and JENNETT, B. (1980) 'Serious head injury in sport', *British Medical Journal*, **281**, pp. 789–91.

LISHMAN, W. A. (1968) 'Brain damage in relation to psychiatric disability after head injury', *British Journal of Psychiatry*, **114**, pp. 373–410.

(1973) 'The psychiatric sequelae of head injury: A review', *Psychological Medicine*, **3**, pp. 304–18.

LIVINGSTON, M. G. (1985) 'Families who care', *British Medical Journal*, **2**, pp. 919–20.

(1986) 'Assessment of need for coordinated approach in families with victims of head injury', *British Medical Journal*, **293**, pp. 742–4.

(1987) 'Head injury: The relatives' response', *Brain Injury*, **1**, pp. 33–9.

LIVINGSTON, M. G. and BROOKS, D. N. (1988) 'The burden on families of the brain injured: A review', *Journal of Head Trauma Rehabilitation*, **3**, 4, pp. 6–15.

LIVINGSTON, M. G., BROOKS, D. N. and BOND, M. R. (1985a) 'Patient outcome in the year following severe head injury and relatives' psychiatric and social functioning', *Journal of Neurology, Neurosurgery, and Psychiatry*, **48**, pp. 876–81.

(1985b) 'Three months after severe head injury: Psychiatric and social impact on relatives', *Journal of Neurology, Neurosurgery, and Psychiatry*, **48**, pp. 870–5.

LIVINGSTON, M. G. and LIVINGSTON, H. M. (1985) 'The Glasgow Assessment Schedule: Clinical and research assessment of head injury outcome', *International Rehabilitation Medicine*, **7**, pp. 145–9.

LONDON, P. S. (1967) 'Some observations on the course of events after severe injury of the head', *Annals of the Royal College of Surgeons of England*, **41**, pp. 460–79.

LONG, C. J. and NOVACK, T. A. (1986) 'Post-concussion symptoms after head trauma: Interpretation and treatment', *Southern Medical Journal*, **79**, pp. 728–32.

LONG, C. S. and WEBB, W. L., Jr. (1983) 'Psychological sequelae of head trauma', *Psychiatric Medicine*, **1**, pp. 35–77.

LORING, D. W. and PAPANICOLAOU, A. C. (1987) 'Memory assessment in neuropsychology: Theoretical considerations and practical utility', *Journal of Clinical and Experimental Neuropsychology*, **9**, pp. 340–58.

LUNDHOLM, J., JEPSEN, B. N. and THORNVAL, G. (1975) 'The late neurological, psychological, and social aspects of severe traumatic coma', *Scandinavian Journal of Rehabilitation Medicine*, **7**, pp. 97–100.

LURIA, A. R. (1963) *Restoration of Function after Brain Injury*, Oxford, Pergamon.

LURIA, A. R., NAYDIN, V. L., TSVETKOVA, L. S. and VINARSKAYA, E. N. (1969) 'Restoration of higher cortical function following local brain damage', in VINKEN, P. J. and BRUYN, G. W. (Eds) *Handbook of Clinical Neurology*, Vol. 3, *Disorders of Higher Nervous Activity*, Amsterdam, North–Holland, pp. 368–433.

LYNCH, S. and YARNELL, P. R. (1973) 'Retrograde amnesia: Delayed forgetting after concussion', *American Journal of Psychology*, **86**, pp. 643–5.

McFIE, J. (1975) *Assessment of Organic Intellectual Impairment*, London, Academic Press.

MACFLYNN, G., MONTGOMERY, E. A., FENTON, G. W. and RUTHERFORD, W. (1984) 'Measurement of reaction time following minor head injury', *Journal of Neurology, Neurosurgery, and Psychiatry*, **47**, pp. 1326–31.

McGEER, P. L. (1984) 'Aging, Alzheimer's disease, and the cholinergic system', *Canadian Journal of Physiology and Pharmacology*, **62**, pp. 741–54.

McGUIRE, T. L. and SYLVESTER, C. E. (1987) 'Neuropsychiatric evaluation and treatment of children with head injury', *Journal of Learning Disabilities*, **20**, pp. 590–5.

MACIVER, I. N., LASSMAN, L. P., THOMSON, C. W. and McLEOD, I. (1958) 'Treatment of severe head injuries', *Lancet*, **2**, pp. 544–50.

McKINLAY, W. W. and BROOKS, D. N. (1984) 'Methodological problems in assessing psychosocial recovery following severe head injury', *Journal of Clinical Neuropsychology*, **6**, pp. 87–99.

McKINLAY, W. W., BROOKS, D. N. and BOND, M. R. (1983) 'Post-concussional symptoms, financial compensation and outcome of severe blunt head injury', *Journal of Neurology, Neurosurgery, and Psychiatry*, **46**, pp. 1084–91.

McKINLAY, W. W., BROOKS, D. N., BOND, M. R., MARTINAGE, D. P. and MARSHALL, M. M. (1981) 'The short-term outcome of severe blunt head injury as reported by relatives of the injured persons', *Journal of Neurology, Neurosurgery, and Psychiatry*, **44**, pp. 527–33.

McLATCHIE, G., BROOKS, N., GALBRAITH, S., HUTCHISON, J. S. F., WILSON, L., MELVILLE, I. and TEASDALE, E. (1987) 'Clinical neurological examination, neuropsychology, electroencephalography and computed tomographic head scanning in active amateur boxers', *Journal of Neurology, Neurosurgery, and Psychiatry*, **50**, pp. 96–9.

McLEAN, A., Jr., TEMKIN, N. R., DIKMEN, S. and WYLER, A. R. (1983) 'The behavioral sequelae of head injury', *Journal of Clinical Neuropsychology*, **5**, pp. 361–76.

McMILLAN, T. M. and GLUCKSMAN, E. E. (1987) 'The neuropsychology of moderate head injury', *Journal of Neurology, Neurosurgery, and Psychiatry*, **50**, pp. 393–7.

MACPHERSON, P. and GRAHAM, D. I. (1978) 'Correlations between angiographic findings and the ischaemia of head injury', *Journal of Neurology, Neurosurgery, and Psychiatry*, **41**, pp. 122–7.

MAKELA, M. E., FRANKOWSKI, R., GILDENBERG, P. L., GROSSMAN, R. G. and WAGNER, K. A. (1982) 'Comparison of head injury outcome rates at two adjacent hospitals', in GROSSMAN, R. G. and GILDENBERG, P. L. (Eds) *Head Injury: Basic and Clinical Aspects*, New York, Raven Press, pp. 203–12.

MALKMUS, D. (1983) 'Integrating cognitive strategies into the physical therapy setting', *Physical Therapy*, **63**, pp. 1952–9.

MANDLEBERG, I. A. (1975) 'Cognitive recovery after severe head injury: 2. Wechsler Adult Intelligence Scale during post-traumatic amnesia', *Journal of Neurology, Neurosurgery, and Psychiatry*, **38**, pp. 1127–32.

    (1976) 'Cognitive recovery after severe head injury: 3. WAIS Verbal and Performance IQs as a function of post-traumatic amnesia duration and time from injury', *Journal of Neurology, Neurosurgery, and Psychiatry*, **39**, pp. 1001–7.

MANDLEBERG, I. A. and BROOKS, D. N. (1975) 'Cognitive recovery after severe head injury: 1. Serial testing on the Wechsler Adult Intelligence Scale', *Journal of Neurology, Neurosurgery, and Psychiatry*, **38**, pp. 1121–6.

MANDLER, G. (1980) 'Recognizing: The judgment of previous occurrence', *Psychological Review*, **87**, pp. 252–71.

MARSCHARK, M. and HUNT, R. R. (1989) 'A re-examination of the role of imagery in learning and memory', *Journal of Experimental Psychology: Learning, Memory, and Cognition*, **15**, pp. 710–20.

MARSCHARK, M., RICHMAN, C. L., YUILLE, J. C. and HUNT, R. R. (1987) 'The role of imagery in memory: On shared and distinctive information', *Psychological Bulletin*, **102**, pp. 28–41.

MARSCHARK, M. and SURIAN, L. (1989) 'Why does imagery improve memory?' *European Journal of Cognitive Psychology*, **1**, 251–63.

MARSHALL, L. F., BECKER, D. P., BOWERS, S. A., CAYARD, C., EISENBERG, H., GROSS, C. R., GROSSMAN, R. G., JANE, J. A., KUNITZ, S. C., RIMEL, R., TABADDOR, K. and WARREN, J. (1983a) 'The National Traumatic Coma Data Bank. Part 1: Design, purpose, goals, and results', *Journal of Neurosurgery*, **59**, pp. 276–84.

MARSHALL, L. F. and BOWERS, S. A. (1985) 'Outcome prediction in severe head injury', in WILKINS, R. H. and RENGACHARY, S. S. (Eds) *Neurosurgery*, New York, McGraw-Hill, pp. 1605–8.

MARSHALL, L. F., TOOLE, B. M. and BOWERS, S. A. (1983b) 'The National Traumatic Coma Data Bank. Part 2: Patients who talk and deteriorate: Implications for treatment', *Journal of Neurosurgery*, **59**, pp. 285–8.

MARTIN, G. (1974) *A Manual of Head Injuries in General Surgery*, London, Heinemann.

MAXWELL, A. E. (1960) 'Obtaining factor scores on the Wechsler Adult Intelligence Scale', *Journal of Mental Science*, **106**, pp. 1060–2.

MAXWELL, E. (1957) 'Validities of abbreviated WAIS scales', *Journal of Consulting Psychology*, **21**, pp. 121–6.

MAXWELL, W. L., KANSAGRA, A. M., GRAHAM, D. I., ADAMS, J. H. and GENNARELLI, T. A. (1988) 'Freeze-fracture studies of reactive myelinated nerve fibres after diffuse axonal injury', *Acta Neuropathologica*, **76**, pp. 395–406.

MERSKEY, H. and WOODFORDE, J. M. (1972) 'Psychiatric sequelae of minor head injury', *Brain*, **95**, pp. 521–8.

MESSICK, S. (1965) 'The impact of negative affect on cognition and personality', in TOMKINS, S. S. and IZARD, C. E. (Eds) *Affect, Cognition, and Personality: Empirical Studies*, New York, Springer, pp. 98–128.

MEYER, A. (1904) 'The anatomical facts and clinical varieties of traumatic insanity', *American Journal of Insanity*, **60**, pp. 373–441.

MILBERG, W. P., HEBBEN, N. and KAPLAN, E. (1986) 'The Boston Process Approach to neuropsychological assessment', in GRANT, I. and ADAMS, K. H. (Eds) *Neuropsychological Assessment of Neuropsychiatric Disorders*, New York, Oxford University Press, pp. 65–86.

MILLER, E. (1970) 'Simple and choice reaction time following severe head injury', *Cortex*, **6**, pp. 121–7.

(1979) 'The long-term consequences of head injury: A discussion of the evidence with special reference to the preparation of legal reports', *British Journal of Social and Clinical Psychology*, **18**, pp. 87–98.

(1980) 'The training characteristics of severely head-injured patients: A preliminary study', *Journal of Neurology, Neurosurgery, and Psychiatry*, **43**, pp. 525–8.

MILLER, E. and CRUZAT, A. (1981) 'A note on the effects of irrelevant information on task performance after mild and severe head injury', *British Journal of Clinical Psychology*, **20**, pp. 69–70.

MILLER, H. (1961a) 'Accident neurosis: Lecture I', *British Medical Journal*, **1**, pp. 919–25.

(1961b) 'Accident neurosis: Lecture II', *British Medical Journal*, **1**, pp. 992–8.

(1966) 'Mental after-effects of head injury', *Proceedings of the Royal Society of Medicine*, **59**, pp. 257–61.

MILLER, H. and CARTLIDGE, N. (1972) 'Simulation and malingering after injuries to the brain and spinal cord', *Lancet*, **1**, pp. 580–5.

MILLER, H. and STERN, G. (1965) 'The long-term prognosis of severe head injury', *Lancet*, **1**, pp. 225–9.

MILOS, R. (1975) 'Hypnotic exploration of amnesia after cerebral injuries', *International Journal of Clinical and Experimental Hypnosis*, **23**, pp. 103–10.

MILTON, S. B. and WERTZ, R. T. (1986) 'Management of persisting communication deficits in patients with traumatic brain injury', in UZZELL, B. P. and GROSS, Y. (Eds) *Clinical Neuropsychology of Intervention*, Boston, Martinus Nijhoff, pp. 223–56.

MINDERHOUD, J. M., BOELENS, M. E. M., HUIZENGA, J. and SAAN, R. J. (1980) 'Treatment of minor head injuries', *Clinical Neurology and Neurosurgery*, **82**, pp. 127–40.

MINER, M. E., FLETCHER, J. M. and EWING-COBBS, L. (1986) 'Recovery versus outcome after head injury in children', in MINER, M. E. and WAGNER, K. A. (Eds) *Neurotrauma: Treatment, Rehabilitation, and Related Issues, No. 1*, Boston, MA, Butterworths, pp. 223–40.

MITCHELL, D. E. and ADAMS, J. H. (1973) 'Primary focal impact damage to the brainstem in blunt head injuries: Does it exist?' *Lancet*, **2**, pp. 215–8.

MOFFAT, N. (1984) 'Strategies of memory therapy', in WILSON, B. A. and MOFFAT, N. (Eds) *Clinical Management of Memory Problems*, London, Croom Helm, pp. 63–88.

MONTGOMERY, A., FENTON, G. W. and McCLELLAND, R. J. (1984) 'Delayed brainstem conduction time in post-concussional syndrome', *Lancet*, **1**, p. 1011.

MOORE, B. E. and RUESCH, J. (1944) 'Prolonged disturbances of consciousness following head injury', *The New England Journal of Medicine*, **230**, pp. 445–52.

MORRIS, L. W. and LIEBERT, R. M. (1970) 'Relationship of cognitive and emotional components of test anxiety to physiological arousal and academic performance', *Journal of Consulting and Clinical Psychology*, **35**, pp. 332–7.

NAJENSON, T., GROSWASSER, Z., STERN, M., SCHECHTER, I., DAVIV, C., BERGHAUS, N. and MENDELSON, L. (1975) 'Prognostic factors in rehabilitation after severe head injury', *Scandinavian Journal of Rehabilitation Medicine*, **7**, pp. 101–5.

NAJENSON, T., SAZBON, L., FISELZON, J., BECKER, E. and SCHECHTER, I. (1978) 'Recovery of communicative functions after prolonged traumatic coma', *Scandinavian Journal of Rehabilitation Medicine*, **10**, pp. 15–21.

NATIONAL CENTER FOR HEALTH STATISTICS (1984) 'Multiple causes of death in the United States' (*Monthly Vital Statistics Report*, Vol. 32, No. 10, Supp. 2), DHHS Pub. No. (PHS) 84–1120, Hyattsville, MD, Public Health Service.

NATIONAL CENTER FOR HEALTH STATISTICS (1988a) 'Current estimates from the National Health Interview Survey, United States, 1987' (*Vital and Health Statistics*, Series 10, No. 166), DHHS Pub. No. (PHS) 88–1594, Washington, DC, US Government Printing Office.

(1988b) *Vital Statistics of the United States, 1988. Vol. II: Mortality, Part A.* DHHS Pub. No. (PHS) 88–1122, Washington, DC, US Government Printing Office.

NELSON, H. E. (1976) 'A modified card sorting test sensitive to frontal lobe defects', *Cortex*, **12**, pp. 313–24.

NELSON, H. E. and MCKENNA, P. (1975) 'The use of current reading ability in the assessment of dementia', *British Journal of Social and Clinical Psychology*, **14**, pp. 259–67.

NELSON, H. E. and O'CONNELL, A. (1978) 'Dementia: The estimation of premorbid intelligence levels using the New Adult Reading Test', *Cortex*, **14**, pp. 234–44.

NEVIN, N. C. (1967) 'Neuropathological changes in the white matter following head injury', *Journal of Neuropathology and Experimental Neurology*, **26**, pp. 77–84.

NEWCOMBE, F. (1969) *Missile Wounds of the Brain: A Study of Psychological Deficits*, London, Oxford University Press.

(1982) 'The psychological consequences of closed head injury: Assessment and rehabilitation', *Injury*, **14**, pp. 111–36.

NEWCOMBE, F. and ARTIOLA I FORTUNY, L. (1979) 'Problems and perspectives in the evaluation of psychological deficits after cerebral lesions', *International Rehabilitation Medicine*, **1**, pp. 182–92.

NEWCOMBE, F., BROOKS, N. and BADDELEY, A. (1980) 'Rehabilitation after brain damage: An overview', *International Rehabilitation Medicine*, **2**, pp. 133–37.

NEWCOMBE, F., HIORNS, R. W., MARSHALL, J. C. and ADAMS, C. B. T. (1975a) 'Acquired dyslexia: Patterns of deficit and recovery', in *Outcome of Severe Damage to the Central Nervous System*, Ciba Foundation Symposium No. 34 (new series), Amsterdam, Elsevier/Excerpta Medica/North–Holland, pp. 227–44.

NEWCOMBE, F., MARSHALL, J. C., CARRIVICK, P. J. and HIORNS, R. W. (1975b) 'Recovery curves in acquired dyslexia', *Journal of the Neurological Sciences*, **24**, pp. 127–33.

NORRMAN, B. and SVAHN, K. (1961) 'A follow-up study of severe brain injuries', *Acta Psychiatrica Scandinavica*, **37**, pp. 236–64.

NOSEWORTHY, J. H., MILLER, J., MURRAY, T. J. and REGAN, D. (1981) 'Auditory brainstem responses in post-concussion syndrome', *Archives of Neurology*, **38**, pp. 275–8.

OBRZUT, J. E. and HYND, G. W. (1987) 'Cognitive dysfunction and psychoeducational assessment in individuals with acquired brain injury', *Journal of Learning Disabilities*, **20**, pp. 596–602.

ODDY, M. (1984a) 'Head injury and social adjustment', in BROOKS, N. (Ed.) *Closed Head Injury: Psychological, Social, and Family Consequences*, Oxford, Oxford University Press, pp. 108–22.

(1984b) 'Head injury during childhood: The psychological implications', in BROOKS, N. (Ed.) *Closed Head Injury: Psychological, Social, and Family Consequences*, Oxford, Oxford University Press, pp. 179–94.

ODDY, M. and HUMPHREY, M. (1980) 'Social recovery during the year following severe head injury', *Journal of Neurology, Neurosurgery, and Psychiatry*, **43**, pp. 798–802.

ODDY, M., HUMPHREY, M. and UTTLEY, D. (1978a) 'Stresses upon the relatives of head-injured patients', *British Journal of Psychiatry*, **133**, pp. 507–13.

(1978b) 'Subjective impairment and social recovery after closed head injury', *Journal of Neurology, Neurosurgery, and Psychiatry*, **41**, pp. 611–6.

OFFICE OF POPULATION CENSUSES AND SURVEYS (1976–87) *Hospital In-patient Enquiry 1974–1985* (Series MB4, Nos. 1–27), London, Her Majesty's Stationery Office.

(1980–88) *Mortality Statistics 1979–1986: Cause* (Series DH2, Nos. 6–13), London, Her Majesty's Stationery Office.

OLIVEROS, J. C., JANDALI, M. K., TIMSIT-BERTHIER, M., REMY, R., BENGHEZAL, A., AUDIBERT, A. and MOEGLEN, J. M. (1978) 'Vasopressin in amnesia', *Lancet*, **1**, pp. 41–2.

OMMAYA, A. K., FAAS, F. and YARNELL, P. (1968) 'Whiplash injury and brain damage: An experimental study', *Journal of the American Medical Association*, **204**, pp. 285–9.

OMMAYA, A. K., GELLER, A. and PARSONS, L. C. (1971a) 'The effect of experimental head injury on one-trial learning in rats', *International Journal of Neuroscience*, **1**, pp. 371–8.

OMMAYA, A. K., and GENNARELLI, T. A. (1974) 'Cerebral concussion and traumatic unconsciousness: Correlation of experimental and clinical observations on blunt head injuries', *Brain*, **97**, pp. 633–54.

(1976) 'A physiopathologic basis for noninvasive diagnosis and prognosis of head injury severity', in MCLAURIN, R. L. (Ed.) *Head Injuries: Proceedings of the Second Chicago Symposium on Neural Trauma*, New York, Grune and Stratton, pp. 49–75.

OMMAYA, A. K., GRUBB, R. L., Jr. and NAUMANN, R. A. (1971b) 'Coup and contrecoup injury: Observations on the mechanics of visible brain injuries in the rhesus monkey', *Journal of Neurosurgery*, **35**, pp. 503–16.

OMMAYA, A. K. and HIRSCH, A. E. (1971) 'Tolerances for cerebral concussion from head impact and whiplash in primates', *Journal of Biomechanics*, **4**, pp. 13–21.

OMMAYA, A. K., HIRSCH, A. E., FLAMM, E. S. and MAHONE, R. H. (1966) 'Cerebral concussion in the monkey: An experimental model', *Science*, **153**, pp. 211–2.

OMMAYA, A. K. and YARNELL, P. (1969) 'Subdural haematoma after whiplash injury', *Lancet*, **2**, pp. 237–9.

OPPENHEIMER, D. R. (1968) 'Microscopic lesions in the brain following head injury', *Journal of Neurology, Neurosurgery, and Psychiatry*, **31**, pp. 299–306.

ORNE, M. T., SOSKIS, D. A., DINGES, D. F. and ORNE, E. C. (1984) 'Hypnotically induced testimony', in WELLS, G. L. and LOFTUS, E. F. (Eds) *Eyewitness Testimony: Psychological Perspectives*, Cambridge, Cambridge University Press, pp. 171–213.

O'SHANICK, G. J. (1986) 'Neuropsychiatric complications in head injury', in PETERSON, L. G. and O'SHANICK, G. J. (Eds) *Psychiatric Aspects of Trauma (Advances in Psychosomatic Medicine*, Vol. 16), Basel, Karger, pp. 173–93.

OSTROWSKI, A. (1968) *Differential and Integral Calculus*, (trans. ed. CROWE, D. E.), Glenview, IL, Scott, Foresman.

OVERALL, J. E. and GORHAM, D. R. (1962) 'The Brief Psychiatric Rating Scale', *Psychological Reports*, **10**, pp. 799–812.

OVERGAARD, J., CHRISTENSEN, S., HVID-HANSEN, O., HAASE, J., LAND, A. -M., HEIN, O., PEDERSEN, K. K. and TWEED, W. A. (1973) 'Prognosis after head injury based on early clinical examination', *Lancet*, **2**, pp. 631–5.

OWEN-SMITH, M. S. (1981) *High Velocity Missile Wounds*, London, Edward Arnold.

PAIVIO, A. (1971) *Imagery and Verbal Processes*, New York, Holt, Rinehart and Winston.

PANTING, A. and MERRY, P. (1972) 'The long-term rehabilitation of severe head injuries with particular reference to the need for social and medical support for the patient's family', *Rehabilitation*, **38**, pp. 33–7.

PAPANICOLAOU, A. C., LEVIN, H. S., EISENBERG, H. M., MOORE, B. D., GOETHE, K. E. and HIGH, W. M., Jr. (1984) 'Evoked potential correlates of post-traumatic amnesia after closed head injury', *Neurosurgery*, **14**, pp. 676–8.

PARKER, S. A. and SERRATS, A. F. (1976) 'Memory recovery after traumatic coma', *Acta Neurochirurgica*, **34**, pp. 71–7.

PARKINSON, D. (1977) 'Concussion', *Mayo Clinic Proceedings*, **52**, pp. 492–6.

PARSONS, O. A. and PRIGATANO, G. P. (1978) 'Methodological considerations in clinical neuropsychological research', *Journal of Consulting and Clinical Psychology*, **46**, pp. 608–19.

PARTINGTON, M. W. (1960) 'The importance of accident-proneness in the aetiology of head injuries in childhood', *Archives of Diseases in Childhood*, **35**, pp. 215–23.

PAYNE-JOHNSON, J. C. (1986) 'Evaluation of communication competence in patients with closed head injury', *Journal of Communication Disorders*, **19**, pp. 237–49.

PAZZAGLIA, P., FRANK, G., FRANK, F. and GAIST, G. (1975) 'Clinical course and prognosis of acute post-traumatic coma', *Journal of Neurology, Neurosurgery, and Psychiatry*, **38**, pp. 149–54.

PECK, D. F. (1970) 'The conversion of Progressive Matrices and Mill Hill Vocabulary raw scores into deviation IQs', *Journal of Clinical Psychology*, **26**, pp. 67–70.

PERRONE, N. (1972) 'Biomechanical problems related to vehicle impact', in FUNG, Y. C., PERRONE, N. and ANLIKER, M. (Eds) *Biomechanics: Its Foundations and Objectives*, Englewood Cliffs, NJ, Prentice–Hall, pp. 567–83.

PETERSON, L. G. (1986) 'Acute response to trauma', in PETERSON, L. G. and O'SHANICK, G. J. (Eds) *Psychiatric Aspects of Trauma (Advances in Psychosomatic Medicine*, Vol. 16), Basel, Karger, pp. 84–92.

PLUM, F. and POSNER, J. B. (1980) *The Diagnosis of Stupor and Coma*, 3rd ed., Philadelphia, PA, Davis.

PRESSLEY, M., BORKOWSKI, J. G. and JOHNSON, C. J. (1987) 'The development of good strategy use: Imagery and related mnemonic strategies', in MCDANIEL, M. A. and PRESSLEY, M. (Eds) *Imagery and Related Mnemonic Processes: Theories, Individual Differences, and Applications*, New York, Springer–Verlag, pp. 274–97.

PRICE, D. J. E. and MURRAY, A. (1972) 'The influence of hypoxia and hypotension on recovery from head injury', *Injury*, **3**, pp. 218–24.

PRICE, J. R. (1987) 'Sexuality following traumatic brain injury', in MINER, M. E. and WAGNER, K. A. (Eds) *Neurotrauma: Treatment, Rehabilitation, and Related Issues, No. 2*, Boston, MA, Butterworths, pp. 173–80.

PRIFITERA, A. and BARLEY, W. D. (1985) 'Cautions in interpretation of comparisons between the WAIS–R and the Wechsler Memory Scale', *Journal of Consulting and Clinical Psychology*, **53**, pp. 564–5.

PRIFITERA, A. and RYAN, J. J. (1983) 'WAIS–R/WAIS comparisons in a clinical sample', *Clinical Neuropsychology*, **5**, pp. 97–9.

PRIGATANO, G. P. (1978) 'Wechsler Memory Scale: A selective review of the literature', *Journal of Clinical Psychology*, **34**, pp. 816–32.

PRIGATANO, G. P., FORDYCE, D. J., ZEINER, H. K., ROUECHE, J. R., PEPPING, M. and WOOD, B. C. (1984) 'Neuropsychological rehabilitation after closed head injury in young adults', *Journal of Neurology, Neurosurgery, and Psychiatry*, **47**, pp. 505–13.
(1986) *Neuropsychological Rehabilitation after Brain Injury*, Baltimore, MD, Johns Hopkins University Press.

PRITCHARD, W. S. (1981) 'Psychophysiology of P300', *Psychological Bulletin*, **89**, pp. 506–40.

PUBLIC HEALTH SERVICE AND HEALTH CARE FINANCING ADMINISTRATION (1980) *International Classification of Diseases, 9th Revision, Clinical Modification (ICD-9-CM)*. *Vol. 1. Diseases: Tabular List*, 2nd ed., DHHS Pub. No. (PHS) 80-1260, Washington, DC, US Government Printing Office.

PUDENZ, R. H. and SHELDEN, C. H. (1946) 'The lucite calvarium — a method for direct observation of the brain: II. Cranial trauma and brain movement', *Journal of Neurosurgery*, **3**, pp. 487–505.

QUERESCHI, M. Y. (1968) 'The comparability of WAIS and WISC subtest scores and *IQ* estimates', *Journal of Psychology*, **68**, pp. 73–82.

QUINE, S., PIERCE, J. P. and LYLE, D. M. (1988) 'Relatives as lay-therapists for the severely head-injured', *Brain Injury*, **2**, pp. 139–49.

RAGINSKY, B. B. (1969) 'Hypnotic recall of aircrash cause', *International Journal of Clinical and Experimental Hypnosis*, **17**, pp. 1–19.

RAVEN, J. C. (1960) *Guide to the Standard Progressive Matrices*, London, Lewis.
(1962) *Extended Guide to the Mill Hill Vocabulary Scales*, London, Lewis.

REGISTRAR GENERAL SCOTLAND (1987) *Annual Report 1986*, Edinburgh, Her Majesty's Stationery Office.

REILLY, E. L., KELLEY, J. T. and FAILLACE, L. A. (1986) 'Role of alcohol use and abuse in trauma', in PETERSON, L. G. and O'SHANICK, G. J. (Eds) *Psychiatric Aspects of Trauma* (*Advances in Psychosomatic Medicine*, Vol. 16), Basel, Karger, pp. 17–30.

REILLY, P. L., ADAMS, J. H., GRAHAM, D. I. and JENNETT, B. (1975) 'Patients with head injury who talk and die', *Lancet*, **2**, pp. 375–7.

REITAN, R. M. (1966) 'A research program on the phychological effects of brain lesions in human beings', in ELLIS, N. R. (Ed.) *International Review of Research in Mental Retardation*, Vol. 1, New York, Academic Press, pp. 153–218.

(1986) 'Theoretical and methodological bases of the Halstead–Reitan Neuropsychological Test Battery', in GRANT, I. and ADAMS, K. M. (Eds) *Neuropsychological Assessment of Neuropsychiatric Disorders*, New York, Oxford University Press, pp. 3–30.

REITAN, R. M. and DAVISON, L. A. (Eds) (1974) *Clinical Neuropsychology: Current Status and Applications*, Washington, DC, Winston.

RELANDER, M., TROUPP, H. and BJÖRKESTEN, G. AF (1972) 'Controlled trial of treatment for cerebral concussion', *British Medical Journal*, **4**, pp. 777–9.

REYNELL, W. R. (1944) 'A psychometric method of determining intellectual loss following head injury', *Journal of Mental Science*, **90**, pp. 710–9.

RIBOT, T. (1882) *Diseases of Memory: An Essay in the Positive Psychology*, New York, Appleton.

RICHARDSON, F. C. (1963) 'Some effects of severe head injury: A follow-up study of children and adolescents after protracted coma', *Developmental Medicine and Child Neurology*, **5**, pp. 471–82.

RICHARDSON, F. C., O'NEIL, H. F., Jr., WHITMORE, S. and JUDD, W. A. (1977) 'Facto analysis of the test anxiety scale and evidence concerning the components of test anxiety', *Journal of Consulting and Clinical Psychology*, **45**, pp. 704–5.

RICHARDSON, J. T. E. (1978) 'Memory and intelligence following spontaneously arrested congenital hydrocephalus', *British Journal of Social and Clinical Psychology*, **17**, pp. 261–7.

(1979a) 'Mental imagery, human memory, and the effects of closed head injury', *British Journal of Social and Clinical Psychology*, **18**, pp. 319–27.

(1979b) 'Signal detection theory and the effects of severe head injury upon recognition memory', *Cortex*, **15**, pp. 145–8.

(1979c) 'The post-concussional syndrome', in OBORNE, D. J., GRUNEBERG, M. M. and EISER, J. R. (Eds) *Research in Psychology and Medicine. Vol. 1: Physical Aspects: Pain, Stress, Diagnosis and Organic Damage*, London, Academic Press, pp. 331–8.

(1982) 'Memory disorders', in BURTON, A. (Ed.) *The Pathology and Psychology of Cognition*, London, Methuen, pp. 48–77.

(1984a) 'Developing the theory of working memory', *Memory and Cognition*, **12**, pp. 71–83.

(1984b) 'The effects of closed head injury upon intrusions and confusions in free recall', *Cortex*, **20**, pp. 413–20.

(1987) 'Social class limitations on the efficacy of imagery mnemonic instructions', *British Journal of Psychology*, **78**, pp. 65–77.

(1989a) 'Human memory: Psychology, pathology, and pharmacology', in JONES, J. G. (Ed.) *Depth of Anaesthesia (Baillière's Clinical Anaesthesiology*, Vol. 3, No. 3), London, Baillière Tindall, pp. 451–71.

(1989b) 'Knowledge representation', in COLMAN, A. M. and BEAUMONT, J. G. (Eds) *Psychology Survey* 7, Leicester, British Psychological Society and Routledge, pp. 98–126.

(in press) 'Imagery and the brain', in CORNOLDI, C. and McDANIEL, M. A. (Eds) *Imagery and Cognition*, New York, Springer–Verlag.

RICHARDSON, J. T. E. and BADDELEY, A. D. (1975) 'The effect of articulatory suppression in free recall', *Journal of Verbal Learning and Verbal Behavior*, **14**, pp. 623–9.

RICHARDSON, J. T. E. and BARRY, C. (1985) 'The effects of minor closed head injury upon human memory: Further evidence on the role of mental imagery', *Cognitive Neuropsychology*, **2**, pp. 149–68.

RICHARDSON, J. T. E., CERMAK, L. S., BLACKFORD, S. P. and O'CONNOR, M. (1987) 'The efficacy of imagery mnemonics following brain damage', in McDANIEL, M. A. and PRESSLEY, M. (Eds) *Imagery and Related Mnemonic Processes: Theories, Individual Differences, and Applications*, New York, Springer–Verlag, pp. 303–28.

RICHARDSON, J. T. E. and SNAPE, W. (1984) 'The effects of closed head injury upon human memory: An experimental analysis', *Cognitive Neuropsychology*, **1**, pp. 217–31.

RIMEL, R. W., GIORDANI, B., BARTH, J. T., BOLL, T. J. and JANE, J. A. (1981) 'Disability caused by minor head injury', *Neurosurgery*, **9**, pp. 221–8.

RIMEL, R. W. and JANE, J. A. (1983) 'Characteristics of the head-injured patients', in ROSENTHAL, M., GRIFFITH, E. R., BOND, M. R. and MILLER, J. D. (Eds) *Rehabilitation of the Head Injured Adult*, Philadelphia, PA, Davis, pp. 9–21.

ROBERTS, A. H. (1969) *Brain Damage in Boxers: A Study of the Prevalence of Traumatic Encephalopathy among Ex-professional Boxers*, London, Pitman.

(1976) 'Long-term prognosis of severe accidental head injury', *Proceedings of the Royal Society of Medicine*, **69**, pp. 137–40.

(1979) *Severe Accidental Head Injury: An Assessment of Long-Term Prognosis*, London, Macmillan.

ROBERTS, A. K. (1983) *The Effects of Rear Seat Passengers on Front Seat Occupants in Frontal Impacts* (TRRL Laboratory Report 1079), Crowthorne, Berks., Transport and Road Research Laboratory.

ROSE, J., VALTONEN, S. and JENNETT, B. (1977) 'Avoidable factors contributing to death after head injury', *British Medical Journal*, **2**, 615–8.

ROSENBAUM, M., LIPSITZ, N., ABRAHAM, J. and NAJENSON, T. (1978) 'A description of an intensive treatment project for the rehabilitation of severely brain-injured soldiers', *Scandinavian Journal of Rehabilitation Medicine*, **10**, pp. 1–6.

ROSENBAUM, M. and NAJENSON, T. (1976) 'Changes in life patterns and symptoms of low mood as reported by wives of severely brain-injured soldiers', *Journal of Consulting and Clinical Psychology*, **44**, pp. 881–8.

ROSENTHAL, R. (1976) *Experimenter Effects in Behavioral Research*, enlarged ed., New York, Irvington.

ROTH, D. L., HUGHES, C. W., MONKOWSKI, P. G. and CROSSON, B. (1984) 'Investigation of validity of WAIS–R short forms for patients suspected to have brain impairment', *Journal of Consulting and Clinical Psychology*, **52**, pp. 722–3.

ROVIT, R. L. and MURALI, R. (1982) 'Injuries of the cranial nerves', in COOPER, P. R. (Ed.) *Head Injury*, Baltimore, MD, Williams and Wilkins, pp. 99–114.

ROWBOTHAM, G. F., MACIVER, I. N., DICKSON, J. and BOUSFIELD, M. E. (1954) 'Analysis of 1400 cases of acute injury to the head', *British Medical Journal*, **1**, pp. 726–30.

RUBENS, A. B., GESCHWIND, N., MAHOWALD, M. W. and MASTRI, A. (1977) 'Post-traumatic cerebral hemispheric disconnection syndrome', *Archives of Neurology*, **34**, pp. 750–5.

RUESCH, J. (1944a) 'Dark adaptation, negative after images, tachistoscopic examinations and reaction time in head injuries', *Journal of Neurosurgery*, **1**, pp. 243–51.

(1944b) 'Intellectual impairment in head injuries', *American Journal of Psychiatry*, **100**, pp. 480–86.

RUESCH, J. and BOWMAN, K. M. (1945) 'Prolonged post-traumatic syndromes following head injury', *American Journal of Psychiatry*, **102**, pp. 145–63.

RUESCH, J., HARRIS, R. E. and BOWMAN, K. M. (1944) 'Pre- and post-traumatic personality in head injuries', in *Trauma of the Central Nervous System (Research Publications of the Association for Research in Nervous and Mental Disease*, Vol. 24), Baltimore, MD, Williams and Wilkins, pp. 507–44.

RUESCH, J. and MOORE, B. E. (1943) 'Measurement of intellectual functions in the acute stage of head injury', *Archives of Neurology and Psychiatry*, **50**, pp. 165–70.

RUNE, V. (1970) 'Acute head injuries in children: A retrospective, epidemiologic, and electroencephalographic study on primary school children in Umea', *Acta Paediatrica Scandinavica*, **209**, pp. 3–12.

RUSSELL, E. W. (1975) 'A multiple scoring method for the assessment of complex memory functions', *Journal of Consulting and Clinical Psychology*, **43**, pp. 800–9.

(1988) 'Renorming Russell's version of the Wechsler Memory Scale', *Journal of Clinical and Experimental Neuropsychology*, **10**, pp. 235–49.

RUSSELL, G. (1981) 'Educational therapy', in EVANS, C. D. (Ed.) *Rehabilitation after Severe Head Injury*, Edinburgh, Churchill Livingstone, pp. 76–90.

RUSSELL, I. F. (1986) 'Comparison of wakefulness with two anaesthetic regimens: Total i.v. v. balanced anaesthesia', *British Journal of Anaesthesia*, **58**, pp. 965–8.

RUSSELL, W. R. (1932) 'Cerebral involvement in head injury: A study based on the examination of two hundred cases', *Brain*, **55**, pp. 549–603.

(1934) 'The after-effects of head injury', *Edinburgh Medical Journal*, **41**, pp. 129–44.

(1935) 'Amnesia following head injuries', *Lancet*, **2**, pp. 762–3.

(1951) 'Disability caused by brain wounds: A review of 1166 cases', *Journal of Neurology, Neurosurgery, and Psychiatry*, **14**, pp. 35–9.

(1960) 'Injury to cranial nerves and optic chiasm', in BROCK, S. (Ed.) *Injuries of the Brain and Spinal Cord and Their Coverings*, 4th ed., London, Cassell, pp. 118–26.

(1971) *The Traumatic Amnesias*, London, Oxford University Press.

RUSSELL, W. R. and NATHAN, P. W. (1946) 'Traumatic amnesia', *Brain*, **69**, pp. 280–300.

RUSSELL, W. R. and SMITH, A. (1961) 'Post-traumatic amnesia in closed head injury', *Archives of Neurology*, **5**, pp. 16–29.

RUTHERFORD, W. H. (1989) 'Post-concussion symptoms: Relationship to acute neurological indices, individual differences, and circumstances of injury', in LEVIN, H. S., EISENBERG, H. M. and BENTON, A. L. (Eds) *Mild Head Injury*, New York, Oxford University Press, pp. 217–28.

RUTHERFORD, W. H., GREENFIELD, T., HAYES, H. R. M. and NELSON, J. K. (1985) *The Medical Effects of Seat Belt Legislation in the United Kingdom* (Department of Health and Social Security, Research Report No. 13), London, Her Majesty's Stationery Office.

RUTHERFORD, W. H., MERRETT, J. D. and McDONALD, J. R. (1977) 'Sequelae at one year following concussion from minor head injuries, *Lancet*, **1**, pp. 1–4.

RUTHERSFORD, W. H., MERRETT, J. D. and McDONALD, J. R. (1979) 'Symptoms at one year following concussion from minor head injuries', *Injury*, **10**, pp. 225–30.

RUTTER, M. (1981) 'Psychological sequelae of brain damage in children', *American Journal of Psychiatry*, **138**, pp. 1533–44.

RUTTER, M., CHADWICK, O., SHAFFER, D. and BROWN, G. (1980) 'A prospective study of children with head injuries: I. Design and methods', *Psychological Medicine*, **10**, pp. 633–45.

SAHGAL, A. (1984) 'A critique of the vasopressin–memory hypothesis', *Psychopharmacology*, **83**, pp. 215–28.

SALAZAR, A. M., GRAFMAN, J. H., VANCE, S. C., WEINGARTNER, H., DILLON, J. D. and LUDLOW, C. (1986) 'Consciousness and amnesia after penetrating head injury: Neurology and anatomy', *Neurology*, **36**, pp. 178–87.

SAMPSON, H. (1956) 'Pacing and performance on a serial addition task', *Canadian Journal of Psychology*, **10**, pp. 219–25.

(1961) 'Effects of practice on paced performance', *Australian Journal of Psychology*, **13**, pp. 185–94.

SARNO, M. T. (1980) 'The nature of verbal impairment after closed head injury', *Journal of Nervous and Mental Disease*, **168**, pp. 685–92.

SCHACTER, D. L. (1987) 'Implicit expressions of memory in organic amnesia: Learning of new facts and associations', *Human Neurobiology*, **6**, pp. 107–18.

SCHACTER, D. L. and CROVITZ, H. F. (1977) 'Memory function after closed head injury: A review of the quantitative research', *Cortex*, **13**, pp. 150–76.

SCHACTER, D. L. and GLISKY, E. L. (1986) 'Memory remediation: Restoration, alleviation, and the acquisition of domain-specific knowledge', in UZZELL, B. P. and GROSS, Y. (Eds) *Clinical Neuropsychology of Intervention*, Boston, MA, Martinus Nijhoff, pp. 257–82.

SCHILDER, P. (1934) 'Psychic disturbances after head injuries', *American Journal of Psychiatry*, **91**, pp. 155–88.

SCHNEIDER, G. E. (1979) 'Is it really better to have your brain lesion early? A revision of the ''Kennard Principle'' ', *Neuropsychologia*, **17**, pp. 557–83.

SCHOENFELD, T. A. and HAMILTON, L. W. (1977) 'Secondary brain changes following lesions: A new paradigm for lesion experimentation', *Physiology and Behavior*, **18**, pp. 951–67.

SCHWARTZ, B. (1967) 'Hemispheric dominance and consciousness', *Acta Neurologica Scandinavica*, **43**, pp. 513–25.

SCOTTISH HEALTH SERVICE (1987) *Scottish Hospital In-Patient Statistics 1985*, Edinburgh, ISD Publications.

SELECKI, B. R., HOY, R. J. and NESS, P. (1968) 'Neurotraumatic admissions to a teaching hospital: A retrospective survey. Part 2: Head injuries', *Medical Journal of Australia*, **1**, pp. 582–5.

SHAFFER, D., CHADWICK, O. and RUTTER, M. (1975) 'Psychiatric outcome of localized head injury in children', in *Outcome of Severe Damage to the Central Nervous System*, Ciba Foundation Symposium No. 34 (new series), Amsterdam, Elsevier/Excerpta Medica/North-Holland, pp. 191–213.

SHALLICE, T. and WARRINGTON, E. K. (1970) 'Independent functioning of verbal memory stores: A neuropsychological study', *Quarterly Journal of Experimental Psychology*, **22**, pp. 261–73.

SHETTER, A. G. and DEMAKAS, J. J. (1979) 'The pathophysiology of concussion: A review', *Advances in Neurology*, **22**, pp. 5–14.

SHIFFRIN, R. M. and SCHNEIDER, W. (1977) 'Controlled and automatic human information processing: II. Perceptual learning, automatic attending, and a general theory', *Psychological Review*, **84**, pp. 127–90.

SHORES, E. A. (1989) 'Comparison of the Westmead PTA Scale and Glasgow Coma Scale as predictors of neuropsychological outcome following extremely severe blunt head injury', *Journal of Neurology, Neurosurgery, and Psychiatry*, **52**, pp. 126–7.

SHORES, E. A., MAROSSZEKY, J. E., SANDANAM, J. and BATCHELOR, J. (1986) 'Preliminary validation of a clinical scale for measuring the duration of post-traumatic amnesia', *Medical Journal of Australia*, **144**, pp. 569–72.

SILVER, J. R., MORRIS, W. R. and OTFINOWSKI, J. S. (1980) 'Associated injuries in patients with spinal injury', *Injury*, **12**, pp. 219–24.

SILVERMAN, I. (1977) *The Human Subject in the Psychological Laboratory*, New York, Pergamon Press.

SILVERSTEIN, A. B. (1982) 'Two- and four-subtest short forms of the Wechsler Adult Intelligence Scale—Revised', *Journal of Consulting and Clinical Psychology*, **50**, pp. 415–8.

SIMS, A. C. P. (1985) 'Head injury, neurosis, and accident proneness', *Advances in Psychosomatic Medicine*, **13**, pp. 49–70.

SIMS, J. K., EBISU, R. J., WONG, R. K. M. and WONG, L. M. F. (1976) 'Automobile accident occupant injuries', *JACEP* (Journal of the American College of Emergency Physicians), **5**, pp. 796–808.

SISLER, G. and PENNER, H. (1975) 'Amnesia following severe head injury', *Canadian Psychiatric Association Journal*, **20**, pp. 333–6.

SITARAM, N., WEINGARTNER, H., CAINE, E. D. and GILLIN, J. C. (1978) 'Choline: Selective enhancement of serial learning and encoding of low imagery words in man', *Life Sciences*, **22**, pp. 1555–60.

SKILBECK, C. E. and WOODS, R. T. (1980) 'The factorial structure of the Wechsler Memory Scale: Samples of neurological and psychogeriatric patients', *Journal of Clinical Neuropsychology*, **2**, pp. 293–300.

SMITH, A. (1961) 'Duration of impaired consciousness as an index of severity in closed head injuries: A review', *Diseases of the Nervous System*, **22**, pp. 69–74.

(1975) 'Neuropsychological testing in neurological disorders', *Advances in Neurology*, **7**, pp. 49–110.

SMITH, E. (1974) 'Influence of site of impact on cognitive impairment persisting long after severe closed head injury', *Journal of Neurology, Neurosurgery, and Psychiatry*, **37**, pp. 719–26.

SNAITH, R. P., BRIDGE, G. W. K. and HAMILTON, M. (1976) 'The Leeds Scale for the self-assessment of anxiety and depression', *British Journal of Psychiatry*, **128**, pp. 156–65.

SNOEK, J., JENNETT, B., ADAMS, J. H., GRAHAM, D. I. and DOYLE, D. (1979) 'Computerised tomography after recent severe head injury in patients without acute intracranial haematoma', *Journal of Neurology, Neurosurgery, and Psychiatry*, **42**, pp. 215–25.

SNOW, R. B., ZIMMERMAN, R. D., GANDY, S. E. and DECK, M. D. F. (1986) 'Comparison of magnetic resonance imaging and computed tomography in the evaluation of head injury', *Neurosurgery*, **18**, pp. 45–52.

SOLOMON, G. S., GREENE, R. L., FARR, S. P. and KELLY, M. P. (1986) 'Relationships among Wechsler Intelligence and Memory Scale Quotients in adult closed head injured patients', *Journal of Clinical Psychology*, **42**, pp. 318–23.

SPIELBERGER, C. D. (1966) 'Theory and research on anxiety', in SPIELBERGER, C. D. (Ed.) *Anxiety and Behavior*, New York, Academic Press, pp. 3–20.

(1972) 'Anxiety as an emotional state', in SPIELBERGER, C. D. (Ed.) *Anxiety: Current trends in theory and research*, Vol. 1, New York, Academic Press, pp. 23–49.

SPREEN, O. and BENTON, A. L. (1969) *Neurosensory Center Comprehensive Examination for Aphasia: Manual of Directions*, Victoria, BC, Neuropsychology Laboratory, University of Victoria.

SQUIRE, L. R., SLATER, P. C. and CHACE, P. M. (1975) 'Retrograde amnesia: Temporal gradient in very long-term memory following electroconvulsive therapy', *Science*, **187**, pp. 77–9.

STABLEIN, D. M., MILLER, J. D., CHOI, S. C. and BECKER, D. P. (1980) 'Statistical methods for determining prognosis in severe head injury', *Neurosurgery*, **6**, pp. 243–8.

STEADMAN, J. H. and GRAHAM, J. G. (1970) 'Head injuries: An analysis and follow-up study', *Proceedings of the Royal Society of Medicine*, **63**, pp. 23–8.

STEVENS, M. M. (1982) 'Post-concussion syndrome', *Journal of Neurosurgical Nursing*, **14**, pp. 239–44.

STEWART, W., GORDON, B., SELNES, O., TUSA, R., JANKEL, W., ZEGER, S., RANDALL, R. and CELENTANO, D. (1989) 'A prospective study of amateur boxers: Methodological issues', *Journal of Clinical and Experimental Neuropsychology*, **11**, pp. 22–3.

STOKX, L. C. and GAILLARD, A. W. K. (1986) 'Task and driving performance of patients with a severe concussion of the brain', *Journal of Clinical and Experimental Neuropsychology*, **8**, pp. 421–36.

STONE, J. L., LOPES, J. R. and MOODY, R. A. (1978) 'Fluent aphasia after closed head injury', *Surgical Neurology*, **9**, pp. 27–9.

STOVER, S. L. and ZEIGER, H. E. (1976) 'Head injury in children and teenagers: Functional recovery correlated with the duration of coma', *Archives of Physical Medicine and Rehabilitation*, **57**, pp. 201–5.

STRANG, I., MACMILLAN, R. and JENNETT, B. (1978) 'Head injuries in accident and emergency departments at Scottish hospitals', *Injury*, **10**, pp. 154–9.

STRAUSS, I. and SAVITSKY, N. (1934) 'Head injury: Neurologic and psychiatric aspects', *Archives of Neurology and Psychiatry*, **31**, pp. 893–955.

STRICH, S. J. (1956) 'Diffuse degeneration of the cerebral white matter in severe dementia following head injury', *Journal of Neurology, Neurosurgery, and Psychiatry*, **19**, pp. 163–85.

(1961) 'Shearing of nerve fibres as a cause of brain damage due to head injury: A pathological study of twenty cases', *Lancet*, **2**, pp. 443–8.

(1969) 'The pathology of brain damage due to blunt head injuries', in WALKER, A. E., CAVENESS, W. F. and CRITCHLEY, M. (Eds) *The Late Effects of Head Injury*, Springfield, IL, Thomas, pp. 501–26.

STROOP, J. R. (1935) 'Studies of interference in serial verbal reactions', *Journal of Experimental Psychology*, **18**, pp. 643–62.

STRUPP, B. J. and LEVITSKY, D. A. (1985) 'A mnemonic role for vasopressin: The evidence for and against', *Neuroscience and Biobehavioral Reviews*, **9**, pp. 399–411.

STUSS, D. T. and BENSON, D. F. (1984) 'Neuropsychological studies of the frontal lobes', *Psychological Bulletin*, **95**, pp. 3–28.

SUMNER, D. (1964) 'Post-traumatic anosmia', *Brain*, **87**, pp. 107–20.

SUNDERLAND, A., HARRIS, J. E. and BADDELEY, A. D. (1983) 'Do laboratory tests predict everyday memory? A neuropsychological study', *Journal of Verbal Learning and Verbal Behavior*, **22**, pp. 341–57.

(1984a) 'Assessing everyday memory after severe head injury', in HARRIS, J. E. and MORRIS, P. E. (Eds) *Everyday Memory, Actions and Absent-Mindedness*, London, Academic Press, pp. 191–206.

SUNDERLAND, A., HARRIS, J. E. and GLEAVE, J. (1984b) 'Memory failures in everyday life following severe head injury', *Journal of Clinical Neuropsychology*, **6**, pp. 127–42.

SWANN, I. J., MACMILLAN, R. and STRANG, I. (1981) 'Head injuries at an inner city accident and emergency department', *Injury*, **12**, pp. 274–8.

SYMONDS, C. P. (1928) 'Observations on the differential diagnosis and treatment of cerebral states consequent upon head injuries', *British Medical Journal*, **2**, pp. 829–32.

(1937) 'Mental disorder following head injury', *Proceedings of the Royal Society of Medicine*, **30**, pp. 1081–94.

(1940) 'Concussion and contusion of the brain and their sequelae', in BROCK, S. (Ed.) *Injuries of the Skull, Brain and Spinal Cord: Neuro-Psychiatric, Surgical, and Medico-Legal Aspects*, London, Baillière, Tindall and Cox, pp. 69–111.

(1942) 'Discussion on the differential diagnosis and treatment of post-contusional states', *Proceedings of the Royal Society of Medicine*, **35**, pp. 601–7.

(1962) 'Concussion and its sequelae', *Lancet*, **1**, pp. 1–5.

(1966) 'Disorders of memory', *Brain*, **89**, pp. 625–44.

SYMONDS, C. P. and RUSSELL, W. R. (1943) 'Accidental head injuries: Prognosis in Service patients', *Lancet*, **1**, pp. 7–10.

TARLOV, E. (1976) 'Optimal management of head injuries', *International Anesthesiology Clinics*, **14**, pp. 69–94.

TAYLOR, A. R. (1967) 'Post-concussional sequelae', *British Medical Journal*, **3**, pp. 67–71.

(1969) 'The cerebral circulatory disturbance associated with the late effects of head injury: An examination of the underlying pathologic and biochemical changes', in WALKER, A. E., CAVENESS, W. F. and CRITCHLEY, M. (Eds) *The Late Effects of Head Injury*, Springfield, IL, Thomas, pp. 46–54.

TAYLOR, A. R. and BELL, T. K. (1966) 'Slowing of cerebral circulation after concussional head injury', *Lancet*, **2**, pp. 178–80.

TEASDALE, G. (1975) 'Acute impairment of brain function: 1. Assessing "conscious level" ', *Nursing Times*, **71**, pp. 914–7.

TEASDALE, G., GALBRAITH, S. and CLARKE, K. (1975) 'Acute impairment of brain function: 2. Observation record chart', *Nursing Times*, **71**, pp. 972–3.

TEASDALE, G. and JENNETT, B. (1974) 'Assessment of coma and impaired consciousness: A practical scale', *Lancet*, **2**, pp. 81–4.

(1976) 'Assessment and prognosis of coma after head injury', *Acta Neurochirurgica*, **34**, pp. 45–55.

TEASDALE, G. M., KNILL-JONES, R. and JENNETT, W. B. (1974) 'Assessing and recording "conscious level" ', *Journal of Neurology, Neurosurgery, and Psychiatry*, **37**, p. 1286.

TEASDALE, G., KNILL-JONES, R. and VAN DER SANDE, J. (1978) 'Observer variability in assessing impaired consciousness and coma', *Journal of Neurology, Neurosurgery, and Psychiatry*, **41**, pp. 603–10.

TEASDALE, G. and MENDELOW, D. (1984) 'Pathophysiology of head injuries', in BROOKS, N. (Ed.) *Closed Head Injury: Psychological, Social, and Family Consequences*, Oxford, Oxford University Press, pp. 4–36.

TEASDALE, G., MURRAY, G., PARKER, L. and JENNETT, B. (1979a) 'Adding up the Glasgow Coma Score', *Acta Neurochirurgica*, Supp. 28, pp. 13–6.

TEASDALE, G., SKENE, A., PARKER, L. and JENNETT, B. (1979b) 'Age and outcome of severe head injury', *Acta Neurochirurgica*, Supp. 28, pp. 140–3.

TEASDALE, G., SKENE, A., SPIEGELHALTER, D. and MURRAY, L. (1982) 'Age, severity, and outcome of head injury', in GROSSMAN, R. G. and GILDENBERG, P. L. (Eds) *Head Injury: Basic and Clinical Aspects*, New York, Raven Press, pp. 213–220.

TEUBER, H. -L. (1969) 'Neglected aspects of the post-traumatic syndrome', in WALKER, A. E., CAVENESS, W. F. and CRITCHLEY, M. (Eds) *The Late Effects of Head Injury*, Springfield, IL, Thomas, pp. 13–34.

THAL, L. J., MASUR, D. M., BLAU, A. D., FULD, P. A. and KLAUBER, M. R. (1989) 'Chronic oral physostigmine without lecithin improves memory in Alzheimer's disease', *Journal of the American Geriatrics Society*, **37**, pp. 42–8.

THOMSEN, I. V. (1974) 'The patient with severe head injury and his family: A follow-up study of 50 patients', *Scandinavian Journal of Rehabilitation Medicine*, **6**, pp. 180–3.

(1975) 'Evaluation and outcome of aphasia in patients with severe closed head trauma', *Journal of Neurology, Neurosurgery, and Psychiatry*, **38**, pp. 713–8.

(1976) 'Evaluation and outcome of traumatic aphasia in patients with severe verified focal lesions', *Folia Phoniatrica*, **28**, pp. 362–77.

(1977) 'Verbal learning in aphasic and non-aphasic patients with severe head injuries', *Scandinavian Journal of Rehabilitation Medicine*, **9**, pp. 73–7.

(1984) 'Late outcome of very severe blunt head trauma: A 10–15 year second follow-up', *Journal of Neurology, Neurosurgery, and Psychiatry*, **47**, pp. 260–8.

THOMSEN, I. V. and SKINHØJ, E. (1976) 'Regressive language in severe head injury', *Acta Neurologica Scandinavica*, **54**, pp. 219–26.

THORSON, J. (1974) 'Pedal cycle accidents: With special reference to the prevention of injuries caused by falls', *Scandinavian Journal of Social Medicine*, **2**, pp. 121–8.

TIMMING, R., ORRISON, W. W. and MIKULA, J. A. (1982) 'Computerized tomography and rehabilitation outcome after severe head trauma', *Archives of Physical Medicine and Rehabilitation*, **63**, pp. 154–9.

TODOROW, S. and HEISS, E. (1978) 'The "fall-asleep-syndrome": A kind of secondary disturbance of consciousness after head injury in children', in FROWEIN, R. A., WILCKE, O., KARIMI-NEJAD, A., BROCK, M. and KLINGER, M. (Eds) *Head Injuries; Tumors of the Cerebellar Region* (*Advances in Neurosurgery*, Vol. 5), Berlin, Springer–Verlag, pp. 102–4.

TOGLIA, J. U. (1969) 'Dizziness after whiplash injury of the neck and closed head injury: Electronystagmographic correlations', in WALKER, A. E., CAVENESS, W. F. and CRITCHLEY, M. (Eds) *The Late Effects of Head Injury*, Springfield, IL, Thomas, pp. 72–83.

TOOTH, G. (1947) 'On the use of mental tests for the measurement of disability after head injury with a comparison between the results of these tests in patients after head injury and psychoneurotics', *Journal of Neurology, Neurosurgery, and Psychiatry*, **10**, pp. 1–11.

TREISMAN, A. M. (1960) 'Contextual cues in selective listening', *Quarterly Journal of Experimental Psychology*, **12**, pp. 242–8.

TULVING, E. (1972) 'Episodic and semantic memory', in TULVING, E. and DONALDSON, W. (Eds) *Organization of Memory*, New York, Academic Press, pp. 381–403.

TURAZZI, S., ALEXANDRE, A. and BRICOLO, A. (1975) 'Incidence and significance of clinical signs of brainstem traumatic lesions: Study of 2600 head-injured patients', *Journal of Neurosurgical Sciences*, **19**, pp. 215–22.

UZZELL, B. P., ZIMMERMAN, R. A., DOLINSKAS, C. A. and OBRIST, W. D. (1979) 'Lateralized psychological impairment associated with CT lesions in head injured patients', *Cortex*, **15**, pp. 391–401.

VAN REE, J. M., HIJMAN, R., JOLLES, J. and DE WIED, D. (1985) 'Vasopressin and related peptides: Animal and human studies', *Progress in Neuro-Psychopharmacology and Biological Psychiatry*, **9**, pp. 551–9.

VAN ZOMEREN, A. H. (1981) *Reaction Time and Attention after Closed Head Injury*, Lisse, Swets and Zeitlinger.

VAN ZOMEREN, A. H., BROUWER, W. H. and DEELMAN, B. G. (1984) 'Attentional deficits: The riddles of selectivity, speed, and alertness', in BROOKS, N. (Ed.) *Closed Head Injury: Psychological, Social, and Family Consequences*, Oxford, Oxford University Press, pp. 74–107.

VAN ZOMEREN, A. H., BROUWER, W. H. and MINDERHOUD, J. M. (1987) 'Acquired brain damage and driving: A review', *Archives of Physical Medicine and Rehabilitation*, **68**, pp. 697–705.

VAN ZOMEREN, A. H. and DEELMAN, B. G. (1976) 'Differential effects of simple and choice reaction after closed head injury', *Clinical Neurology and Neurosurgery*, **79**, pp. 81–90.

(1978) 'Long-term recovery of visual reaction time after closed head injury', *Journal of Neurology, Neurosurgery, and Psychiatry*, **41**, pp. 452–7.

VAN ZOMEREN, A. H. and VAN DEN BURG, W. (1985) 'Residual complaints of patients two years after severe head injury', *Journal of Neurology, Neurosurgery, and Psychiatry*, **48**, pp. 21–8.

VARNEY, N. R. (1988) 'The prognostic significance of anosmia in patients with closed-head trauma', *Journal of Clinical and Experimental Neuropsychology*, **10**, pp. 250–4.

VIGOUROUX, R. P., BAURAND, C., NAQUET, R., CHAMENT, J. H., CHOUX, M., BENAYOUN, R., BUREAU, M., CHARPY, J. P., CLAMENS-GUEY, M. J. and GUEY, J. (1971) 'A series of patients with cranio-cerebral injuries studied neurologically, psychometrically, electroencephalographically, and socially', in *Head Injuries: Proceedings of an International Symposium*, Edinburgh, Churchill Livingstone, pp. 335–41.

VON MONAKOW, C. (1914) *Die Lokalisation im Grosshirn und der Abbau der Funktion durch kortikale Herde*, Wiesbaden, Bergmann. Excerpt published 1969 as 'Diaschisis' (trans. G. HARRIS) in PRIBRAM, K. H. (Ed.) *Brain and Behaviour: 1. Mood, States and Mind. Selected Readings*, Harmondsworth, Middx., Penguin Books, pp. 27–36.

VON WOWERN, F. (1966) 'Post-traumatic amnesia and confusion as an index of severity in head injury', *Acta Neurologica Scandinavica*, **42**, pp. 373–8.

WACKS, M. R. and BIRD, H. A. (1970) 'Massive gross pulmonary embolism of cerebral tissue following severe head trauma', *Journal of Trauma*, **10**, pp. 344–8.

WADDELL, P. A. and GRONWALL, D. M. A. (1984) 'Sensitivity to light and sound following minor head injury', *Acta Neurologica Scandinavica*, **69**, pp. 270–6.

WALSH, K. W. (1978) *Neuropsychology: A Clinical Approach*, Edinburgh, Churchill Livingstone.

WALTON, R. G. (1982) 'Lecithin and physostigmine for post-traumatic memory and cognitive deficits', *Psychosomatics*, **23**, pp. 435–6.

WARD, A. A., Jr. (1966) 'The physiology of concussion', *Clinical Neurosurgery*, **12**, pp. 89–111.

WARRINGTON, E. K., JAMES, M. and MACIEJEWSKI, C. (1986) 'The WAIS as a lateralizing and localizing diagnostic instrument: A study of 656 patients with unilateral cerebral lesions', *Neuropsychologia*, **24**, pp. 223–9.

WARRINGTON, E. K., LOGUE, V., and PRATT, R. T. C. (1971) 'The anatomical localisation of selective impairment of auditory verbal short-term memory', *Neuropsychologia*, **9**, pp. 377–87.

WARRINGTON, E. K. and SHALLICE, T. (1970) 'The selective impairment of auditory verbal short-term memory', *Brain*, **92**, pp. 885–96.

WASTERLAIN, C. G. (1971) 'Are there two types of post-traumatic retrograde amnesia?' *European Neurology*, **5**, pp. 225–8.

WAUGH, N. C. and NORMAN, D. A. (1965) 'Primary memory', *Psychological Review*, **72**, pp. 89–104.

WECHSLER, D. (1917) 'A study of retention in Korsakoff psychosis', *Psychiatric Bulletin of the New York State Hospital*, **2**, pp. 403–51.

    (1941) *The Measurement of Adult Intelligence*, 2nd ed., Baltimore, MD, Williams and Wilkins.

    (1944) *The Measurement of Adult Intelligence*, 3rd ed., Baltimore, MD, Williams and Wilkins.

    (1945) 'A standardized memory scale for clinical use', *Journal of Psychology*, **19**, pp. 87–95.

    (1949) *Wechsler Intelligence Scale for Children*, New York, Psychological Corporation.

    (1955) *Wechsler Adult Intelligence Scale*, New York, Psychological Corporation.

    (1981) *Wechsler Adult Intelligence Scale — Revised*, New York, Psychological Corporation.

    (1987) *Manual for the Wechsler Memory Scale — Revised*, San Antonio, TX, Psychological Corporation.

WEDDELL, R., ODDY, M. and JENKINS, D. (1980) 'Social adjustment after rehabilitation: A two year follow-up of patients with severe head injury', *Psychological Medicine*, **10**, pp. 257–63.

WEIGHILL, V. E. (1983) ' "Compensation neurosis": A review of the literature', *Journal of Psychosomatic Research*, **27**, pp. 97–104.

WEINGARTNER, H., CAINE, E. D. and EBERT, M. H. (1979a) 'Encoding processing, learning, and recall in Huntington's disease', in CHASE, T. N., WEXLER, N. S. and BARBEAU, A. (Eds) *Huntington's Disease (Advances in Neurology*, Vol. 23), New York, Raven Press, pp. 215–26.

    (1979b) 'Imagery, encoding, and retrieval of information from memory: Some specific encoding–retrieval changes in Huntington's disease', *Journal of Abnormal Psychology*, **88**, pp. 52–8.

WEISBERG, L. A. (1979) 'Computed tomography in the diagnosis of intracranial disease', *Annals of Internal Medicine*, **91**, pp. 87–105.

WEISSMAN, M. M., PRUSOFF, B. A., THOMPSON, W. D., HARDING, P. S. and MYERS, J. K. (1978) 'Social adjustment by self-report in a community sample and in psychiatric outpatients', *Journal of Nervous and Mental Disease*, **166**, pp. 317–26.

WEST, J. R., DEADWYLER, S. A., COTMAN, C. W. and LYNCH, G. S. (1976) 'An experimental test of diaschisis', *Behavioral Biology*, **18**, pp. 419–25.

WESTON, M. J. and WHITLOCK, F. A. (1971) 'The Capgras syndrome following head injury', *British Journal of Psychiatry*, **119**, pp. 25–31.

WHITAKER, J. (1976) *Motor Cycle Safety: Accident Survey and Rider Injuries* (TRRL Supplementary Report 239), Crowthorne, Berks., Transport and Road Research Laboratory.

    (1980) *A Survey of Motorcycle Accidents* (TRRL Laboratory Report 913), Crowthorne, Berks., Transport and Road Research Laboratory.

WHITE, A. C., ARMSTRONG, D. and ROWAN, D. (1987) 'Compensation psychosis', *British Journal of Psychiatry*, **150**, pp. 692–4.

WHITMAN, S., COONLY-HOGANSON, R. and DESAI, B. (1984) 'Comparative head trauma experiences in two socioeconomically different Chicago-area communities: A population study', *American Journal of Epidemiology*, **119**, pp. 186–201.

WILLIAMS, M. (1969) 'Traumatic retrograde amnesia and normal forgetting', in TALLAND, G. A. and WAUGH, N. C. (Eds) *The Pathology of Memory*, New York, Academic Press, pp. 75–80.

WILLIAMS, M. and ZANGWILL, O. L. (1952) 'Memory defects after head injury', *Journal of Neurology, Neurosurgery, and Psychiatry*, **15**, pp. 54–8.

WILLIAMS, P. L. and WARWICK, R. (1975) *Functional Neuroanatomy of Man*, Edinburgh, Churchill Livingstone.

WILMOT, C. B., COPE, N., HALL, K. M. and ACKER, M. (1985) 'Occult head injury: Its incidence in spinal cord injury', *Archives of Physical Medicine and Rehabilitation*, **66**, pp. 227–31.

WILSON, B. (1984) 'Memory therapy in practice', in WILSON, B. A. and MOFFAT, N. (Eds) *Clinical Management of Memory Problems*, London, Croom Helm, pp. 89–111.

(1987a) *Rehabilitation of Memory*, New York, Guilford Press.

(1987b) 'Single case experimental designs in neurological rehabilitation', *Journal of Clinical and Experimental Neuropsychology*, **9**, pp. 527–44.

(1989) 'Models of cognitive rehabilitation', in WOOD, R. L. and EAMES, P. (Eds) *Models of Brain Injury Rehabilitation*, London, Chapman and Hall, pp. 117–41.

WILSON, J. A., PENTLAND, B., CURRIE, C. T. and MILLER, J. D. (1987) 'The functional effects of head injury in the elderly', *Brain Injury*, **1**, pp. 183–8.

WINDLE, W. F., GROAT, R. A. and FOX, C. A. (1944) 'Experimental structural alterations in the brain during and after concussion', *Surgery, Gynaecology, and Obstetrics*, **79**, pp. 561–72.

WINOGRON, H. W., KNIGHTS, R. M. and BAWDEN, H. N. (1984) 'Neuropsychological deficits following head injury in children', *Journal of Clinical Neuropsychology*, **6**, pp. 269–86.

WOLKOWITZ, O. M., TINKLENBERG, J. R. and WEINGARTNER, H. (1985) 'A psychopharmacological perspective of cognitive functions: II. Specific pharmacologic agents', *Neuropsychobiology*, **14**, pp. 133–56.

WOOD, R. L. (1979) 'The relationship of brain damage, measured by computerised axial tomography, to quantitative intellectual impairment', in OBORNE, D. J., GRUNEBERG, M. M. and EISER, J. R. (Eds) *Research in Psychology and Medicine. Vol. 1: Physical Aspects: Pain, Stress, Diagnosis and Organic Damage*, London, Academic Press, pp. 339–46.

WOOD, R. L. and EAMES, P. (1981) 'Application of behaviour modification in the rehabilitation of traumatically brain-injured patients', in DAVEY, G. (Ed.) *Applications of Conditioning Theory*, London, Methuen, pp. 81–101.

WOO-SAM, J., ZIMMERMAN, I. L., BRINK, J. D., UYEHARA, K. and MILLER, A. R. (1970) 'Socio-economic status and post-trauma intelligence in children with severe head injuries', *Psychological Reports*, **27**, pp. 147–53.

WORLD HEALTH ORGANIZATION (1977) *Manual of the International Statistical Classification of Diseases, Injuries, and Causes of Death*, Vol. 1, Geneva, World Health Organization (London, Her Majesty's Stationery Office).

WRIGHTSON, P. and GRONWALL, D. (1981) 'Time off work and symptoms after minor head injury', *Injury*, **12**, pp. 445–54.

YARNELL, P. R. and LYNCH, S. (1970) 'Retrograde memory immediately after concussion', *Lancet*, **1**, pp. 863–4.

(1973) 'The "ding": Amnestic states in football trauma', *Neurology*, **23**, pp. 196–7.

ZATORRE, R. J. and MCENTEE, W. J. (1983) 'Semantic encoding deficits in a case of traumatic amnesia', *Brain and Cognition*, **2**, pp. 331–45.

ZIMMERMAN, R. A., BILANIUK, L. T., BRUCE, D., DOLINSKAS, C., OBRIST, W. and KUHL, D. (1978a) 'Computed tomography of pediatric head trauma: Acute general cerebral swelling', *Radiology*, **126**, pp. 403–8.

ZIMMERMAN, R. A., BILANIUK, L. T. and GENNARELLI, T. (1978b) 'Computed tomography of shearing injuries of the cerebral white matter', *Radiology*, **127**, pp. 393–6.

Index of Authors

Index